PULMONARY THROMBOEMBOLISM

PULMONARY

THROMBOEMBOLISM

Edited by

KAZI MOBIN-UDDIN, M.B.B.S.

Assistant Professor of Surgery
Division of Cardio-Thoracic Surgery
University of Kentucky College of Medicine
Consultant, Cardio-Thoracic Surgery
Veteran's Administration Hospital
Lexington, Kentucky

With a Foreword by

Ward O. Griffen, Jr., M.D.
Lexington, Kentucky

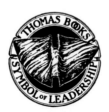

CHARLES C THOMAS • PUBLISHER
Springfield • Illinois • U.S.A.

Published and Distributed Throughout the World by

CHARLES C THOMAS • PUBLISHER

BANNERSTONE HOUSE

301-327 East Lawrence Avenue, Springfield, Illinois, U.S.A.

© 1975, by CHARLES C THOMAS • PUBLISHER

ISBN 0-398-03227-0

Library of Congress Catalog Card Number: 74-8152

Printed in the United States of America

Library of Congress Cataloging in Publication Data

Main entry under title:

Pulmonary thromboembolism.

"Edited proceedings of a symposium entitled 'Pulmonary thromboembolism—new concepts,' sponsored by the Department of Surgery and the Office of Continuing Education, University of Kentucky, College of Medicine, and held at the University Hospital in Lexington, Kentucky."

1. Pulmonary embolism—Congresses. I. Mobin-Uddin, Kazi, 1930-   ed. II. Kentucky. University. Dept. of Surgery. III. Kentucky. University. College of Medicine. Office of Continuing Education. [DNLM: 1. Pulmonary embolism—Congresses. WG420]

Library of Congress Cataloging in Publication Data

P98 1973]
RC776.P85P83   616.1'35   74-8152
ISBN 0-398-03227-0

CONTRIBUTORS

Richard D. Allen, M.D., Fellow, Cardiovascular Division, Department of Medicine, University of Kentucky College of Medicine, Lexington, Kentucky.

John S. Belko, M.S., Biochemist-in-charge Veteran's Administration Hospital, West Roxbury, Massachusetts.

Robert L. Berger, M.D., Professor of Surgery, Chairman, Department of Cardio-Thoracic Surgery, Boston University Medical Center, Boston, Massachusetts.

Dennis A. Bloomfield, M.B., M.R.C.P., M.R.C.P.E., Assistant Professor of Medicine, New York State University, Downstate Medical Center, and Director, Cardiopulmonary Laboratory, Maimonides Medical Center, Brooklyn, New York.

Lester R. Bryant, M.D., Sc.D., Professor of Surgery, Chief, Cardio-Thoracic Surgery, University of Kentucky College of Medicine, Lexington, Kentucky.

J. F. Cade, M.D., Assistant Professor, Department of Medicine, McMaster University, Hamilton, Ontario, Canada.

Christine M. Cole, M.S., Biometrician, Coordinating Center, Urokinase Pulmonary Embolism Trial, National Heart and Lung Institute, Bethesda, Maryland.

William W. Coon, M.D., Professor of Surgery, University of Michigan School of Medicine, Ann Arbor, Michigan.

James E. Dalen, M.D., Associate Professor of Medicine, Harvard Medical School, Senior Associate in Medicine, Peter Bent Brigham Hospital, Boston, Massachusetts.

James A. Deweese, M.D., Professor of Surgery, University of Rochester School of Medicine, Rochester, New York.

Marcus Dillon, M.D., Professor of Surgery, Division of Cardio-Thoracic Surgery, University of Kentucky College of Medicine, Lexington, Kentucky.

v

Annette L. Edelstein, Research Assistant, Surgical Research Laboratories, The Medical College of Pennsylvania, Philadelphia, Pennsylvania.

Geoffrey Evans, M.B.B.S., Associate Professor of Surgery, McMaster University Medical Center, Hamilton, Ontario, Canada.

W. Robert Felix, Jr., M.D., Assistant Professor of Surgery, The Medical College of Pennsylvania, Philadelphia, Pennsylvania.

William D. Fullen, M.D., Assistant Professor of Surgery, Director, Trauma Service, University of Cincinnati Medical Center, Cincinnati, Ohio.

A. S. Gallus, M.D., Assistant Professor, Department of Medicine, McMaster University, Hamilton, Ontario, Canada.

Jack Hirsh, M.D., Professor of Medicine and Pathology, McMaster University Medical Center, Hamilton, Ontario, Canada.

Thomas M. Hyers, M.D., Formerly Medical Liaison Officer, Urokinase Pulmonary Embolism Trial, National Heart and Lung Institute, Bethesda, Maryland.

Johannes Ipsen, M.D., Professor of Medical Statistics & Epidemiology, Department of Community Medicine, School of Medicine, University of Pennsylvania, Philadelphia, Pennsylvania.

Allan M. Lansing, M.D., Ph.D., F.R.C.S. (C), Professor of Surgery, University of Louisville School of Medicine, Louisville, Kentucky.

Kevin M. McIntyre, M.D., Assistant Chief, Cardiology, Veteran's Administration Hospital, West Roxbury, and Assistant Professor of Medicine, Harvard Medical School, Boston, Massachusetts.

Charles R. Memhardt, B.S., Head, Vascular Disease Research, The Kendall Research Center, Barrington, Illinois.

Andrianne J. Millett, (Medical Student) Pulmonary Division, Department of Medicine, University of Kentucky College of Medicine, Lexington, Kentucky.

Kazi Mobin-Uddin, M.B.B.S., Assistant Professor of Surgery, Division of Cardio-Thoracic Surgery, University of Kentucky College of Medicine, Lexington, Kentucky.

William O. Myers, M.D., Department of Thoracic and Cardiovascular Surgery, Marshfield Clinic, Marshfield, Wisconsin.

Jacqueline A. Noonan, M.D., Professor and Chairman, Department of Pediatrics, University of Kentucky College of Medicine, Lexington, Kentucky.

John R. O'Brien, M.A., D.M., M.R.C.P., F.R.C.PATH., Consultant Haematologist, St. Mary's General Hospital, Portsmouth, England. Clinical Reader in Experimental Haematology, Southampton University.

Alton Ochsner, M.D., Senior Consultant, Ochsner Clinic and Alton Ochsner Medical Foundation and Emeritus Professor of Surgery, Tulane University School of Medicine, New Orleans, Louisiana.

Joseph A. O'Donnell, M.D., F.R.C.S (I), Teaching Fellow in Surgery, University of Massachusetts Medical School, Worcester, Massachusetts.

Richard P. O'Neill, M.D., Associate Professor of Medicine, Pulmonary Division, Department of Medicine, University of Kentucky College of Medicine, Lexington, Kentucky.

Joseph C. Parker, Jr., M.D., M.S., Associate Professor of Pathology, Chief of Surgical Pathology, Department of Pathology, University of Kentucky College of Medicine, Lexington, Kentucky.

Robert B. Penman, M.D., Professor of Medicine, Chief, Pulmonary Division, Department of Medicine, University of Kentucky College of Medicine, Lexington, Kentucky.

George L. Popky, M.D., Associate Professor of Radiology, The Medical College of Pennsylvania, Philadelphia, Pennsylvania.

Jefferson F. Ray III, M.D., Department of Thoracic and Cardiovascular Surgery, Marshfield Clinic, Marshfield, Wisconsin.

Stanley M. Rogoff, M.D., Professor of Radiology, University of Rochester School of Medicine, Rochester, New York.

Arthur A. Sasahara, M.D., Chief, Cardiopulmonary Section, Veteran's Administration Hospital, West Roxbury, and Associate Professor of Medicine, Harvard Medical School, Boston, Massachusetts.

Richard D. Sautter, M.D., Department of Thoracic and Cardiovascular Surgery, Marshfield Clinic, Marshfield, Wisconsin.

G.V.R.K. Sharma, M.D., Chief, Pulmonary Section, Veteran's Administration Hospital, West Roxbury, and Instructor in Medicine, Harvard Medical School, Boston, Massachusetts.

Bernard Sigel, M.D., Professor of Surgery, The Medical College of Pennsylvania, Philadelphia, Pennsylvania.

Donald Silver, M.D., Professor of Surgery, Duke University Medical Center, Durham, North Carolina.

Allan L. Simon, M.D., Professor of Diagnostic Radiology, Yale University School of Medicine, New Haven, Connecticut.

John A. Spittell, M.D., Professor of Medicine, Mayo Graduate School of Medicine, Division of Cardiovascular Diseases, Mayo Clinic, Rochester, Minnesota.

H. William Strauss, M.D., Assistant Professor of Radiology, Medicine and Radiation Health, Johns Hopkins Medical Institutions, Baltimore, Maryland.

Borys Surawicz, M.D., Professor of Medicine, Chief, Cardiovascular Division, University of Kentucky College of Medicine, Lexington, Kentucky.

Joe R. Utley, M.D., Associate Professor of Surgery, Division of Cardio-Thoracic Surgery, University of Kentucky College of Medicine, Lexington, Kentucky.

Henry N. Wagner, Jr., M.D., Professor of Medicine, Radiology and Radiation Health, The Johns Hopkins Medical Institutions, Baltimore, Maryland.

H. Brownell Wheeler, M.D., Professor and Chairman, Department of Surgery, University of Massachusetts School of Medicine, Worcester, Massachusetts.

FOREWORD

PULMONARY EMBOLISM is one of the few conditions for which there is no recognizable description in the Bible. This is not surprising since venous thrombosis was not described in medical writings before the thirteenth century, and pulmonary circulation of blood was not discovered until Harvey described it in 1628. Even then more than 200 years went by before Hélie gave a clear clinical description of a case of pulmonary embolism which was verified at autopsy. A few years later Paget described blood clots in the pulmonary arteries, and in one case he observed similar clots in the femoral vein. At about the same time Virchow with his usual systematic study demonstrated conclusively that pulmonary embolism was secondary to venous thrombosis.

After these investigations, general textbooks as well as works devoted specifically to embolic diseases continued to build on the work of Virchow, but even into the latter part of the nineteenth century the condition was still considered to be fatal. However, in 1890 Welch recognized pulmonary embolism (or thrombosis) could occur as a chronic illness for which there was little specific treatment. He did mention Trendelenburg's operation although the account published by Trendelenburg did not appear until 1907.

During this same period there were some early experimental works on pulmonary emboli using mercury, wax and fresh blood clots. In fact, Panum in 1864 recognized that pulmonary embolism could occur in dogs without causing symptoms, and that the emboli could undergo complete dissolution within the pulmonary artery. In 1920 Dunn reported on the reflex physiologic effects of small pulmonary emboli in goats thus stimulating interest in the physiologic and pharmacologic approach to a practical clinical treatment of pulmonary embolism. Meanwhile blood clotting was being investigated and its mechanism gradually elucidated. Thus began a new avenue of approach to thromboembolic disease. With the advent of clinically applicable anticoagulant drugs thirty years ago, much of the human experimental investigations centered on treatment of established venous thrombosis or pulmonary embolism by appropriate manipulation of blood clotting.

Still episodes of pulmonary embolism occurred subsequent to peripheral venous thrombosis either despite adequate anticoagulation or in cases of "silent" leg thrombosis. These events have stimulated the studies of the past three or four decades. The first area of investigation was that of man-

ix

agement of the patient with a pulmonary embolism. Following the sugges-
tion of Homans to ligate the femoral or iliac veins in such cases, the concept
of inferior vena caval ligation came into vogue. Plication and clipping of
the inferior vena cava were subsequently advocated in order to prevent the
peripheral edema of legs which sometimes occurred after vena caval ligation. All of these caval interruption procedures require a surgical operation
in a patient who was often quite ill. Thus means were sought for a less
stressful but equally effective method of caval ligation and led to the
development of an intracaval umbrella by Dr. Mobin-Uddin. This device
could be placed into an appropriate position in the vena cava by exposing
the jugular vein in the neck under local anesthesia and inserting the
umbrella in a transvenous technique. The second area of study was means
of detecting venous thrombosis early in order to prevent the tragedy of
pulmonary embolism. Several noninvasive detection methods have been
advocated as well as venography in suspect cases. Some workers have advocated another approach of preventive regimen of mini heparin therapy
throughout the operative experience. In the meantime search for more
effective, safer anticoagulants continues.

The multifaceted investigational efforts and intense interest in this
entire field simply emphasizes the fact that the problem has not been
solved yet. In April 1973 we were honored to have a number of experts in
the field of thromboembolic disease and pulmonary embolus join members
of the faculty of the University of Kentucky College of Medicine in a
symposium on pulmonary embolism—new concepts. Dr. Mobin-Uddin, as
the program chairman, encouraged the participants to delve into the old
and the new, the theoretical and the practical. Thus the program ran the
gamut of hypercoagulable states, pulmonary microembolism and thromboembolism in children through modern techniques of identifying silent deep
vein thrombosis and recent as well as established techniques of diagnosing
pulmonary embolism to means of preventing pulmonary embolism and the
pharmacologic and surgical therapy for established pulmonary embolism.
The symposium was well-attended and greatly received. Dr. Mobin-Uddin
and the participants were urged to publish the material. Thus has come
this present publication which is a most welcome, up-to-date treatise on
the subject of venous thrombosis and pulmonary embolism.

WARD O. GRIFFEN, JR., M.D.

PREFACE

Tʜɪs ᴘᴜʙʟɪᴄᴀᴛɪᴏɴ represents the edited proceedings of a symposium entitled "Pulmonary Thromboembolism—New Concepts," sponsored by the Department of Surgery and the Office of Continuing Education, University of Kentucky, College of Medicine and held at the University Hospital in Lexington, Kentucky.

In recent years we have witnessed spectacular advances in the diagnosis, prevention and management of patients with venous thromboembolic disease. The Lexington conference on thromboembolism was organized to review the present state of the art and to examine the new techniques and developments in this area.

An outstanding international known faculty was assembled for this three-day meeting. The superb quality of the presentations and the discussions following each allowed for the free exchange of information and ideas and were greatly responsible for the success of this conference. Publication of this book will enable a sharing of this valuable information and experience. Special "workshops" were organized to provide an opportunity for the participants to learn the new technique of transvenous caval interruption by the umbrella filter.

I am most grateful to the faculty for its participation and for providing the manuscripts for publication in this book. I wish to express deep appreciation to Drs. Frank R. Lemon, Associate Dean, and Dr. Ronald D. Hamilton, Director, Office of Continuing Education, University of Kentucky Medical Center, for their guidance, encouragement and valuable suggestions. The success of this symposium was the result of the excellent administrative management provided by them and their able associates. Special thanks is extended to Miss Joy Greene of the Continuing Education Office for a job well done.

I wish to thank Ed Spaw, Chief Technician, Cardio-Thoracic Laboratory, and Del Henderson, R.T., Associate-In-Radiology, and their associates in so efficiently organizing the wet clinics.

Appreciation is due to Mrs. Janet Haynes, Mrs. Yvonne Biederman and Mrs. Charles Chappell for their untiring efforts in the preparation of the manuscripts of this book.

I gratefully acknowledge the financial support of the program provided by the Eli Lilly Company of Indianapolis, Indiana; and of Edwards Laboratories, Santa Ana, California. The dog filters and applicators for use in the laboratory session were also provided by the Edwards Laboratories.

Kᴀᴢɪ Mᴏʙɪɴ-Uᴅᴅɪɴ

xi

CONTENTS

SECTION I

VENOUS THROMBOSIS

SECTION II

PULMONARY THROMBOEMBOLISM—PATHOPHYSIOLOGY

SECTION III

PULMONARY THROMBOEMBOLISM—DIAGNOSIS

PULMONARY THROMBOEMBOLISM

SECTION I

VENOUS
THROMBOSIS

Chapter 1

THE PATHOGENESIS OF VENOUS THROMBOSIS

John R. O'Brien

Introduction

I SHALL ASSUME, with the best authorities[10] that pathogenesis means the mode of origin and development of a morbid condition and that it includes remote predisposing factors studied epidemiologically and also the local events and mechanisms brought into play. The definition of thrombosis is much more difficult as it is impossible to say when a thrombus begins. The scene may be set at birth if there is a strong family predisposition; or it might be said to begin at the earliest reversible event which perhaps occurs in all of us all the time. Are clinically silent thrombi included? Perhaps worst of all: is there only one kind of thrombosis or, as I suspect, many different kinds precipitated by different events?

Having now given myself permission to range far and wide I shall first briefly review the pathology—what we find in sections. The incidence and predisposing factors will be surveyed for clues about possible mechanisms. I shall then follow Virchow's triad and consider the vessel wall, its contents, namely red cells, white cells and platelets and plasma, and the hydrodynamic situation; my aim will be to try to understand the mechanism involved. Excellent detailed reviews already exist, see for example Hume et al.,[7] Hampton[6] and Foster et al.[4] In my allotted space I can only summarize and bring the argument up to date. I shall then summarize five different areas of my recent work which is relevant to this topic.

HISTOLOGY

The characteristic feature of macroscopic and microscopic examination of thrombi is their variability. They can be rough or smooth, greyish-white through pink to the usual clotted blood color, and they come in all sizes and shapes. Histologically there are four basic characteristics. First the inhomogeneity of a thrombus: it is usually seen to be formed of layers. The remaining characteristics consist of the three types of material to be found:

5

(1) areas of closely packed platelets (the white head); (2) tightly packed bands or areas of fibrin; and (3) the red thrombus consisting of large masses of red cells caught in a more or less loose network of fibrin (the red tail).

While experimental damage to the intima undoubtedly leads to thrombus formation, it is striking that most descriptions of naturally occurring thrombi do not find intimal damage. Polymorphys often surround an area of platelet deposition and clearly they play some part. Indeed the detection of isotopically tagged WBC has been suggested as a method of localizing thrombi.[9]

I cannot look at a fixed section of a thrombus without trying to work out how it arose. Very clearly it is formed as a result of profoundly differing local conditions. The authorities seem unable to agree whether the initial lesion is a deposit of fibrin or a platelet mass. While thrombin could play a part in the formation of a platelet mass there are a dozen other possible mechanism for platelet disposition. However if fibrin is seen, this must indicate that at some stage in the local evolution, thrombin was present locally at sufficient concentration and for sufficient time to convert fibrinogen to fibrin. If stationary blood clots, a fine network of fibrin holds vast numbers of red cells in the clot. Thus if the section shows a red thrombus it can be concluded that, at that particular site at the time of formation, the blood flow was minimal or nonexistent. The bands of packed fibrin can only be formed in rapidly flowing blood. A sufficient concentration of thrombin must exist locally to clot the fibrinogen yet the flow be sufficient to "defibrinate" the blood as it passes.

There emerges a kaleidoscopic pattern of change in the microenvironment. We need to know the time scale of these various events and what determines that in one area of a thrombus at one time platelets are deposited and at another time (how much later?) fibrin and even later, when there is relative stasis, a red clot. The latter stages of organization, recanalization and lysis of thrombi will not be discussed. This histological appreciation sets the scene; most of this article is devoted to considering what events lead up to and produce these findings.

The photomicrographs emphasize the variety of appearances and hence the variety of local events. They are of a small recent thrombus 1 cm long found at post mortem in a valve cusp in a leg vein, and are stained by a picro-Mallory method. Plate 1 shows the vessel wall at the bottom with the media stained blue and with, in fact, little or no damage to the intima. The thrombus forming downstream, i.e. from left to right, has gross histological differences in different parts (Plate 1). At a higher power (Plate 2) it can be seen that all the blue granular material is platelets and that there are areas—one is shown here—where there is an exclusive deposition of platelets (with a very few leucocytes). Plate 3 shows that the reddy-orange stranded material is fibrin; again there has been a time and place where almost pure fibrin is deposited. This must result from thrombin activity but in turbulent blood producing the confused fibrin pattern. The absence of red cells indicates that conditions were appropriate for the blood to be "defibrinated" as it passed. In another area (Plate 4) almost pure red cells have been trapped. Plate 5 shows two adjacent areas: one consisting of red cells and the other almost exclusively of polymorphs (with a few platelets). This emphasizes the extreme proximity between two parts of the thrombus obviously caused by completely different local conditions. All these many different appearances were evidently produced by very different conditions which existed, probably at different times, but in close proximity and all in an area 1 cm long. Plate 6, with a mixed picture and the appearance of *swirl* due to red fibrin strands being laid down along the direction of blood flow, emphasizes again the importance of the hydro-dynamic situation which may change often, and probably determines the balance of other factors influencing the deposition of fibrin, platelets, red cells or polymorphs.

INCIDENCE AND PREDISPOSING FACTORS

Most of the information discussed under this heading will almost inevitably apply to the manifestation of clinical disease. As suggested in the introduction, thrombi detected by other methods could have a very different incidence and pathogenic pattern: for example, thrombi detected by ^{125}I labelled fibrinogen and/or phlebography are between four and ten times more common than the clinically overt disease. It is pertinent to ask what determines which of the many clinically silent ^{125}I detectable thrombi become clinically manifest. Thus links or discrepancies between these two ways of diagnosing thrombosis are particularly relevant.

There seems fairly good evidence that the incidence of thrombosis or at least pulmonary embolism has increased sharply since 1940 at least in England; but there are the usual difficulties about ascertainment and comparability of figures. Certainly in 1967 thrombosis in all its forms was recorded on death certificates about twice as often as cancer, and a number of comparisons suggest that venous thrombosis is seen far more often in the Western Europeans than in Africa or India but as pointed out by Murphy[11] it is very difficult to apportion these differences if they exist between genetic and environmental predisposing causes.

Table 1-I enumerates some factors that are generally considered to increase the chance of venous thrombosis. The validity of the evidence for each of these factors will not be discussed nor the extent of interaction between these factors. However some general points of interest relative to

mechanisms emerge. Blood Group A and a familial predisposition for
example must have a permanent effect and hint at a permanent thrombotic diathesis; yet presumably alone they will not cause a thrombus unless
there are additional local and/or general precipitating factors. There are
acquired long-term factors like the Pill and malignancy; again they must
exert a long-term predisposition and presumably potentiate a local precipitating event. Operations do produce systemic changes in the blood, as
well as altering the blood flow to the legs, so they could well contribute to
systemic as well as local factors. Then, as perhaps the proximate causes are
approached there are conditions affecting the blood flow; pregnancy and
other conditions lead to sluggish flow. These factors could have local,
short-term effects. All these factors must contribute indirectly to the final
event to some extent and the mechanisms involved certainly deserve detailed study. Nevertheless none of these factors explains why a thrombus
occurs at one particular site. The isotopically labelled fibrinogen technique
shows that usually there is only one thrombus, less frequently two or three
separate incidents, but never is thrombosis initiated extensively throughout
the venous system. Thus, even though a thrombus may subsequently grow
and extend widely, the initiating event must occur locally at a particular
site with a particular set of local circumstances.

TABLE 1-I

SOME FACTORS PREDISPOSING TO VENOUS THROMBOSIS

Operations
    especially if long on hips or pelvis.
Poor Blood Flow
    Varicose veins
    Obstructed venous return
    Lack of movement—bed rest, stroke.
Childbirth
Females during reproductive period
Increased age
Malignancy
Use of "the Pill"
Blood Group A
Smoking
Familial predisposition
High blood viscosity
Obesity
High platelet count (perhaps)

LOCAL MECHANISMS

The Vessel Wall

While platelets do not stick readily or perhaps at all to intact healthy

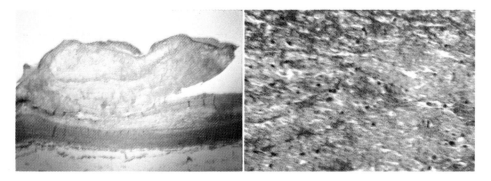

PLATE 1   PLATE 2

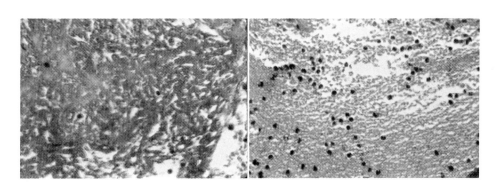

PLATE 3   PLATE 4

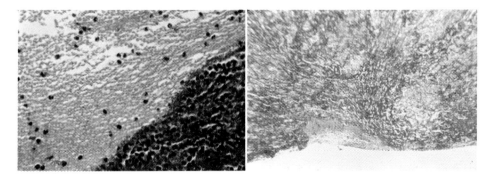

PLATE 5   PLATE 6

vascular endothelium, there is no doubt that if the endothelium is damaged, the subjacent stroma and especially the exposed collagen will induce platelet adhesion. Once platelets are stuck to collagen the release mechanism occurs whereby ADP is liberated from the stuck platelets which makes other platelets entering the area of high ADP concentration extremely sticky: thus platelets pile up to form a mass that may cause eddies. The adherent platelets also expose platelet Factor III which facilitates clotting. Thus the scene, with variations, is set for thrombus formation. However, careful search of thrombosed vessels usually fails to reveal an area of damage. Mild hypoxia is insufficient and it seems unlikely that, for example, operation patients sustain endothelial damage, although they often develop thrombosis. Nevertheless, Begent and Born[1] have shown experimentally that minute amounts of ADP once in the lumen, delivered in fact by iontophoresis, can initiate platelet deposition. It is also of great interest that they also show that blood velocity plays a major part.

The Contents

A great deal of research time has been devoted to finding an abnormality in the *plasma*, a "hypercoagulable state" which might account for the fibrin deposition that occurs at least in some part of almost every thrombus. It has already been pointed out that thrombin could be the primum movens, either causing fibrin deposition or activating the platelets. High levels of Factor VIII, activated Factor Xa and other clotting abnormalities have been incriminated. But there is no agreed abnormality, except perhaps the increase in heparin neutralizing activity. This activity *in vivo* probably does not inactivate heparin since little or no heparin exists in plasma. It may be a coincidental byproduct of platelet activation or it may have some important, as yet ill understood function.

A high *red cell* count undoubtedly predisposes to thrombosis, and it has two effects. The blood is more viscid and so the circulation is slowed. The red cells tend to take a center position in laminar flow in the veins and the smaller platelets are, as it were, jostled to the periphery. There is little evidence that the high ADP content of red cells ever gets a chance to influence platelet function. The *white cells* are regularly found even early in thrombus formation and, labelled, they have been used to detect thrombosis.[9] (The author found excess polymorphs in a "thrombus" in a heart-lung filter after thirty minutes in the circulation.) They may contribute in various ways and perhaps activate the fibrinolytic system at a later stage.

The platelets play a major role; some would argue *the* major role in the initiation even of a venous thrombus. (Their contribution to arterial thrombosis is even greater but is not considered here.) If the endothelium is intact, then the problem is how are the first platelets attracted and why do

they adhere. Once the first platelet has stuck the accretion of more platelets and the release of ADP and the influence of this mass by inducing
turbulence and the exposure of PF3 have already been mentioned as good
reasons for the development of a thrombosis.

What is the initiating mechanism? If the majority of thrombi begin in
valve cusps as has been claimed[7] then certainly the hydrodynamic peculi-
arities in a cusp pocket must be implicated. Electron micrographs exist
showing focal concentrations of ten to one hundred platelets in blood
vessels in the relative absence of red cells. This must indicate a "silting
out" of platelets presumably in a vortex. If there is a vortex, then there are
more and gentler collisions and there is time for the activation of clotting
factors before they are swept downstream and time for platelets to develop
membrane change and become more "sticky."

The Hydrodynamic Situation

The last paragraph has already emphasized what is probably the major
factor determining the localization of a thrombus, namely local, perhaps
transitory changes in the hydrodynamic pattern leading to vortices and
permitting the initiation of trace local amounts of thrombin or ADP and
probably allowing platelets to aggregate and/or to stick to the endothelium.
(See for example Mustard et al.[12] who consider blood flow and thrombus
formation, and an excellent review of Goldsmith.[5])

MECHANISMS REVEALED BY TREATMENT

The suggested mechanisms outlined above are to some extent specula-
tion; the way that indirect and remote factors have an effect is largely
unknown. The finding in thrombosis of abnormalities of coagulation or of
platelet function when these are clearly defined, and the functions tested
well understood, should lead to better understanding of the processes
involved. But at present, understanding of the mechanism inhibited by
successful treatment is probably the most powerful *in vivo* method of
understanding the thrombotic mechanism(s).

The indendione anticoagulants can act only by inhibiting blood coagulation. While there is no doubt they significantly decrease the chance of
thrombosis, yet many treated cases still develop DVT. Since these drugs
are only moderately effective, it can be concluded confidently that fibrin
formation by thrombin plays a definite part in thrombus formation but that
the local concentration of thrombin is only little affected by the mild therapeutic inhibition of systemic coagulation.

Aspirin has no effect whatsoever on the development of postoperative
venous thrombosis.[17] From this it can confidently be claimed that the release mechanism in platelets, which is grossly inhibited by aspirin plays an

insignificant part in this type of thrombosis. Even fully aspirinated platelets can undergo the release process if sufficiently strongly stimulated by collagen (but not by adrenaline), so a very strong local stimulus in a thrombus might stimulate some release. Nevertheless it still follows that if release played an important part, some degree of inhibition of thrombosis would be expected, and it was not found.

Heparin in small doses (5000 U b.d.) profoundly decreases the incidence of postoperative DVT[8] at least when these are diagnosed by the ^{125}I-fibrinogen method. This fact holds a vital clue to the mechanism involved. The heparin concentration is too low to exert a significant antithrombin effect. It has been shown that a natural anti-Xa is stimulated by heparin.[20] Perhaps this is the mechanism involved. Activated Factor X had already been suggested as the cause of at least experimental "hypercoagulable states" in which stasis induces thrombosis of a kind.[19] The regular finding of increased anti-heparin activity (Platelet Factor 4) in many forms of thrombosis may be a related phenomenon. This clinically useful finding with its intriguing but incompletely understood message about the thrombotic mechanism has been discussed elsewhere.[12,13]

PERSONAL OBSERVATIONS

Predisposing Factors

Three hundred and three patients were entered into the trial of aspirin for the prevention of postoperative thrombosis using the [125]Iodine labelled fibrinogen technique to detect thrombi.[18] Aspirin proved to have no effect but seventy-four patients developed thrombosis and we could compare the incidence of possible predisposing factors in the thrombotic group with the group who did not thrombose. Males, older patients, those whose operations lasted a long time, who had varicose veins, those with malignancy and those undergoing some big operations, e.g. transabdominal G.U. operations (46%)—but not transurethral G.U. operations (7%)—all showed a significant increase in risk. Patients of blood group O and B had less thrombosis but this was not significant. Many of these factors are interrelated, nevertheless age and duration of operation showed up on all types of analysis.

These results emphasize once again the complexity of pathogenesis. Here are totally dissimilar factors which almost certainly act via very different pathways. Perhaps the mechanisms involved and even the final morphology of the thrombi might be different. On the other hand, the dissimilar factors could act finally through a common pathway and produce identical thrombi. If some test of a function involved before the final event is found to be abnormal in dissimilar situations, say, in old age and during operations, then it would suggest that a final common path exists.

Site and Day of Onset

Almost 70 percent of the thrombi were present by the first postoperative day, i.e. at the time the legs were first scanned. About 15 percent occurred on the second day and very few thereafter.[16] Thus the operation clearly played a major part in the production of thrombosis and bed rest, even though early ambulation is encouraged, can have had little effect.

It is also of importance that the great majority of the thrombi were first detected in the calf and remained localized to this site. In 167 patients there were eighty-six thrombi (some patients had multiple thrombi); and 53 percent of the thrombi were in the lower calf, 35 percent in the upper calf and only 12 percent were detected in the thigh.

There is a striking difference between the number of patients with thrombi detected by the ^{125}I-method and the day of onset, and those with clinically evident disease. Less than one in four patients diagnosed by the isotope method had any clinical signs at all, which emphasizes again the need for specifying most carefully what lesion one is discussing.

Continuous Monitoring

We wanted to know exactly when a thrombus forms and how long this takes and whether and when it subsequently increases in size (further deposition) or decreases in size (thrombolysis). Accordingly a machine was devised to monitor continuously the signals over the leg veins after injecting ^{125}I-labelled fibrinogen. For each leg this consists of two light splints, one for the thigh and one for the calf, holding two Geiger Muller tubes. These eight monitors from both legs are counted serially and the signals appropriately modified are printed out on a time chart. Each monitor is counted for five minutes once every forty minutes. This machine has been shown to detect thrombi—it works—but this study is in its early stages.

Abnormalities of Fibrinogen

Doctors Fletcher and Alkjaersig of St. Louis have perfected and now automated[2] a method using gel (Biogel 5M) exclusion chromatography for separating on a Molecular Weight basis the single fibrinogen molecules (MW 330,000), the large complexes of fibrinogen (MW 450,000 to 1,000,000) and fibrin degradation products and fibrinogen derivatives (MW 257,000 or less).

Normally in health only the monospecies fibrinogen molecule was found but these workers claimed that the above modified forms of fibrinogen circulated in the presence of thrombosis. The MRC study in which many patients were scanned for thrombosis detected by the ^{125}I-fibrinogen method, provided an excellent opportunity for examining this claim. Samples from those patients with and without thrombosis were accordingly sent to Dr. Fletcher.

In a combined study[2] we were able to show that prior to operation, a small number of patients already had an abnormal fibrinogen pattern. They may well have had a thrombus in relation to their illness (many had carcinoma of the lung); so these patients are discarded from the analysis. When the patients with a normal fibrinogen pattern before operation are considered, then the correlation between an abnormal fibrinogen pattern and the ^{125}I test was excellent. With two unexplained exceptions all patients who developed ^{125}I-thrombosis also developed abnormal fibrinogen patterns. Of the patients who remained postoperatively normal by Fletcher's test, only one showed ^{125}I-thrombosis. There were a number who developed an abnormal fibrinogen pattern but who had no evidence of ^{125}I-thrombosis in the legs; but they could well have had thrombosis elsewhere (see Table 1-II).

TABLE 1-II

RADIO-IODINATED FIBRINOGEN

Chromatography	Thrombosis is present	Thrombosis is absent
Abnormal	41	7
Normal	2	31

These findings show that in postoperative patients the development of modified fibrinogen molecules strongly suggests that a thrombus has formed. There was insufficient evidence to show whether this fibrinogen abnormality was the cause or the result, but it remains a very sensitive test and an intriguing observation. It also clearly implicates systemic circulating fibrinogen and also the whole system of clotting and fibrinolysis in the events relating to local thrombus formation. It is, however, odd that the fibrinogen half-life is probably similar whether a thrombus develops or not.[15]

Postoperative Platelet Function Changes

As well as studying changes in fibrinogen molecules after thrombosis, we also carried out a battery of platelet function tests before and after the operation.[17] Thus it was possible retrospectively to look at the preoperation results and divide them into those from patients who subsequently thrombosed and those who did not. Changes occurring in patients with thrombosis after the operation might be due to the operation or the result of the thrombus, but changes occurring before are likely to be related to the cause and cannot be the result of thrombosis.

Comparing preoperative patients who developed thrombosis with those who did not, the aggregation to ADP was significantly *less* pre- and postoperatively in patients who thrombosed. Aggregation with adrenaline, thrombin and collagen showed a similar trend, i.e. less aggregation in thrombotics, but fewer significant differences emerged. The heparin/thrombin clotting time was shorter, indicating more heparin neutralization by thrombotics than by those who did not thrombose. This difference was not significant, but the thrombotics differed very significantly from apparently healthy controls.

The Russell Viper Venom (Stypven) accelerated clotting time was shorter in the thrombosis than in nonthrombotics, strongly suggesting that more phospholipid was available.

In summary, the most striking change is the decreased aggregating efficiency of platelets in the plasma of those patients who developed thrombosis. Thrombotics may have a little more phospholipid exposed in plasma and on their platelets. This unexpected result has been considered[13, 14] but remains unexplained. Certainly as yet, they throw no new light on the patholgenesis of thrombosis.

In myocardial infarction the stressed template bleeding time is apparently significantly shorter, suggesting more active platelets.[15] Its application to venous thrombosis might help clarify the part platelets play.

Conclusion

In conclusion I reiterate my original difficulty, namely, the difficulty of knowing what we are talking about! The more closely we look, the more difficult it is to define thrombosis and there is a proportionate difficulty in considering which of the many postulated, and in some cases, demonstrated pathways are involved. Epidemiology will suggest possible mechanisms. Experimental thrombosis may help clarify the picture. But I believe that successful therapy itself, duly studied and understood, may help us most in our efforts to understand, treat and prevent venous thrombosis.

REFERENCES

1. Begant, N. and Born, G. V. R.: Growth rate *in vivo* of platelet thrombi produced by iontophoresis of ADP as a function of mean blood flow velocity. *Nature,* 227:926, 1970.
2. Fletcher, A. P. and Alkjaersig, N.: Blood screening methods for the diagnosis of venous thrombosis. *Millbank Mem Fund Q,* 50:1, pt. 2, 170, 1972.
3. Fletcher, A. P., Alkjaersig, N., O'Brien, J. R. and Tulevski, V. G.: Blood hypercoagulability and thrombosis. *Trans Assoc Am Physicians,* 83:159-167, 1970.
4. Foster, C. S., Genton, E., Henderson, M., Sherry, S. and Wessler, S.: The epidemiology of venous thrombosis. *Millbank Mem Fund Q,* 50:1, pt. 2, 1972.

5. Goldsmith, H. L.: In Spaet, T. H. (Ed.): *Progress in Haemostasis and Thrombosis.* New York, Grune & Stratton, 1972, pp. 97-141.

6. Hampton, J. R. and Mitchell, J. R. A.: In Biggs, R. (Ed.): *Human Blood Coagulation, Haemostasis and Thrombosis.* Oxford, Blackwell, 1972, pp. 477-496.

7. Hume, M., Sevitt, S. and Thomas, D.: *Venous Thrombosis and Pulmonary Embolism.* Cambridge, Mass., Harvard University Press, 1970.

8. Kakkar, V. V., Field, E. S., Nicholaides, A. N., Flute, P. T., Wessler, S. and Yin, E. T.: Low doses of heparin in prevention of deep vein thrombosis. *Lancet,* 2:669, 1971.

9. Kwaan, H. C. and Grumet, G.: The use of 51 Cr-labelled leucocytes in the detection of venous thrombosis. Third Congress Int. Soc. Thrombosis and Haemostasis, Washington, 1972, p. 400.

10. MacNulty, A. S.: *Butterworth's Medical Dictionary.* London, Butterworth, 1965.

11. Murphy, E. A.: Genetic and haematologic factors in venous thrombosis. *Millbank Mem Fund Q, 50:*1, pt. 2, 71-85, 1972.

12. Mustard, J. F., Jorgensen, L. and Packham, M. A.: *Thromb et Diath Haem,* Suppl 54, 151, 1973.

13. O'Brien, J. R.: The Mechanisms of Venous Thrombosis: Anticoagulants, Aspirin and Heparin. *Mod Concepts Cardiovasc Dis, 42:*11-15, 1973a.

14. ————: Heparin and platelets and venous thrombosis. *Am Heart J.* In press, 1973b.

15. O'Brien, J. R., Etherington, M., Jameson, S., Klaber, M. and Ainsworth, J.: Stressed template bleeding-time and other platelet function tests in myocardial infarction. *Lancet, 1:*694-696, 1973.

16. O'Brien, J. R., Tulevski, V. and Heady, J. A.: Rate of fibrinogen turnover in thrombosis. *Lancet, 2:*445, 1972.

17. O'Brien, J. R., Tulevski, V. G., Etherington, M., Madgwick, T., Alkjaersig, N. and Fletcher, A.: Platelet function studies before and after operation and thrombosis. *J Lab Clin Med, 83:*342, 1974.

18. Report of the Steering Committee of a Trial Sponsored by the Medical Research Council: Effect of aspirin on postoperative venous thrombosis. *Lancet, 2:*441, 1972.

19. Wessler, S. and Yin, E. T.: Experimental hypercoagulable states induced by factor X. Comparison of the nonactivated and activated forms. *J Lab Clin Med, 72:*256, 1968.

20. Yin, E. T., Wessler, S. and Stoll, P. J.: Identity of plasma activated factor X inhibitor with anti-thrombin III and heparin cofactor. *J Biol Chem, 246:*3712-3719, 1971.

Chapter 2

DOPPLER ULTRASOUND METHOD IN DIAGNOSIS OF DEEP VEIN THROMBOSIS

Bernard Sigel, W. Robert Felix, Jr.,

George L. Popky and Johannes Ipsen

D OPPLER ULTRASOUND blood flow detection provides a relatively simple method for detecting deep venous thrombosis in the lower limbs. This technique can also be used for determining the competency of valves in the deep veins, thereby providing supportive evidence for the diagnosis of the postphlebitic syndrome. Examination may be performed quickly at the bedside. We have now performed over 12,000 Doppler ultrasound examinations in over 7,000 patients. In this presentation, we wish to briefly describe the method, document its accuracy, and emphasize its strengths and weaknesses.

METHOD

The principle of the Doppler ultrasound blood velocity detector is based on the fact that blood flow may be sensed through intact skin by the shift in frequency produced by the backscatter of high frequency sound from moving red cells. A continuous wave signal of a frequency between five and ten megaHertz is introduced into the tissue. Because ultrasound does not readily traverse a gaseous medium, an acoustical coupling gel is applied between the transducer and the skin. The transducer is composed of two ceramic crystals set adjacent and usually at a slight angle to each other. One crystal transmits the sound and the other receives the backscattered signal. The difference in frequency between the transmitted and received signal produced by the Doppler shift is an index of the velocity of the red cells. As used transcutaneously, this device cannot precisely measure flow velocity because the angle between the transducer and the blood vessel cannot be determined precisely. However, it can be used to sense flow. The Doppler frequency shift, between transmitted and received signals, is provided as an audio signal which can readily be heard by earphones or loud-speaker.*

Most instruments employ a filter to remove the lower frequency noise. This is helpful in arterial flow detection because the flow is rapid; how-ever, flow in slower moving streams, such as veins, may not be detectable. The absence of a signal from a vessel does not necessarily mean that no flow is occurring. The absence of a signal can also mean slow flow which may be quite normal in veins. To overcome this limitation, we introduced the principle of manually compressing the extremity to produce a pulse wave or augmentation flow wave which propagates up and down the deep venous system at greater velocity than the flow of blood in veins. Propaga-tion of this wave distally is damped by normally functioning valves. Propa-gation centrally may be ultrasonically detected proximal to the site of compression as a transient augmented flow signal which we have termed Augmented or A-sound. This A-sound may be superimposed on a spontane-ous flow signal or S-sound which is cyclical with the respiration. In the diagnosis of venous disease, we rely on the use of augmented flow signals as heard through a loudspeaker. The examiner determines whether the A-sound is present, diminished, or absent. Our technique has been de-scribed in detail previously;[1,3] consequently, only a brief summary will be given here.

The Doppler ultrasound examination is used in conjunction with the clinical examination for venous disease. We first inspect and palpate the lower extremities. Then we employ the ultrasound detector. The ultra-sound examination may be complete or partial depending on whether we are interested in detecting occlusion and incompetent valves or occlusion alone. Usually we perform the complete examination initially. Subsequently, if reexamination is desired within a few days of the first examination, we perform only a partial examination to determine the occurrence of venous thrombosis in the intervening period.

In order to assess the deep venous system of the lower limb for both occlusion and incompetent valves, ultrasound examination is performed at three locations: (1) common femoral vein; (2) posterior tibial vein; and (3) popliteal vein. The examination is performed with the patient supine in bed or on an examining table. The head of the bed should be slightly raised to maintain a larger pool of venous blood in the lower extremities.

The common femoral vein at the inguinal ligament is examined first. The transducer is applied over the vein just medial to the femoral artery pulse. An S-sound is usually present in phase with the patient's respiration. The

*Supported by grants from the National Heart & Lung Institute (Public Health Service) No. HL-11774, The John A. Hartford Foundation, and by Part I Research Funds of the Veterans Administration.

lower thigh is compressed manually and the examiner notes the occurrence of the A-sound (Fig. 2-1). With the position of the transducer maintained, augmentation maneuvers are repeated by calf compression and finally by dorsiflexion of the foot.

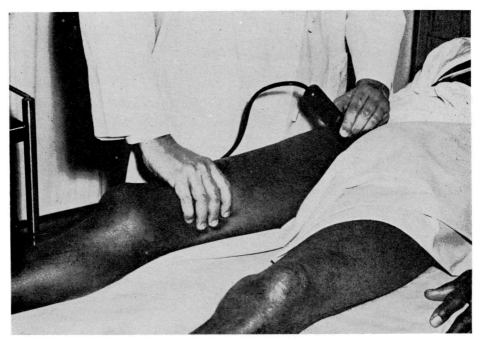

Figure 2-1.   Elicitation of distal positive femoral A-sound by lower thigh compression. See text for explanation. (By permission of *Archives of Surgery*.)

The posterior tibial vein is examined posterior to the medial malleolus. The calf at the junction of the mid and lower third is compressed first and the presence of an A-sound determined. Following release, the examiner again notes the presence of an A-sound. Subsequently, the procedure is repeated distal to the transducer with compression and release of the foot.

After the femoral and posterior tibial veins are examined in the opposite extremity, the patient is turned to a prone position for examination of the popliteal veins. To best examine the popliteal vein, a pillow or other prop is placed beneath the leg to permit 10 to 15° flexion of the knee. Full hyper-extension of the leg can obliterate the S-sound in the popliteal flow prob-ably indicating an impairment of flow. The popliteal vein signal is either with or lateral to the artery signal. The lower calf is compressed and released and the presence of A-sounds noted. Compression proximal to the transducer is performed at the lower third, middle third, and upper third of the thigh.

If there is interest only in determining the presence of occlusion the examination may be limited to the common femoral vein sites with compression of the thigh, leg and dorsiflexion of the foot.

The Doppler ultrasound diagnosis of occlusion is made by the absence or marked diminution of augmented flow signals at the femoral vein produced by distal compression. If the femoral augmented flow signals following lower thigh compression are normal but absent or reduced from calf compression, we interpret the examination as revealing *leg vein occlusion*. If the augmented flow sound from thigh compression is also abnormal, our ultrasound diagnosis becomes *femoral vein occlusion*. We grade the extent of occlusion as *partial* or *complete* depending on the elicitation of diminished or absent femoral augmented sounds. For the diagnosis of occlusion, we rely entirely upon femoral augmented flow sounds produced by distal compression.

Incompetence of valves is determined by the occurrence of two types of augmented flow sounds which normally should not be present. Release of manual compression distal to the monitoring transducer will produce an augmented flow signal if the valves are incompetent. Augmented sounds at the popliteal vein produced by compressing the mid and upper thirds of the thigh indicate incompetence of the femoral vein valves.

ACCURACY OF DOPPLER ULTRASOUND DETECTION OF VENOUS DISEASE

We performed a validative study to correlate the ultrasound method with phlebography or operative and autopsy findings and to compare it with clinical examination.[3] Among the first 500 patients examined by us, we obtained confirmation of findings by phlebography in 139 and by operation or autopsy in eight. In these 147 patients, information was available on 248 extremities because phlebograms were usually performed bilaterally. A number of patients examined by phlebography had negative findings on clinical and ultrasound examination but were suspected of having recent pulmonary embolism.

In our validative study, results were expressed in terms of sensitivity and specificity. Sensitivity is defined as the number of positive extremities obtained divided by the actual number of extremities proven to have venous occluson by phlebography or anatomic confirmation. Specificity is defined as the number of negative extremities observed divided by the number of extremities proven to be nonoccluded. Comparison of Doppler ultrasound and clinical methods to validating examinations in the diagnosis of deep venous occlusion revealed the following findings:

	Ultrasound Examination	*Clinical Examination*
Sensitivity	63/83 Extremities = 75.9%	45/83 Extremities = 54.2%
Specificity	150/165 Extremities = 90.9%	106/165 Extremities = 64.2%

Comparison of Doppler ultrasound and clinical methods were also compared to phlebography in the diagnosis of incompetent deep valves with the following results:

	Ultrasound Examination	*Clinical Examination*
Sensitivity	55/72 Extremities = 76.4%	37/72 Extremities = 52.8%
Specificity	84/124 Extremities = 67.7%	98/124 Extremities = 79.0%

In order to quantitate better the limitation of the ultrasound method, we reassessed the sensitivity in terms of the estimated duration of the venous thrombosis and the location of venous occlusion.

The accuracy of the ultrasound technique in terms of the duration of the venous thrombosis was estimated by assessing the chronicity of the vein occlusion in the venograms. By employing an arbitrary set of criteria for "new" and "old" occlusion, we estimated the sensitivity of the ultrasound diagnosis in diagnosing "new" occlusion as 78.1 percent, and in detecting "old" occlusion as 67.5 percent.

The sensitivity of the ultrasound technique in relation to the distribution of the thrombi within the deep veins also was determined. Sensitivity was 60.7 percent (17 of 28 extremities) in the extremities with leg vein occlusion alone. Where the femoral vein was occluded, the sensitivity was 83.6 percent. Thus, the Doppler ultrasound technique is more accurate in detecting femoral vein rather than calf vein occlusion.

Conclusions

Doppler ultrasound examination for diagnosing venous disease in the lower extremities is useful as a screening and surveillance procedure. In particular, it should be used in conjunction with clinical evaluation.

The procedure is most useful in detecting recent occlusion involving the femoral and popliteal veins. It is less accurate in diagnosing calf vein occlusion. Thus, ultrasound detection is most applicable for the diagnosis of established rather than incipient thrombosis involving the major deep veins of the proximal lower extremity. This is the stage of deep venous thrombosis most commonly associated with life-threatening pulmonary embolism. Bearing these limitations in mind, the technique has a number of advantages. These include its noninvasive nature which provides a safe, simple, inexpensive procedure which is well accepted by patients.

REFERENCES

1. Sigel, B., Popky, G. L., Wagner, D. K., Boland, J. P., Mapp, E. M. and Feigl, P.: A Doppler ultrasound method for diagnosing lower extremity venous disease. *Surg Gynecol Obstet*, *127*:339, 1968.

2. Sigel, B., Felix, Jr., W. R., Popky, G. L. and Ipsen, J.: Diagnosis of lower limb venous thrombosis by Doppler ultrasound technique. *Arch Surg, 104*:174, 1972.

3. Sigel, B., Popky, G. L., Mapp, E. M., Feigl, P., Felix, Jr., W. R. and Ipsen, J.: Evaluation of Doppler ultrasound examination: Its use in diagnosis of lower extremity venous disease. *Arch Surg, 100*:535, 1970.

DISCUSSION

Dr. Murphy (Lexington): Will Doppler technique detect both complete and partial occlusions?

Dr. Sigel: Yes, it will pick up both types.

Question: Can you actually quantitate the degree of occlusion in the veins?

Dr. Sigel: That is pretty difficult to judge, because all we have is a venogram and it is pretty tough to tell just how much of the vein is occluded by the venogram. Plus the fact that one of the reasons for getting the false negative, that is getting a normal Doppler signal in the presence of occlusion, it may not only be the fact that there is only a partial occlusion, but because there are alternate channels so that it is difficult to decide that point. I believe that the reason why the results are less good in calf veins, the occlusion particularly if only one or two tributory systems are involved, is that the pulse wave can propagate up the open system and produce a normal signal.

Question: What kinds of instruments are there and what is their cost?

Dr. Sigel: There are a number of manufacturers making this and the simpler forms, that is without fancy write-outs that are the continuous wave directional Doppler ultrasound unit. I will show you some results with that unit later on. Here one can record on two channels and get forward flow and reverse flow or one can sum the effect and get a single line which, if you have 90 percent flow in one direction and 10 percent flow in the other direction, appears at 80 percent in one direction. The third type of Doppler is the so-called pulse Doppler ultrasound detector and this combines the principle of the Doppler ultrasound with the pulse echo ultrasound that you are all familiar with which is used for scanning mid-lines and things like this. By combining these two principles, it is possible to get blood flow velocity information at various depths so that one can say go across the flow stream. These are the three types that you should be aware of. The later type, the pulse Doppler is more sophisticated and most expensive and it is still a fairly good research tool to a large extent. The other two are more readily available and I guess they are finding greater application. The cost varies from around three to four hundred dollars for the simplest non-directional device to several thousands of dollars for the pulsed Doppler.

Dr. Kucera (Florida): We have a Doppler and we have used it for a lot of arterial occlusive disease and find it very helpful, but this produces a rather loud, harsh sound and I'm wondering how you can hear a low venous hum when this vein is in the same neighborhood as the loud arterial noise.

Dr. Sigel: The augmentation maneuver produces a signal which is so loud and characteristic that it actually temporarily drowns out the arterial signal. This makes it very easy to assess venous patency.

Question: Does venography lead to complications such as venous thrombosis?

Dr. Sigel: To determine that venographically would be very difficult because it is tough to convince a patient to have a second venogram. What we are now doing as a matter of fact is the venous examination before and after venograms and arteriograms. One of the interesting things is following venogram we have not picked up occlusion. Following arteriography there is a transient occlusion that worried us at first, but we think now it is just simply due to the swelling and extravasation that may occur, but it doesn't behave like the venous thrombosis and goes away.

Dr. Hirsh: Can you pick up isolated iliac vein thrombosis?

Dr. Sigel: We really stop at the inguinal ligament in our routine examination. We have not had really too much experience with looking for iliac vein thrombosis. We are really looking for a very simple test that we can allow nurses and technicians to do.

Chapter 3

IMPEDANCE PLETHYSMOGRAPHY IN THE DIAGNOSIS OF DEEP VEIN THROMBOSIS

H. Brownell Wheeler

Joseph A. O'Donnell[*]

IMPEDANCE PLETHYSMOGRAPHY is a convenient and sensitive method for measuring changes in the venous blood volume of the leg. By demonstrating a decreased volume response to temporary venous outflow obstruction, impedance plethysmography can reliably diagnose venous thrombosis. This chapter outlines the theory and current practice of this new diagnostic technique.

Relationship Between Blood Volume and Electrical Impedance

Blood is a good conductor of electricity. The amount of blood present in the leg affects its electrical conductivity. When blood volume *increases*, the impedance (or resistance) to passage of an electrical current *decreases*. Conversely, when blood volume decreases, the electrical resistance rises.

There is a constant mathematical relationship between voltage, resistance and current, in accordance with Ohm's law (voltage = current x resistance). If the current strength is held constant, changes in voltage reflect changes in resistance. If a constant current is passed through the lower leg, changes in voltage indicate changes in the resistance of the leg due to changes in blood volume. These blood volume changes can be recorded with great sensitivity by connecting skin electrodes to appropriate instrumentation. This indirect method for measuring blood volume changes was initially described by Nyboer[9] as a means for evaluating peripheral arterial blood flow. He introduced the term "impedance plethysmography," and we have subsequently used the term "impedance phlebography"[11,12] to describe

---

[*]We would like to acknowledge our deep indebtedness to Dr. Karl Benedict, Jr. and the members of the Department of Radiology at St. Vincent Hospital. This study would not have been possible without the technically excellent phlebograms which they performed.

the use of impedance measurements for the study of venous blood volume changes.

Effect of Thrombosis on Venous Pressue-Volume Relationships

When a person is lying supine, the pressure in the deep leg veins slightly exceeds the pressure in the great veins of the pelvis and abdomen. If the intraabdominal pressure increases until it exceeds that of the leg veins, venous return from the legs stops. There is then a progressive increase in venous pressure and volume in the leg. When the abdominal venous pressure falls to normal, there is prompt venous outflow and a rapid decrease in leg venous pressure and volume.

Intraabdominal pressure normally fluctuates during respiration. Even during shallow respiration, small fluctuations in pressure can be measured in the inferior vena cava. These pressure changes in the inferior vena cava result in correspondingly changes in the pressure and volume of blood in the leg veins. If a deep breath is taken, the respiratory venous volume excursion in the leg is increased.[2] The response becomes even more pronounced if a Valsalva maneuver is carried out.

Changes in intraabdominal pressure can also be produced experimentally by inflating a pneumatic cuff around the abdomen. The venous volume increase in the leg is similar to that observed during respiration but the pressure increment is more easily controlled, since it does not depend upon patient cooperation. Pressure-volume responses in the lower leg can be observed even more conveniently by placing a pneumatic cuff around the thigh.

If thrombosis is present, the normal relationships between venous pressure and volume are altered. Venous run-off is slower because of mechanical obstruction to venous outflow. This venous outflow obstruction also results in a greater resting venous volume and less capacity of the venous system to expand. Accordingly, there is a smaller volume increase in response to respiration or application of a pneumatic cuff. The more extensive the thrombosis, the less marked is the initial volume response. In recent complete thrombosis of the femoral vein, there is practically no volume response to deep breathing or application of a thigh cuff.

Alterations in the volume response of the venous system to temporary venous outflow obstruction are most marked in the early stages of venous thrombosis. As time goes by, the response usually improves, even when venography shows clot to be still present. This improvement may be due to the development of collateral venous channels. It may also be due in part to the gradual disappearance of venous spasm associated with fresh thrombosis.

PROCEDURE

Four circumferential electrodes are placed around the calf. The inner two electrodes are placed approximately ten cm apart, encompassing the maximum volume of the calf muscles. A weak alternating current is then passed through the outer two electrodes. The current strength is so weak as to be imperceptable to the subject. The frequency ($25KH_z$) is so high as to be incapable of stimulating the heart. The voltage changes in the electrical field are recorded, reflecting changes in the electrical resistance due to fluctuations in blood volume.*

Patients are studied in the supine position with the leg slightly externally rotated and flexed approximately 40° at the knee. This position is usually assumed naturally if the patient is asked to shift his weight to the hip on the side being studied.

The purpose of the examination is to observe the venous volume response in the calf to temporary venous outflow obstruction. In most patients venous outflow obstruction is easily induced by any maneuver which increases the intraabdominal pressure. Normal deep breathing causes fluctuations in intraabdominal pressure and usually produces clear-cut venous volume variations in the calf. If the patient is asked to take a maximum inspiration and hold it for approximately ten seconds, there is a marked rise in the venous volume in the calf. With expiration, there is a prompt fall in venous volume. In some patients, an increase in intraabdominal pressure may be achieved more easily by asking the patient to strain, as though moving his bowels, or to carry out a Valsalva maneuver.

These breathing maneuvers are a simple and useful means of assessing normal venous dynamics. However, they have certain limitations. Breathing maneuvers require patient cooperation. In senile, critically ill, or uncooperative patients, it may be impossible to have the patient carry out any maneuver which significantly increases abdominal pressure. The test is easiest to perform in patients who are both cooperative and relatively healthy.

The venous pressure increase produced by any voluntary respiratory maneuver is difficult to standardize. In practice, one must rely upon obtaining the *maximum* venous volume change which can be produced. The magnitude of this response will depend not only upon the state of the venous system, but also upon the patient's efforts. In patients who are unable to make a maximum respiratory effort, the respiratory increment in venous pressure may be so slight as to give an apparent false positive

---

*The impedance measuring equipment employed in these studies was kindly supplied by Codman, Inc., Randolph, Mass. 02368.

response. The examiner must pay close attention to the respiratory effort of the individual being tested and evaluate the venous volume response in relation to the respiratory effort observed. Some patients cannot be tested reliably because of their inability to produce an adequate increase in intra-abdominal pressure.

Because the change in blood volume with any respiratory maneuver is relatively small, abnormal tracings may be produced easily by technical artifacts. The most important technical artifact is the positioning of the leg. If the knee is fully extended, there is mechanical compression of the popliteal vein in some individuals. If the leg is elevated, the venous volume response to breathing is diminished. The leg must be flat or slightly dependent for the breathing test (unlike the pressure cuff test). A tourniquet effect resulting in an abnormal test may also be produced by tight clothing or elastic undergarments. A high percentage of false positive examinations will occur when these technical factors are not closely controlled, as well as when the patients do not make a respiratory effort which generates a significant increase in abdominal pressure. The procedure employed in breathing tests has been described in more detail elsewhere.[12]

A more reproducible venous outflow obstruction can be produced by a pneumatic tourniquet placed around the thigh or abdomen. The examiner can control both the degree of pressure transmitted to the venous system and the duration for which it is maintained. The method is applicable to patients who are unable to cooperate with respiratory maneuvers. The observed change in blood volume is considerably greater than with the breathing test.

In performing the test, a 7-inch wide thigh pressure cuff is inflated to a pressure of forty-five cm H_2O for forty-five seconds. This normally produces a marked increase in venous volume, with a rapid run-off following release of the pressure. The response is markedly accentuated if the leg is elevated approximately $20°$ prior to testing.

Elevation empties the veins of the lower leg and therefore increases the capacity of the venous system to expand when a thigh tourniquet is applied. In the flat position, the leg veins are filled to a variable degree, depending in part upon the resting venous pressure. Some patients give a borderline pressure cuff response with the legs flat, but a normal test with the legs slightly elevated.

If an abnormal test is obtained, the examiner should repeat the test with careful attention to any technical details which might influence the results. Such technical details include any delay in the emptying of the pneumatic cuff, as well as the position of the leg and any other factors which also influence the results of the deep breathing test. In the absence of any adverse technical factors, it can be assumed that any abnormal

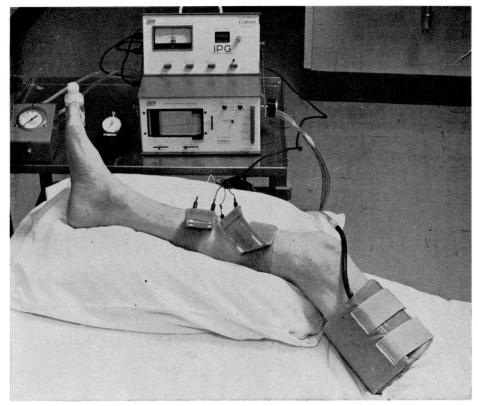

Figure 3-1.   Impedance plethysmography using a pneumatic cuff around the thigh.

pressure cuff test is due to thrombosis or other pathological obstruction of the venous system.

INTERPRETATION

The great majority of impedence examinations are obviously normal or abnormal upon even cursory study. There is a great discrepancy between the volume response of a normal patient and that of a patient with significant venous thrombosis.

RESPIRATORY TEST. A normal breathing test usually shows spontaneous small impedance excursions due to normal respiration. It always shows a significant venous volume increase with *maximum* inspiration and a prompt run-off with expiration. The maximum respiratory excursion (MRE) should exceed 0.3 percent of the resting baseline impedance within ten seconds. In patients with recent venous thrombosis, this normal respiratory response is dramatically damped. The MRE in such patients is usually less than 0.15 percent of resting baseline impedance. However,

Impedance Response to Venous Occlusion

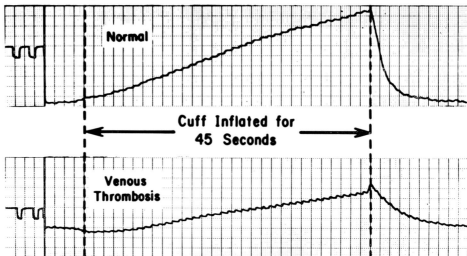

Figure 3-2.   Calf impedance response to inflation and release of a thigh tourniquet. The discrepancy between normal and abnormal tracings often exceeds that depicted.

Venous Occlusive Impedance Plethysmography
Mean and Standard Deviation

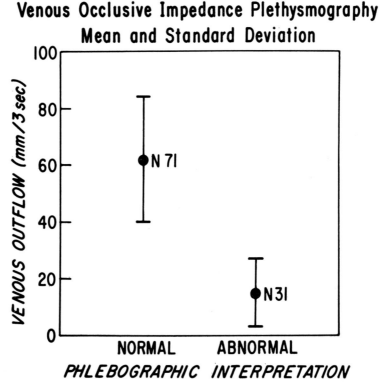

Figure 3-3.   Maximum venous outflow (mm impedance change) after release of thigh tourniquet.

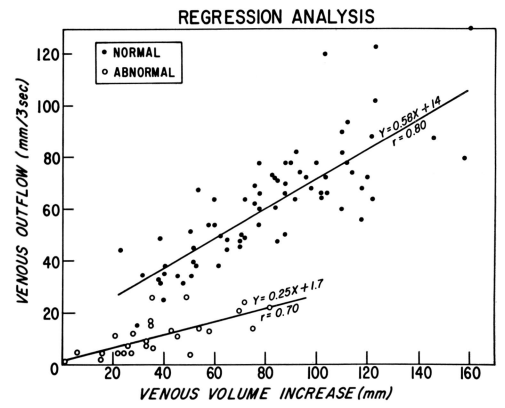

REGRESSION ANALYSIS

Figure 3-4. Regression analysis of initial venous volume increase and subsequent venous outflow in patients with normal and abnormal venograms.

patients with old venous thrombosis and well-developed collateral circulation sometimes have normal respiratory excursions. The pressure cuff test in such patients often indicates an impaired rate of venous outflow. The combination of a normal breathing test and an abnormal pressure cuff test is characteristic of patients with old thrombosis and persistent main vessel occlusion, but with well-developed collateral circulation.

THIGH CUFF TEST. The pressure cuff test normally shows a marked increase in venous volume following inflation of the thigh tourniquet, with an extremely rapid outflow following release of the tourniquet. Interpretation depends upon measurement of (a) the initial volume increase and (b) the subsequent rate of venous outflow. The rapidity of outflow during the first two or three seconds is particularly useful in the diagnosis of venous thrombosis.

In normal patients, the venous outflow within three seconds following release of the thigh tourniquet usually exceeds 75 percent of the total venous volume increase occurring during the entire forty-five seconds of cuff inflation. However, normal patients with a large initial volume increase may be unable to clear 75 percent of this large volume of blood within three seconds. The rapidity and magnitude of venous outflow are best interpreted by also considering the magnitude of the initial volume increase.

CLINICAL EXPERIENCE

The initial results reported with impedance plethysmography using breathing maneuvers showed a correlation with venograms in excess of 90%.[11, 12] This favorable experience was confirmed by other workers (Gazzaniga et al., 1972), but was not universal. One group of investigators reported a high incidence of false positive examinations.[4, 5] Another group found no false positive results, but reported several false negative examinations, particularly in calf vein clots.[10]

In reviewing the overall experience employing impedance plethysmography with breathing maneuvers, it is apparent that the conduct of the examination and the selection of patients are of paramount importance in the accuracy of results obtained. If an adequate respiratory effort is made and if there are no technical factors influencing the test, false positive results are extremely uncommon. False negative results with the breathing test are equally rare in patients with *recent* clots affecting the venous system from the popliteal vein to the inferior vena cava, although *old* thrombosis of these vessels with well-developed collateral circulation may give normal or nearly normal breathing tests. It seems likely that the percentage of false negative results will increase as the size of the clot decreases and its location is confined to smaller tributaries. When impedance plethysmography is done on a patient population with a high percentage of small calf vein clots, a moderate number of false negative examinations may be expected.

The pressure cuff technique appears to be less subject than the breathing test to technical artifacts and problems related to patient cooperation. At present we rely primarily upon pressure cuff testing with the leg in the 20° elevated position, but we still continue to employ the breathing test whenever the patient is able to cooperate.

Combining the breathing and pressure cuff tests in a recent series of 140 consecutive venograms led to a correction prediction of venographic findings in 96 percent of patients. There were two false positive examinations, presumably due to technical factors. Both tests were subsequently repeated and found to be normal. There were four false negative examinations, all in patients with a single calf vein clot less than six cm in length. This high diagnostic accuracy was observed in patients clinically suspected of venous thrombosis. Most of these patients had fairly extensive disease, or else none at all. The accuracy of the method in screening routine postoperative patients for small clots confined to one or two calf muscle veins would doubtless be lower.

DISCUSSION

Symptoms suggesting thrombophlebitis are common in clinical practice, and the diagnosis on clinical grounds alone is notoriously unreliable. A rapid and accurate procedure to evaluate patients suspected of thrombophlebitis is urgently needed, and impedance plethysmography appears to meet this need. The great majority of patients clinically suspected of thrombophlebitis can be readily evaluated at the bedside by impedance measurements. In the occasional dubious case, X-ray phlebography can be employed.

Impedance plethysmography may also be useful in screening patient populations thought to be at high risk from thromboembolic disease. It is well known that extensive thrombosis may exist in the venous system in the absence of clinical signs or symptoms. The majority of patients who die from pulmonary embolism have no prior signs or symptoms to suggest the diagnosis. In patient groups where pulmonary embolism is known to be a significant risk factor, routine screening with impedance measurements may provide a convenient, noninvasive way to detect the presence of occult deep vein thrombosis prior to the onset of pulmonary embolism.

Impedance plethysmography may also be employed to follow the course of deep vein thrombosis and to evaluate the indications for continued anticoagulant therapy. If clot lysis occurs and the deep veins regain patency, impedance tests return to normal. On the other hand, if there is propagation of the thrombus, the impedance tracings become more abnormal. Study of sequential impedance tracings therefore provides a means of following the course of the disease. When impedance results return to normal, it seems logical to assume that anticoagulants may be discontinued with more safety than when impedance tests show persistent thrombosis.

The venous volume response in the lower leg to application of a pneumatic tourniquet at the thigh has also been reported employing other types of plethysmography.[1,3,6,8] These studies confirm that pressure cuff testing can provide good diagnostic accuracy in patients with venous thrombosis. It seems likely that measurements of venous volume will become a widely employed diagnostic procedure for venous thrombosis because of the simplicity and safety for the patient, as well as the diagnostic accuracy obtained.

Summary

Impedance plethysmography is a noninvasive diagnostic procedure which can detect the presence of thrombosis in the major veins draining the lower leg with > 95 percent reliability. Its accuracy in the diagnosis of small clots in calf veins remains to be established. The method is safe and simple for the patient and can be carried out at the bedside.

The procedure depends upon observation of the venous volume response in the lower leg to changes in proximal venous pressure. These venous pressure changes can be produced either by respiratory maneuvers or by application of a pneumatic cuff to the thigh or abdomen. The pneumatic cuff technique is more widely applicable because it does not require patient cooperation and because it provides a more reproducible test response. A combination of the breathing test and the pressure cuff test has demonstrated an overall reliability of 96 percent in predicting the findings of subsequent venograms in patients clinically suspected of deep vein thrombosis (134/140 consecutive venograms).

REFERENCES

1. Barnes, R. W., Collicott, P. E., Mozersky, D. J., Sumner, D. S. and Standness, D. E., Jr.: Noninvasive quantitation of maximum venous outflow in acute thrombophlebitis. *Surgery*, 72:971-979, 1972.
2. Brecher, G. A.: *Venous Return.* New York, Grune & Stratton, Inc., 1956.
3. Cranley, J. J., Gay, A. Y., Grass, A. M. and Simeone, F. A.: A plethysmographic technique for the diagnosis of deep venous thrombosis of the lower extremities. *Surg Gynecol Obstet, 136*:385-394, 1973.
4. Deuvaert, F. E., Dmochowski, J. R. and Couch, N. P.: Positional factors in venous impedance plethysmography. *Arch Surg, 106*:43-55, 1973.
5. Dmochowski, J. R., Adams, D. F. and Couch, N. P.: Impedance measurement in the diagnosis of deep venous thrombosis. *Arch Surg, 104*:170-173, 1972.
6. Eriksson, E.: Plethysmographic studies of venous diseases of the legs. *Acta Chir Scand Suppl, 398*:33-42, 1968.
7. Gazzaniga, A. B., Pacella, A. F., Bartlett, R. H. and Geraghty, T. R.: Bilateral impedance rheography in the diagnosis of deep vein thrombosis of the legs. *Arch Surg, 104*:515-519, 1972.
8. Hallbook, T. and Gothlin, J.: Strain gauge plethysmography and phlebography in diagnosis of deep venous thrombosis. *Acta Chir Scand, 137*:37-52, 1971.
9. Nyboer, J.: *Electrical Impedance Plethysmography.* Springfield, Ill., Charles C Thomas Publisher, 1970.
10. Steer, M. L., Spotnitz, A. J., Cohen, S. I., Paulin, S. and Salzman, E. W.: Limitations of impedance phlebography for diagnosis of venous thrombosis. *Arch Surg, 106*:44-48, 1973.
11. Wheeler, H. B., Mullick, S. C., Anderson, J. N., and Pearson, D.: Diagnosis of occult deep vein thrombosis by a noninvasive bedside technique. *Surgery,* 70:20-28, 1971.
12. Wheeler, H. B., Pearson, D., O'Connell, D. and Mullick, S. C.: Impedance phlebography: Technique, interpretation, and results. *Arch Surg, 104*:164-169, 1972.

Chapter 4

^{125}I-FIBRINOGEN SCANNING

A. S. Gallus and J. Hirsh

PULMONARY EMBOLISM is the commonest preventable cause of death in hospitalized patients.[1,2] Anticoagulant treatment of clinically apparent pulmonary embolism reduces mortality from this disease.[3] However, more than half the patients with massive pulmonary embolism do not have preceding clinical signs of minor venous thromboembolism[4,5] even though postmortem examination shows that most patients who die of pulmonary embolism have associated leg vein thrombosis.[6]

Theoretically, reduction in morbidity and mortality from venous thromboembolism could be achieved (1) by improved prophylaxis of venous thromboembolism (this is discussed elsewhere in the symposium) or (2) by early diagnosis of subclinical leg vein thrombosis. ^{125}I-fibrinogen scanning is the most promising currently available method for detecting subclinical leg vein thrombosis.[7-12]

Detection of venous thrombosis by radio-iodine labelled fibrinogen scanning depends on incorporation of circulated labelled fibrinogen into the thrombus, which is then detected by measuring the increased overlying surface radioactivity with an isotope detector. The feasibility of this technique was demonstrated in animals[13-15] and man[15-17] in the early 1960's but the method has been extensively evaluated only recently.[7-12]

Fibrinogen scanning can be used in two ways. First, it can be used expectantly in patients who do not have venous thrombosis but who are at high risk of developing venous thrombosis. For expectant scanning the labelled fibrinogen is injected at the start of the high risk period and the patient is then scanned repeatedly to detect the thrombosis as it develops. Second, it can be used diagnostically to detect established venous thrombosis. In diagnostic scanning the labelled fibrinogen is injected after thrombus formation and the test becomes positive if fibrinogen is deposited onto the established thrombus or if the thrombus extends.

The use of fibrinogen carries a theoretical risk of transmitting serum

33

hepatitis. In practice, this risk is virtually eliminated if the fibrinogen is prepared from a small number of carefully screened donors.

We prepare fibrinogen from plasma of four volunteer blood donors who have not transmitted hepatitis during five years of frequent blood donation and who are hepatitis associated antigen negative by a complement fixation assay and by radioimmunoassay.[12] Fibrinogen is prepared by ammonium sulphate precipitation of plasma[18] and is labelled with [125]Iodine by a jet iodination technique.[19] The labelled fibrinogen prepared in this way is more than 95 percent clottable and has a clottable radioactivity of between 95 and 98 percent. Free iodide is removed from the labelled fibrinogen by ion exchange and the labelled fibrinogen is then passed through filters of 0.45 and 0.22 micron pore size.[12] The labelled fibrinogen is stored in 100 micro curie single dose aliquots in sterile rubber topped glass containers which are kept at $-70°C$ until used. The batches of ^{125}I-fibrinogen are dispensed only after sterility is confirmed by bacteriological tests.

We have now fibrinogen scanned over 1,000 patients, and, like other workers who have also used fibrinogen obtained from a restricted pool of accredited blood donors,[11, 20] have not found jaundice after fibrinogen scanning.[11, 12, 20] In addition, we have not noted any pyrogenic reactions or other side effects after ^{125}I-fibrinogen injection.

The choice of [125]Iodine over [131]Iodine to label fibrinogen is one of convenience. The longer half-life (60 days) of [125]Iodine leads to a longer shelf life of the labelled fibrinogen than when [131]Iodine is used. There is also greater difference of activity between thrombus and flowing blood since the [125]Iodine in a thrombus decays with the half-life of the isotope, while that in the circulating blood decays with the half-life of fibrinogen which is approximately four days. Total body radiation is less with [125]Iodine and the softer radiation permits the use of lighter counting equipment.[11] However, the tissue penetration of [125]Iodine is less and its energy spectrum does not permit scanning with a gamma camera or rectilinear scanner. For this reason, recent attempts have been made to use [131]Iodine labelled fibrinogen for this purpose[21] but the results of these studies are still very preliminary.

SCANNING TECHNIQUE

Patients are scanned with a ratemeter[12] with their legs elevated to 15°. Readings are taken over both legs and recorded as a percentage of the surface radioactivity obtained over the heart. The surface radioactivity is measured over the femoral vein at seven to eight cm intervals starting at the inguinal ligament and at similar intervals over the medial and posterior aspects of the calf and popliteal fossa. Venous thrombosis is suspected if there is an increase in the ratemeter readings of more than 20 percent at any point compared with readings over adjacent points on the same leg, over the same point on the previous day and over the corresponding point on the opposite leg. Venous thrombosis is diagnosed if the scan remains abnormal at a repeat examination and the abnormality persists for more than 24 hours.[7, 8, 11]

Expectant Fibrinogen Scanning

Venography has shown that the clinical signs and symptoms of calf vein thrombosis are unreliable. Thus, up to 50 percent of patients with clinically suspected calf vein thrombosis do not have venographically demonstrable thrombosis[6] while up to 50 percent of patients with venographically demonstrated leg vein thrombosis have clinically normal legs.[22] We have also demonstrated poor correlation between clinical signs of venous thrombosis and phlebography (Table 4-I).

TABLE 4-I

RESULTS OF VENOGRAPHY IN 120 PATIENTS PRESENTING WITH CLINICAL SYMPTOMS AND SIGNS SUGGESTIVE OF LEG VEIN THROMBOSIS (SWELLING, TENDERNESS, PAIN)

Results of Venography	Patients
Calf vein thrombosis	27
Popliteal vein thrombosis	5
Femoral vein thrombosis	29
Normal venogram	59

Incidence of Positive ^{125}I-Fibrinogen Scans in High Risk Patients

Expectant fibrinogen scanning has confirmed the high incidence of subclinical leg vein thrombosis found either by venography[22] or at autopsy in sick hospital patients.[23] The incidence of positive fibrinogen scans in high risk patients is shown in Table 4-II.[8, 11, 12, 24-36] The majority of these thrombi are limited to the calf and are clinically silent.

TABLE 4-II

INCIDENCE OF ABNORMAL FIBRINOGEN SCANS IN HIGH-RISK PATIENTS

Diagnosis	Incidence	References
Elective surgery:		
Major general abdominal surgery	14%-33%	8,11,12,24-28
Thoracic surgery	26%-65%	28,29
Gynecological surgery	11%-18%	11,30
Retropubic prostatectomy	28%-50%	11,31
Transurethral resection	4%	11
Emergency surgery:		
Hip fracture	48%-74%	11,12,32
Childbirth:	3%	11
Medical:		
Myocardial infarction	23%-38%	12,33-35
Stroke	60%	36

Correlation of ^{125}I-Fibrinogen Scanning with Venography

Comparison of ^{125}I-fibrinogen scanning with phlebography has been made by a number of investigators.[7, 8, 11, 24, 26, 30, 37-41] The results of these comparisons are shown in Table 4-III. The agreement between ^{125}I-fibrinogen technique and venography is approximately 92 percent.

TABLE 4-III

A COMPARISON OF THE RESULTS OF EXPECTANT ^{125}I-FIBRINOGEN SCANNING AND VENOGRAPHY

Fibrinogen scan Venogram	Abnormal		Normal		Results agree
	+	−	+	−	
a) *General surgery and medical patients*					
Legs: Flanc et al. (1968)	17	1	0	7	24/25
Negus et al. (1968)	26	2	0	29	55/57
Lambie et al. (1970)	40	4	2	16	56/62
Milne et al. (1971)	18	5	0	12	30/35
Gallus et al. (1973)	58	3	3	49	107/113
Subtotal	159	15	5	113	272/292 (93%)
Patients: Tsapogas et al. (1971)	11	0	1	83	94/95
Kakkar (1972)	32	4	2	50	82/88
Gallus et al. (1973)	40	1	3	12	52/56
Subtotal	83	5	6	145	228/239 (95%)
b) *Hip surgery:*					
Legs: Pinto (1970)	20	2	0	3	23/25
Field et al. (1973)	29	7	2	25	54/63
Gallus et al. (1973)	38	5	3	24	62/70
Subtotal	87	14	5	52	139/158 (88%)
Patients: Hume and Gurewich (1972)	10	2	0	0	10/12
Gallus et al. (1973)	31	1	1	7	38/40
Subtotal	41	3	1	7	48/52 (92%)

Limitations of ^{125}I-Fibrinogen Scanning

The most important limitation of this technique is its inability to detect the presence of venous thrombi above the inguinal ligament and its relative insensitivity to thrombi in the upper thigh.

High levels of leg radioactivity in the absence of deep venous thrombosis are seen with superficial thrombophlebitis, hematomas, cellulitis, arthritis, and edema.

The scanning time is limited by the *in vivo* survival of the fibrinogen. After a single injection of 100 micro curies counting is possible for approximately seven days. If the patient is still at risk a second and, if indicated, a third injection can be given to prolong scanning time for up to twenty-one days.

The Clinical Relevance of Thrombosis Detected with *125I-Fibrinogen Scanning*

The clinical relevance of ^{125}I-fibrinogen scanning has been questioned. Thus it has been reported that only eight of seventy-two patients presenting with pulmonary embolism had abnormal ^{125}I-fibrinogen scans, while forty of these patients had iliofemoral vein thrombosis detected by femoral venography.[42] It was therefore suggested that the majority of these patients with pulmonary embolism had thrombosis confined to the iliofemoral venous segment where it is undetectable by ^{125}I-fibrinogen scanning. However, these patients already had venous thrombosis of indeterminate age when ^{125}I-fibrinogen scanning was commenced, so results cannot be extrapolated to those of expectant ^{125}I-fibrinogen scanning. In addition, all patients had ^{131}I-macro-aggregated human serum albumin lung scans, which reduce the sensitivity of ^{125}I-fibrinogen leg scanning for some days,[43] and the leg veins were not examined with ascending venography; so the true incidence of distal leg vein thrombosis which could have been detected with expectant ^{125}I-fibrinogen scanning is not known in these patients.

On the other hand, prospective studies of high risk patients scanned expectantly have shown a very low risk of pulmonary embolism in patients with a normal fibrinogen scan, and a considerably higher risk in patients in whom the scan was positive (Table 4-IV). Kakkar[11] has presented evidence that the majority of thrombi commence in the soleal sinuses of the calf, and has suggested that proximal thrombi form as an extension from these calf vein thrombi. If this is so, then the lack of sensitivity of fibrinogen scanning to thrombi above the inguinal ligament becomes a minor limitation. He has also presented evidence that the risk of clinical pulmonary embolism from untreated asymptomatic postoperative calf vein thrombi detected with expectant fibrinogen scanning is extremely low, but that the risk of embolism from thrombi in the popliteal or femoral vein is approximately 40 percent.[44] He has therefore suggested that fibrinogen scan detected asymptomatic popliteal or femoral vein thrombi should be treated with anticoagulants while calf vein thrombi do not need treatment as long as scanning is continued. It is likely, then, that ^{125}I-fibrinogen scanning does detect the majority of patients who are at risk of clinically significant pulmonary embolism, although there is little doubt from postmortem studies that some pulmonary emboli are associated with isolated thrombosis in veins outside the range of scanning.[6]

We have attempted to resolve this controversy by performing a detailed comparison of expectant fibrinogen scanning and venography in patients with abnormal and normal scans after general surgery or suspected myo-

TABLE 4-IV

PULMONARY EMBOLISM IN PATIENTS NOT RECEIVING PROPHYLAXIS BUT
STUDIED WITH EXPECTANT FIBRINOGEN SCANNING

Fibrinogen Scan	*Abnormal*	*Normal*
a) *General Surgery*		
Kakkar et al. (1969)	4/40	0/92
Lambie et al. (1970)	0/49	0/62
Williams (1971)*	0/12	0/17
Hills et al. (1972)*	2/30	0/110
Bonnar & Walsh (1972)*	1/15	0/125
Gordon-Smith et al. (1972)	0/21	0/29
Kakkar et al. (1972)*	0/17	0/22
Nicolaides et al. (1972)*	0/29	0/93
Gallus et al (1973)*	1/40	2/280
Subtotal	8/253 (3.2%)	2/830 (0.2%)
b) *Medical Patients*		
Murray et al. (1970)	4/13	0/37
Nicolaides et al. (1971)	0/7	0/26
Warlow et al. (1972)	4/18	0/12
Haudley et al. (1972)	1/6	0/20
Gallus et al. (1973)*	0/7	0/31
Subtotal	9/51 (17.5%)	0/126 (0.0%)
c) *Hip Surgery*		
Pinto (1970)	0/8	0/17
Field et al. (1972)	0/30	0/20
Gallus et al. (1973)*	0/14	1/18
	0/52 (0.0%)	1/55 (1.8%)

*Patients treated with anticoagulants after diagnosis of popliteal or femoral vein thrombosis.

cardial infarction, and after hip surgery. The purpose of this investigation
was to determine (1) the usefulness of fibrinogen scanning for making
therapeutic decisions and (2) the frequency of isolated iliofemoral and
femoral vein thrombosis in high risk patients.

Results were analyzed separately in 137 unoperated limbs of fifty-six
patients without hip surgery and forty patients after hip surgery, and in
the forty operated legs of the patients after hip surgery; since in the latter
group extravascular accumulation of ^{125}Iodine labelled fibrin due to operative bleeding increases surface radioactivity over the operated thigh and
makes the scan uninterpretable in that area.

Patients were selected for venography as well as scanning in three ways.
Initially venography was performed in patients with normal and abnormal
scans to validate the scanning technique. Subsequently, venography was
only performed on patients with abnormal scans but bilateral venography
was done even if only one leg showed scan evidence of venous thrombosis.

More recently, all patients scanned after hip surgery had venograms as well as scans to detect femoral vein thrombosis on the operated side.

Eighty-three of the 138 scans on unoperated limbs were abnormal, fifty-two were normal and three showed equivocal evidence of vein thrombosis. Venography confirmed fifty-two of fifty-nine suspected calf vein thrombi, four of twelve suspected popliteal vein thrombi, and all eight suspected femoral vein thrombi. Three scan detected popliteal area thrombi were in superficial veins. Falsely abnormal scans in the popliteal area of two limbs were due to inflammation of the knees in a patient with rheumatoid arthritis. Scanning missed one small calf vein thrombus, two popliteal vein thrombi and one small femoral vein thrombus. Thus, use of scanning alone to make therapeutic decisions according to the principles outlined by Kakkar[44] would have produced a therapeutic error in eleven of 138 scans (8%). No leg with a normal scan had iliac or high femoral vein thrombosis.

Venography of forty operated legs scanned after hip surgery confirmed the presence of fourteen of fifteen calf and six of ten popliteal vein thrombi suggested by scanning. In two patients with abnormal scans in the popliteal area and normal popliteal veins there was hematoma extending to the back of the knee from the operation site. Although the scan was uninterpretable over the operated thigh, seven of the nine legs with femoral vein thrombosis undetectable by scanning because of the surgical bleeding had scan evidence of associated calf or popliteal vein thrombosis.

Thus, expectant fibrinogen scanning in patients without leg surgery appears to be a reliable method of detecting venous thrombi limited to the calf. It is less reliable for detecting thrombi in the popliteal area and the resulting therapeutic error can be minimized by performing venography on patients with a suspected diagnosis of popliteal vein thrombosis before deciding on long-term anticoagulant treatment. Although scanning seemed very reliable for detecting femoral vein thrombosis, the series was small and our present feeling is that venography should also be performed on patients with scan detected femoral vein thrombosis.

Despite the severe limitations of fibrinogen scanning in patients with hip surgery, it appears that the occurrence of femoral and popliteal vein thrombosis is unusual in the operated leg without associated calf vein thrombosis detectable with fibrinogen scanning. Thus, if calf vein thrombosis in the operated limb had been used as an indication for venography, eleven of thirteen popliteal and femoral vein thrombi would have been detected. It is clear that scanning cannot be used to make therapeutic decisions after hip surgery but the strong association of scan detectable calf and popliteal vein thrombosis with femoral vein thrombosis in the operated leg does allow scanning to be used as an indication for venography in these patients.

The majority of discrepancies between venography and expectant fibrinogen scanning can be explained by hematoma, inflammation, or incomplete visualization of veins by venography. However, a small proportion of patients have abnormal scans and completely normal venograms for no apparent reason.

We have investigated possible causes of discrepancy between venograms and scanning in an experimental thrombosis model in dogs.[52] Venous thrombosis was produced in foreleg veins of thirty-six dogs after preinjection of ^{125}I dog-fibrinogen. Blood was aspirated from a segment of vein isolated between two tourniquets into a syringe containing thrombin and was then reinjected into the vein. The thrombus so produced was retained in the leg vein by a proximal stenosis. Results of fibrinogen scanning were then compared with those of venography and of direct examination of the thrombus after dissection and opening of the vein. The correlation between venography and direct examination of the vein was better than 95 percent. The correlation between fibrinogen scanning and venography was 100 percent when a thrombus was present but it was found that fibrinogen scans remained positive for up to forty-eight hours after spontaneous lysis of the thrombus or embolization of the thrombus. Examination of the vein wall after embolization showed marked endothelial damage and extensive fibrin deposition at the site of the previous thrombosis. These results are compatible with the view that a normal venogram in the presence of an abnormal fibrinogen scan may sometimes indicate embolization of thrombus which had been present and caused an inflammatory reaction in the vein wall.

Exceptant fibrinogen scanning has been used to evaluate a variety of prophylatic methods described in Chapter 22, "Low Dose Heparin Prophylaxis." It has also been used to investigate the possibility that there may be changes in blood tests before and just after surgery which predict the risk of postoperative vein thrombosis.[45-49] If such blood tests exist they could be used to select patients for prophylaxis and special diagnostic techniques. We have performed fourteen tests of hemostasis and fibrinolytic activity in seventy-three patients before and after elective major surgery. Twenty-seven of these patients developed postoperative vein thrombosis detected with fibrinogen scanning and the results of tests were compared in patients with and without thrombosis. Of the tests done before surgery only the partial thromboplastin time showed a statistically significant difference between patients with and without thrombosis. Patients with a long preoperative partial thromboplastin time were found to have a low risk of venous thrombosis while patients with a short partial thromboplastin time had a moderately increased risk of thrombosis. Of the tests done on the first postoperative day, the partial thromboplastin time, antiplasmin assay, and fibrin split product titre showed statistically significant differences between patients with and without thrombosis. Thus, patients with a long partial thromboplastin time still had a low risk of subsequent thrombosis while patients with a short partial thromboplastin time had a relatively high risk of postoperative thrombosis and patients with thrombosis also had a slightly increased level of serum fibrin split products. Tests done after the first postoperative day until the seventh day showed no difference between patients with and without thrombosis.[56]

Diagnostic Scanning

Fibrinogen scanning is less reliable when it is used to detect established thrombosis because the test only becomes positive if fibrinogen is still being deposited onto the thrombus or if the thrombus extends. The reported incidence of abnormal fibrinogen scans in patients with venographically proven thrombosis is approximately 70 percent,[7, 11, 50, 51] except for one study which showed a considerably lower incidence.[42] We have found an incidence of 80 percent. The factors which determine whether or not an established thrombus will be detected by scanning include the age of the thrombus, whether or not it is totally occlusive, and whether or not the patient is being treated with anticoagulants.[51] A further limitation of the use of ^{125}I-fibrinogen scanning to diagnose established venous thrombosis is that it may take up to forty-eight hours for the scan to become abnormal. For these reasons, venography is the best way of rapidly confirming clinically suspected venous thrombosis. However, we have found scanning to be very useful for detecting extension of venographically proven thrombosis in patients who are either not treated with anticoagulants or treated with relatively low doses of anticoagulants because of a high risk of bleeding.

REFERENCES

1. Morrell, M. T. and Dunnill, M. S.: The postmortem incidence of pulmonary embolism in a hospital population. *Br J Surg, 55*:347-352, 1968.
2. Modan, B., Sharon, E. and Jelin, N.: Factors contributing to the incorrect diagnosis of pulmonary embolic disease. *Chest, 62*:388-393, 1972.
3. Barritt, D. W. and Jordan, S. C.: Anticoagulant drugs in the treatment of pulmonary embolism. A controlled trial. *Lancet, 1*:1309-1312, 1960.
4. Miller, G. A. H. and Sutton, G. C.: Acute massive pulmonary embolism. Clinical and hemodynamic findings in 23 patients studied by cardiac catheterization and pulmonary angiography. *Br Heart J, 32*:518-523, 1970.
5. McDonald, I. G., Hirsh, J., Hale, G. S. and O'Sullivan, E. F.: Major pulmonary embolism: A correlation of clinical findings, haemodynamics, pulmonary angiography and pathological physiology. *Br Heart J, 34*:356-364, 1972.
6. Hume, M., Sevitt, S. and Thomas, D. P.: *Venous Thrombosis and Pulmonary Embolism.* Cambridge, Mass., Harvard University Press, 1970, pp. 1-456.
7. Flanc, C., Kakkar, V. V. and Clarke, M. B.: The detection of venous thrombosis of the legs using ^{125}I-labelled fibrinogen. *J Surg, 55*:742-747, 1968.

8. Negus, D., Pinto, D. J., LeQuesne, L. P., Brown, N. and Chapman, M.: ^{125}I-labelled figrinogen in the diagnosis of deep-vein thrombosis and its correlation with phlebography. *Br J Surg, 55*:835-839, 1968.

9. Kakkar, V. V., Howe, C. T., Nicolaides, A. N., Renney, J. T. G. and Clarke, M. B.: Deep vein thrombosis of the leg. Is there a "high risk" group? *Am J Surg, 120*:527-530, 1970.

10. Browse, N. L., Clapham, W. F., Croft, D. N., Jones, D. J., Lea Thromas, M., Olwen Thomas, J.: Diagnosis of established deep vein thrombosis with the ^{125}I-fibrinogen uptake test. *Br Med J, 4*:325-328, 1971.

11. Kakkar, V. V.: The diagnosis of deep vein thrombosis using the ^{125}I-fibrinogen test. *Arch Surg, 104*:152-159, 1972.

12. Gallus, A. S., Hirsh, J., Tuttle, R. J., Trebilcock, R., O'Brien, S. E., Carroll, J. J., Minden, J. H. and Hudecki, S. M.: Small subcutaneous doses of heparin in prevention of venous thrombosis. *N Engl J Med, 288*:545-557, 1973.

13. Hobbs, J. T. and Davies, J. W. L.: Detection of venous thrombosis with ^{131}I-labelled fibrinogen in the rabbit. *Lancet, 2*:134-135, 1960.

14. Hobbs, J. T.: External measurement of fibrinogen uptake in experimental venous thrombosis and other local pathological states. *Br J Exp Pathol, 43*:48-58, 1962.

15. Palko, P. O., Nanson, S. M. and Fedoruk, S. O.: The early detection of deep venous thrombosis using ^{131}I-tagged human fibrinogen. *Can J Surg, 7*:215-226, 1964.

16. Nanson, E. M., Palko, P. O., Dick, A. A. and Fedoruk, S. O.: Early detection of deep venous thrombosis of the legs using ^{131}I-tagged human fibrinogen: A clinical study. *Ann Surg, 162*:438-445, 1965.

17. Atkins, P. and Hawkins, L. A.: Detection of venous thrombosis in the legs. *Lancet, 2*:1217-1219, 1965.

18. Regoeczi, E.: Fibrinogen catabolism: kinetics of catabolism following sudden elevation of the pool with exogenous fibrinogen. *Clin Sci, 38*:111-121, 1970.

19. McFarland, A. S.: *In vivo* behavior, of ^{131}I-fibrinogen. *J Clin Invest, 42*:346-361, 1963.

20. Croft, D.: ^{125}I-fibrinogen and hepatitis. *N Engl J Med, 284*:1159, 1971.

21. Dugan, M. A., Kozar, J. T. and Charles, N. D.: Radioactive labelling of deep venous thrombi using Iodine-131 fibrinogen. Proc. III Congress. The International Society on Thrombosis and Hemostasis 394, 1972.

22. Culver, D., Crawford, J. S., Gardiner, J. H. and Wiley, A. M.: Venous thrombosis after fracture of the upper end of the femur: A study of incidence and site. *J Bone Joint Surg, 52B*:61-69, 1970.

23. Sevitt, S. and Gallagher, N. J.: Prevention of venous thrombosis and pulmonary embolism in injured patients. *Lancet, 2*:981-989, 1959.

24. Tsapogas, M. J., Goussous, H., Peabody, R. A., Karmody, A. M. and Eckert, C.: Postoperative venous thrombosis and the effectiveness of prophylactic measures. *Arch Surg, 103*:561-567, 1971.

25. Harvey Kemble, J. V.: Incidence of deep vein thrombosis. *Br J Hosp Med, 6*:721-726, 1971.

26. Milne, R. M., Griffiths, J. M. T., Gunn, A. A. and Ruckley, C. V.: Postoperative deep venous thrombosis. A comparison of diagnostic techniques. *Lancet, 2*:445-447, 1971.

27. Sripad, S., Antcliffe, A. C. and Martin, P.: Deep vein thrombosis in two district hospitals in Essex. *Br J Surg, 58*:563-565, 1971.

28. Nicolaides, A. N., Dupont, P. A., Desai, S., Lewis, J. D., Douglas, J. N., Dodsworth, H., Furides, L., Luck, R. J. and Jamieson, C. W.: Small doses of subcutaneous heparin in preventing deep venous thrombosis after major surgery. *Lancet*, 2:890-893, 1972.

29. O'Brien, J. R., Tulevski, V. and Etherington, M.: Two *in vivo* studies comparing high and low aspirin dosage. *Lancet*, 1:399-400, 1971.

30. Bonnar, J. and Walsh, J.: Prevention of thrombosis after pelvic surgery by British dextran 70. *Lancet*, 1:614-616, 1972.

31. Gordon-Smith, I. C., Hickman, J. A. and Masri, S. H.: The effect of the fibrinolytic inhibitor epsilon-amino caproic acid on the incidence of deep-vein thrombosis after prostatectomy. *Br J Surg*, 59:522-524, 1972.

32. Wood, E. H., Prentice, C. R. M. and McNicol, G. P.: Association of fibrinogen-fibrin related antigen (F. R. antigen) with post-operative deep vein thrombosis and systemic complications. *Lancet*, 1:166-169, 1972.

33. Murray, T. S., Lorimer, A. R., Cox, F. C. and Lawrie, T. D. V.: Leg vein thrombosis following myocardial infarction. *Lancet*, 2:792-793, 1970.

34. Nicolaides, A. N., Kakkar, V. V., Renney, J. T. G., Kidner, P. H., Hutchinson, D. C. S. and Clarke, M. B.: Myocardial infarction and deep-vein thrombosis. *Br Med J*, 1:432-434, 1971.

35. Maurer, B. J., Wray, R. and Shillingford, J. P.: Frequency of venous thrombosis after myocardial infarction. *Lancet*, 2:1385-1387, 1971.

36. Warlow, C., Ogston, D. and Douglas, A. S.: Venous thrombosis following strokes. *Lancet*, 1:1305-1306, 1972.

37. Lambie, J. M., Mahaffy, R. G., Barber, D. C., Karmody, A. M., Scott, M. M. and Matheson, N. A.: Diagnostic accuracy in venous thrombosis. *Br Med J*, 2:142-143, 1970.

38. Gallus, A. S., Inwood, M. J., Hirsh, J., Tuttle, R., Turpie, A. G. G. and Stolberg, ...: In preparation, 1973.

39. Pinto, D. J.: Controlled trial of an anticoagulant (warfarin sodium) in the prevention of venous thrombosis following hip surgery. *Br J Surg*, 57:349-352, 1970.

40. Field, E. S., Nicolaides, A. N. Kakkar, V. V. and Crellin, R. Q.: Deep vein thrombosis in patients with fractures of the femoral neck. *Br J Surg*, 59:377-379, 1972.

41. Hume, M. and Gurewich, V.: Peripheral venous scanning with ^{125}I-tagged fibrinogen. *Lancet*, 1:845, 1972.

42. Mavor, G. E., Mahaffy, R. G., Walker, M. G., Duthie, J. S., Dhall, D. P., Gaddie, J. and Reid, G. F.: Peripheral venous scanning with ^{125}I-tagged fibrinogen. *Lancet*, 1:661-663, 1972.

43. Warlow, C. and Douglas, A. S.: ^{125}I-labelled fibrinogen test: Effect of ^{131}I-albumin. *Lancet*, 2:1196, 1972.

44. Kakkar, V. V., Howe, C. T., Flanc, C. and Clarke, M. B.: Natural history of postoperative deep-vein thrombosis. *Lancet*, 2:230-233, 1969.

45. Negus, D., Pinto, D. J. and Brown, N.: Platelet adhesiveness in postoperative deep-vein thrombosis. *Lancet*, 1:220-224, 1969.

46. Becker, J.: The relation of platelet adhesiveness to postoperative venous thrombosis of the legs. *Acta Chi Scand*, 138:781-786, 1972.

47. O'Brien, J. R., Etherington, H., Jamieson, S. and Klaber, M. R.: Platelet function in venous thrombosis and low dosage heparin. *Lancet*, 1:1302-1305, 1972.

48. Becker, J.: Fibrinolytic activity in the blood and its relation to postoperative venous thrombosis of the lower limbs. *Acta Chir Scand, 138*:787-792, 1972.
49. Mansfield, A. O.: Alteration in fibrinolysis associated with surgery and venous thrombosis. *Br J Surg, 59*:754-757, 1972.
50. Browse, N. L., Clapham, W. F., Croft, D. N., Jones, D. J., Lea Thomas, M. and Olwen Williams, J.: Diagnosis of established deep vein thrombosis with the ^{125}I-fibrinogen uptake test. *Br Med J, 4*:325-328, 1971.
51. Konttinen, Y. P., Stenman, U.-H. and Schuman, S.: Peripheral scanning with ^{125}I-tagged fibrinogen in pulmonary embolism. *Lancet, 2*:972, 1972.
52. Kerrigan, G. N. W., Buchanan, M. R., Cade, J. F., Regoeczi, E. and Hirsh, J.: Investigation of the mechanism of false positive ^{125}I-labelled fibrinogen scans. (In Preparation) 1973.

DISCUSSION

Dr. O'Brien: Dr. Hirsh, I enjoyed your paper very much. Could I say one thing about superficial and deep venous thrombosis and I^{125} scanning? May I point out the important effect of depth of the lesion on the extent of the signal. If the thrombosis is near the surface it will produce a quite disproportionate excess of counts, above the background count due to the blood in the normal blood vessels. Indeed, the inverse square applies. If you have a thrombosis near the surface on one side of the legs and you scan immediately over this side the excess counts will be high. If you then scan the dimetrically side of the leg, then since the excess signals from the thrombus have to pass right through the leg excess counts will be virtually negligible. If excess counts from opposite sides of the leg are the same, this very strongly suggests that the thrombus is symmetrically placed between the two points. In fact you can triangulate; you can take counts from three places and triangulate and plot out exactly where the thrombus is.

Dr. Smith (Des Moines) You've had a lot of experience with this method and evidently have followed quite a few patients. Could I ask you what percentage of emboli you would estimate come from the legs and what percentage come from the pelvis?

Dr. Hirsh: This is a very important question and one that is difficult to answer with accuracy. Data from autopsy studies suggests that approximately 70 to 80 percent of emboli arise from leg veins but the interpretation of this data is open to question since the presence of a thrombus at a particular site in a patient with pulmonary embolism at autopsy does not prove that the thrombus was the site of origin of the embolus. Another approach to this question is provided by data gathered from the literature on the incidence of pulmonary embolism in patients who have been scanned prospectively. There was a 4.5 percent incidence of pulmonary embolism in approximately 300 patients who had positive leg scans and only a 0.3 percent incidence of pulmonary embolism in over 1,000 patients with negative scans. This does not necessarily prove that the embolus arose from the site of the positive scan but does suggest that the vast majority of pulmonary emboli are associated with leg vein thrombosis rather than isolated iliac or pelvic vein thrombosis.

Question: In some of Kakkar's early work, he reported the finding that a large percentage of patients who develop postoperative thrombi develop them on the first postoperative day and that many of these thrombi subsequently disappeared over the next two or three days. I am not aware that these were documented by venography and wonder if there is a difference between this group of patients and those in which thrombi gradually increase in size over the next three to four days.

Dr. O'Brien: I think it is most important to consider how you will document these. The heart count day after day decreased rapidly with the rapid physiological turnover of fibrinogen. If a thrombus stays constant then the local excess counts due to the thrombus equally stays constant (you can ignore the isotopic decay for over a week or so) then if this is expressed as a percentage of the heart count, the percentage obviously will increase dramatically. However, if you in fact measure and record the absolute excess counts locally this will usually be found to decrease slowly. I fully accept that on occasions it does decrease dramatically in which case either embolization or lysis has occurred. I think it most important to define precisely which way these scansion techniques are recorded and to appreciate fully the significance of the answers.

Dr. Hirsh: I think that the issue in question is: Can one detect which of the 40 to 50 percent of patients who develop scan evidence of thrombosis after surgery will have thrombi which extend? To my knowledge, there are no methods currently available that enable us to detect this group, but, hopefully, prospective studies such as the one that I have described in which serial blood tests are documented and compared in scan positive and scan negative individuals may help to answer this question.

Chapter 5

PHLEBOGRAPHY IN THROMBOEMBOLISM

James A. DeWeese and Stanley M. Rogoff

THE SUPERFICIAL VEINS of the lower extremity can usually be visualized and palpated without difficulty. The deep veins of the leg, however, are hidden within their muscular compartments. Phlebography provides means of visualizing these deep veins.

It is helpful to have an understanding of some of the physiologic principles of venous drainage from the leg to understand the methods of performing phlebography and to evaluate the phlebograms obtained. Since the venous pressure is lower in the deep veins than in the superificial veins, the flow of blood is normally from the superficial system to the deep system. The unidirectional flow of blood from the superficial to the deep system and then toward the heart is guaranteed by the presence of valves in the veins. Muscular activity and the resultant action of the muscle pump further empties the blood from the veins and further decreases the pressure within the deep veins and accentuates the flow of blood from the super-ficial to the deep system. In other words, blood or the radiopaque in the superficial vein of any part of the lower extremity will find its way into the deep system unless there is obstruction of the deep vein by thrombus, pressure or ligature, which increases the venous pressure in these deep veins. The flow of blood is then through collateral veins to the thigh or pelvis above the site of obstruction where venous pressures are lower.

Berberich and Hirsch described the feasibility of injecting a radio-opaque substance into a vein and demonstrating it roentgenographically in 1923.[5] Bauer, and also Daugherty and Homans in 1940 visualized the veins of the entire leg with an injection into a foot vein.[3, 11] Bauer found that by placing a tight tourniquet around the ankle that he could obtain a better visualization of the deep veins, particularly in the presence of deep venous thrombi. There have been continued modifications and improvements in the contrast materials and there are several that are now safe and effective. The volume of opaque injected is important. Felder and Murphy demonstrated that a significantly greater number of veins was visualized when forty ml of contrast material was injected and Rabinov and Paulin have advocated using as much as 125 ml to visualize the entire extremity.[12, 18] Scott and Roach, and also Greitz, demonstrated that with the patient in a semierect position emptying of opaque from the veins was delayed.[13, 20] The fact that all contrast materials have a specific gravity greater than that of blood, serves to accentuate this delay and provides better visualization of the valves. Greitz pointed out that following exercise, more veins in the lower leg, as well as the upper leg, could be visualized as the opaque was propelled toward the heart.[13] We evaluated a technique of performing phlebograms utilizing the above mentioned principles in 1958.[6] In the past fifteen years over 2,000 phlebograms were performed, of which over 500 were performed in the presence of acute deep venous thrombosis.

Method (Fig. 5-1)

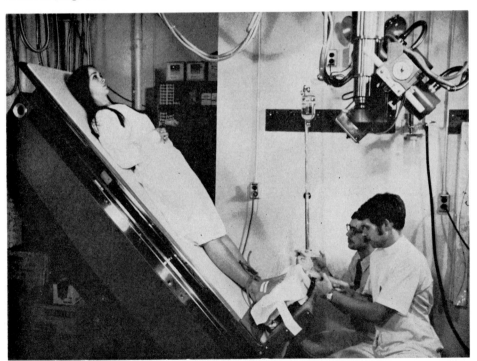

Figure 5-1. The patient is positioned on a tilt-table with the head 45 degrees from the horizontal. A needle is inserted into superficial vein on the dorsum of the foot. A tourniquet is tightly placed around the ankle. Fifty cc of a radio-opaque material is injected into each leg and a long film exposed.

(1) The patient is placed in a semierect position, 45 degrees from the horizontal. The procedure is usually performed bilaterally at the same time.

(2) a number 20-gauge needle is inserted percutaneously into any vein on the dorsum of the foot. In rare instances a cut-down is necessary and a polyethylene tubing inserted. A slow infusion of isotonic sodium chloride solution is begun through a three-way stop cock. (3) A rubber tourniquet is applied tightly around the ankle. (4) Fifty milliliters of a suitable radio-opaque material is injected over a one minute period. (5) A long 14 x 34-inch film is exposed. (6) The tourniquet is released and the patient raises himself on his toes three to five times. (7) A second long radiograph is exposed. (8) In most instances the cassette tray and X-ray tube are then shifted as rapidly as possible to make a third 14 x 17-inch radiograph of the pelvic region. (9) After the third radiograph has been made the patient is placed in a horizontal position and isotonic sodium chloride solution infused rapidly through the needle in the foot to help clear the opaque substance from the veins.

MODIFICATIONS IN TECHNIQUE

It is sometimes necessary to repeat the studies to obtain information not found on the first set of films. Examples of such situations and suggested modifications are as follows: (1) *Suspected massive iliofemoral venous thrombosis.* With extensive obstruction of the deep veins and marked elevation of venous pressures, it is advisable to place the patients only fifteen degrees from the horizontal position and to ask them to raise themselves on their toes five to ten times in order to propel the radio-opaque into the thigh and pelvis. (2) *Lack of significant filling of calf veins.* On some occasions the tourniquet is applied too tightly and if there is insufficient filling of the calf veins removal of the tourniquet may increase the number of vessels opacified. In other instances lack of filling of the deep veins is secondary to obstruction, particularly in the region of the popliteal fascia. In those instances application of a second tourniquet just below the knee may force more opaque into the deep system. (3) *Lack of filling of thigh veins.* Lowering the head of the table so that the patient is only thirty degrees or fifteen degrees from the horizontal may increase the filling of the thigh and pelvic veins. In other instances it is possible to obtain the same effect by having the patient raise himself on his toes at least ten times. (4) *Lack of filling of pelvic veins.* Increased opacification of the pelvic veins may be obtained by lowering the head of the table so that the patient is only fifteen degrees from the horizontal or having him plantar flex several times. A tight tourniquet or blood pressure cuff can be applied to the thigh and after the dye is injected the tourniquet or blood pressure cuff can be rapidly removed which allows the dye to pass rapidly into the pelvic region. (5) *Visualization of the inferior vena cavae.* Although faint visualization of the inferior vena cava may be obtained by the above techniques, it is preferable to introduce a needle or catheter percutaneously directly

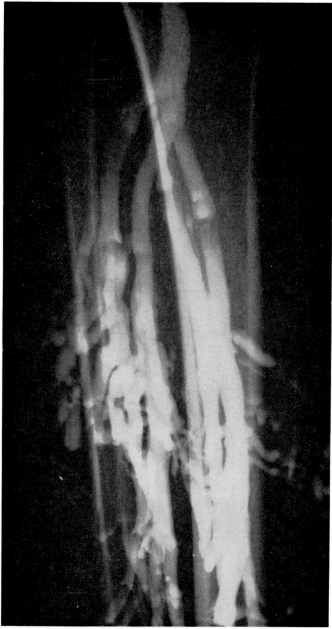

Figure 5-2. *Normal calf veins.* The double posterior tibial, peroneal, and anterior tibial veins are visualized entering the popliteal vein below the level of the knee joint. The vein walls are smooth and valves are visible. Perforating veins with competent valves preventing reflux filling of the superficial veins are visualized.

into the common femoral veins and inject thirty ml of radio-opaque material rapidly into these veins with the patient in a position fifteen degrees from the horizontal with the head elevated.

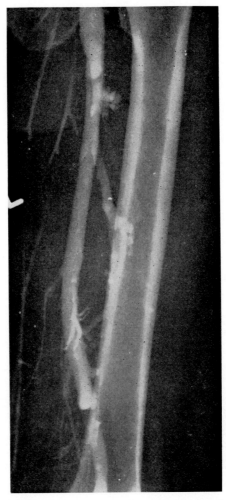

Figure 5-3. *Normal thigh veins.* The popliteal and superficial femoral and common femoral veins are visualized with their usual bulges at the site of the valves. There is a communication in the lower thigh between the superficial femoral and deep femoral vein which is, therefore, visualized.

OTHER TECHNIQUES. Our own experience has been almost exclusively with the method and modifications just described. Other authors have advocated very different basic methods, including avoidance of weight-bearing and/or tourniquets,[18] or the routine use of fluoroscopy and multiprojectional spot-filming[16] or the judicious use of multiple tourniquets or the routine injection of a radio-opaque bolus much larger than thirty mls.[15, 16, 17] We cannot yet comment on advantages or disadvantages of such methods as substitutes for our own, except to estimate that they may improve its accuracy but also add to the complexity of performing the examination.

NORMAL PHLEBOGRAM

Lower Leg (Fig. 5-2)

It is possible to visualize all or part of the anterior tibial, peroneal, and posterior tibial veins which are the main deep venous channels in the lower leg. These veins are usually double. They present a uniform tapering outline and several valves are always present. The sural veins, which are smaller veins draining the gastrocnemius muscle and which usually enter the popliteal ring directly, are frequently seen. Short segments of perforators ending at a competent valve without filling the superficial vein are also frequently seen.

Upper Leg (Fig. 5-3)

The calf veins empty into the popliteal vein a few centimeters above or below the knee joint. The popliteal vein becomes the superficial femoral in the lower thigh and is joined by the deep femoral vein in the groin to become the common femoral vein. The popliteal, superficial femoral, and common femoral veins are also visualized in most studies or can be visualized by using a modification of the basic technique. The deep femoral vein is visualized in approximately one half of the cases because of a communication between the superficial femoral and deep femoral veins in the lower thigh. The vessels are smooth-walled and of uniform caliber except for some minimal dilatation at the site of valves. The greater saphenous vein may or may not be seen. Following exercise, the opaque is emptied from the majority of the veins in the calf and even in the thigh and frequently only small amounts of opaque are visualized in the cusps of the normal valves. In both the lower leg and upper leg one frequently sees veins running in a transverse direction communicating between deep veins and in some instances between deep veins and superficial veins. In addition, collaterals running in a longitudinal direction are occasionally visualized even in normal extremities.

ACUTE THROMBOSIS

The unequivocal diagnosis of acute venous thrombosis is based on: (1) the presence of well defined filling defects in heavily opacified veins; (2) the demonstration of these defects on at least two radiographs. The defects are frequently globular and in some instances, however, they appear serpentine and seem to be waving in the proximal blood stream. Smaller bubble-like defects are frequently seen distal to a thrombus defect or distal to a segment of obstructed vein. If one or more calf veins is not visualized this cannot be considered diagnostic of thrombosis since even in normal extremities these veins are sometimes not all visualized. Nonvisualization of the femoral vein, on the other hand, particularly if there is good opacifica-

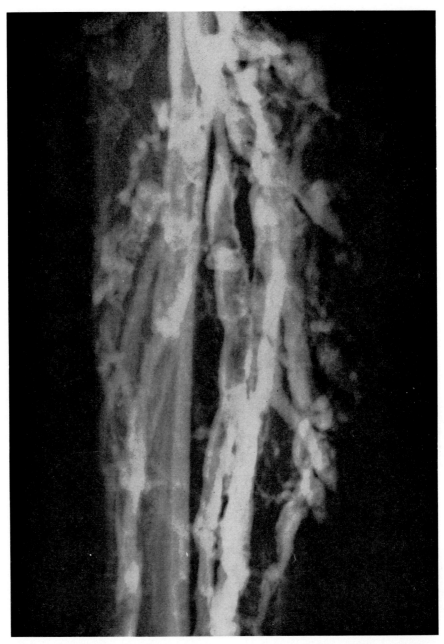

Figure 5-4. *Lower leg venous thrombosis.* A large globular filling defect in a well-opacified peroneal vein is visualized in the center of the picture. Distally in the same vein, small bubble defects of smaller thrombi are visualized. A serpentine defect can be seen in the adjacent anterior tibial vein. A similar defect can also be seen in the posterior tibial vein overlying the tibia in the upper portion of the picture.

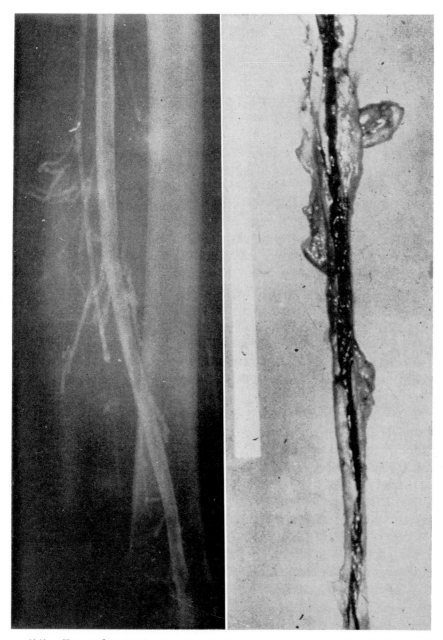

Figure 5-5. *Femoral vein thrombosis.* A long serpentine thrombus in the popliteal and femoral vein which does not completely occlude the vein is identified in the phlebogram on the left. At postmortem examination the femoral vein was removed and the long thrombus identified, as seen on right.

tion of the proximal and distal veins in the presence of collaterals, is considered evidence of thrombotic obstruction.

Thrombi can be differentiated from streaming artifacts by their shape and by the sharpness of their outlines. The streaming artifacts also vary with exercise whereas the thrombus defects remain constant following exercise on the second film. We have had the opportunity to explore many of the veins at the time of a venous thrombectomy, venous interruption, or at postmortem examination and the diagnosis of venous thrombosis was confirmed in all instances.

Lower Leg Thrombosis (Fig. 5-4)

Venous thrombosis confined to the lower leg usually involves only one or two of the three major veins. The clots are usually not completely obstructive and since the veins are usually double, there appears to be very adequate flow of the radio-opaque material through the deep veins and into the popliteal vein. Clots are also frequently visualized in the perforating veins. On occasion, they appear to propagate into the popliteal vein as long serpentine filling defects.

Femoral Vein Thrombosis (Fig. 5-5)

In patients in whom thrombi are visualized in the femoral veins there are also usually thrombi in the calf veins. Rarely there is localized and segmental involvement of the femoral vein beginning in the region of the adductor magnus tendon and extending to the common femoral vein. This appearance is remarkably similar to that seen in the arterial system and suggests the possibility that this particular type of thrombosis may be related to mechanical trauma at the adductor tendon level. When the superficial femoral vein is completely occluded there is extensive collateral flow. Much of the flow is through the greater saphenous vein but in addition, there are always communications between the lower leg veins and the deep femoral vein. In the acute stage, but even more frequently in the post-thrombotic stage, small veins are seen paralleling the course of the femoral vein, presumably venae comitantes. Since the femoral vein is occasionally bifid, the thrombosis may be localized to one half of the double vein.

Iliofemoral Venous Thrombosis (Figs. 5-6 and 5-7)

When the proximal extent of thrombosis is in the iliac veins, approximately 50 percent of the extremities also demonstrate extensive obstruction of the lower leg veins and femoral veins suggesting that the thrombosis has ascended from the lower leg. However, in the other 50 percent there is significant thrombosis in the iliac and proximal femoral veins but minimal or no evidence of disease distally. This suggests that the disease originates proximally in these patients. This supposition can be confirmed at the time of iliofemoral venous thrombectomy in many of these patients. The clots which are removed from the iliac vein are more adherent and pathologically older than the distal thrombi. The greater saphenous vein is usually the most prominent collateral vein visualized to the level of the groin and numerous small collaterals are usually seen in the pelvis. In some extremities the deep femoral vein remains at least partially patent to the level of the common femoral vein.

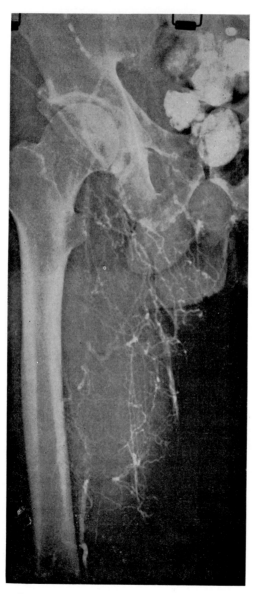

Figure 5-6. *Iliofemoral venous thrombosis.* There is lack of filling and therefore, total obstruction of the femoral and external iliac veins. Numerous small collaterals are visualized, however, and these collaterals do extend into the pelvis and to the opposite iliac vein.

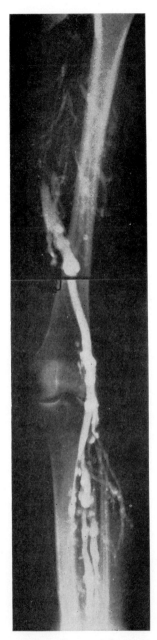

Figure 5-7. *Iliofemoral venous thrombosis.* There is complete obstruction of the iliac and proximal femoral vein such that only collaterals are visualized in the upper thigh. On the other hand, the popliteal and the calf veins which are visualized appear free of thrombus.

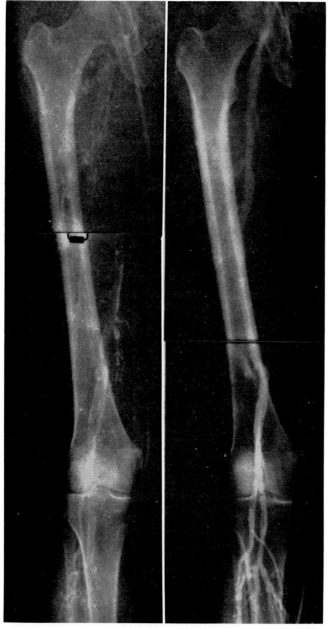

Figure 5-8. *Post-thrombotic changes.* The phlebogram on the left was taken at the time of acute iliofemoral venous thrombosis and large filling defects are identified in the popliteal, femoral, and deep femoral veins. The greater saphenous vein is serving as an important collateral. The phlebogram on the right was obtained six months later. The superficial femoral vein remains obstructed. The venous drainage is through a recannalized popliteal vein and its communication with the deep femoral vein. These patent veins do show changes of an irregular wall, lack of dilatation, and the scarcity of valves typical of post-thrombotic changes.

Post-Thrombotic Changes (Fig. 5-8)

The phlebographic appearance of veins which have contained thrombi has been described by Bauer, Grietz, and others.[4, 13] We have also had the opportunity to follow serially the phlebographic appearance of veins containing thrombi through their healing phase. Phlebograms obtained on patients one or two weeks after phlebograms demonstrated thrombi in calf veins will frequently appear normal if the patient receives anticoagulants.[10] This same phenomenon may be observed in the popliteal and femoral veins if the clots are nonobstructive. It must be assumed in these instances that the clots either have embolized, have been lysed, or that they have become adherent and organized to the wall of the vein without producing sufficient inflammatory changes to alter the regularity of the wall of the vein or to render the valves incompetent. More frequently the scars of a previous thrombosis can be identified by the irregularity of the wall of the vein and the absence of valves. These veins do not become dilated presumably because of thickening of the wall of the vein by fibrosis. On other occasions, the thrombosed vein may remain obstructed and only collaterals or venous bypasses are visualized. The dilated collaterals also do not appear to have valves.

CLINICAL USES OF PHLEBOGRAPHY

Diagnosis of Acute Deep Venous Thrombosis

It is difficult to make an accurate clinical diagnosis of deep venous thrombosis. The reason for this is two-fold. In the first place, thrombi may be present in the absence of significant clinical findings and in the second place, other conditions frequently mimic the signs and symptoms of acute thrombosis.

Autopsy series have confirmed the fact that many patients die of acute pulmonary emboli without the presence of venous thrombosis being recognized prior to death. Presumably about 80 percent of these individuals harbored thrombi in the veins of the lower extremity which embolized and caused the death. The studies of Kakkar and others have demonstrated that thrombi are frequently present in the dep veins of the calf following elective operations (27.8%); hip fractures (54%); prostatectomies (23.8%); and myocardial infarctions (19%).[14] Phlebography has been of considerable help to us in making the positive diagnosis of deep venous thrombosis in the presence of minimal signs or symptoms.[8]

On the other hand, there are clinical conditions which can be confused with deep venous thrombosis. These conditions include rupture of the medial slip of the gastrocnemius muscle or plantaris muscle, acute lymphedema, cellulitis, knee joint effusion or hemorrhage, and hysteria. We have observed patients with the above mentioned diagnosis who have received anticogulants without phlebography being performed. This aggravated the situation for many of these patients, particularly those with bleeding into the knee joint or into the soft tissues of the leg. The use of anticoagulants has been avoided in many similar patients by performing phlebograms and finding no evidence of venous thrombi.[6]

Evaluation of Other Diagnostic Tests

There have recently appeared a number of new techniques for diagnosing venous thrombosis. One of the most promising of these is the use of radio-iodinated fibrinogen. Following the intravenous injection of the material, radioscans are made over the site of suspected thrombosis which identify areas of increased radioactivity. Unfortunately, the test is not accurate in the region of the pelvis or upper thigh nor over areas with recent incisions or trauma because of increased background activity. In addition, the test is positive only when the thrombus is forming or is propagating.[14] The Doppler ultrasound technique and the impedance phlebography technique have been found to be useful in the diagnosis of thrombosis which has caused significant obstruction of major veins in the lower extremity. Unfortunately, venous thrombi are frequently not obstructing or involve only minor deep veins and the flow of blood may not be significantly affected.[21, 22] Phlebography is still considered the most accurate method for making the diagnosis and the value of any new technique is measured by comparing it with phlebography.

Determination of Source of Pulmonary Emboli

Autopsy series have indicated that venous thrombosis can be identified in the lower extremities of over 80 percent of patients with pulmonary emboli. Phlebograms have been used to identify these thrombi with proven or suspected pulmonary emboli. In our institution the test has most frequently been performed when a patient has had recurrent pulmonary emboli despite adequate anticoagulation. The phlebograms have either confirmed the presence of major deep venous thrombosis, identified the presence of small unsuspected thrombi, or ruled out the presence of significant thrombi in the lower extremity. It has, therefore, been possible to select logically the site of venous interruption for the failures of anticoagulation. Unilateral or bilateral femoral vein interruption has been performed on patients with thrombi localized to the lower leg or thigh, whereas inferior vena caval interruption has been performed on those with iliac vein involvement or in those with suspected pelvic vein involvement because no thrombi were identified in the lower extremity.[1, 2]

Evaluation of Methods of Therapy

Phlebography has provided objective means for evaluating the effects of various forms of therapy including anticoagulants, thrombolytic drugs, partial interruptions, and ligations of veins, and venous thrombectomies.

The ability of heparin to prevent the propagation of acute deep venous thrombosis and the virtual disappearance of small thrombi, presumably secondary to natural fibrinolysis during the course of heparin therapy, has been documented.[10]

The affect of Streptokinase or other materials which activate the natural thrombolytic processes has also been documented by phlebograms.[17]

Phlebograms have been performed on sixteen patients who had ligation of their femoral vein and thirteen of these patients were found to have progression of their distal thrombosis. On the other hand, there was progression of distal thrombosis in only eight of nineteen extremities in which the femoral vein was partially interrupted.[1] Phlebograms obtained on seven patients who had ligation of their inferior vena cava indicated that six of the seven had progression of their distal thrombosis. Postoperative phlebograms were obtained on eleven patients who had partial interruption of their inferior vena; none of these patients demonstrated progression of their distal thrombosis and the site of partial interruption was patent in seven of eleven cases.[2]

Phlebograms were performed on twenty-seven patients following venous thrombectomy of their iliac and femoral veins. Five of the phlebograms demonstrated patent veins and visible valves in the major veins. Eight of the phlebograms demonstrated patency of most but not all of the major veins known to be occluded prior to surgery and valves were visible in many of the veins. Phlebograms on eight of the extremities demonstrated patency of some veins known to be occluded prior to surgery but residual or recurrent thrombosis was still present. In six extremities the thrombosis was equal to or greater than that seen on the preoperative study.[9, 10]

COMPLICATIONS

There have been remarkably few complications following performance of phlebography. When the technique was first used patients were placed in a semierect position sixty degrees from the horizontal. Fainting would frequently occur following the elevation of the table or during the injection of the radio-opaque. By positioning the patient only forty-five degrees from the horizontal, elevating the head of the table slowly, carefully explaining the technique to the patient, and using less irritating radio-opaque contrast materials, fainting has virtually been eliminated. The incidence of urticaria, flushing, or vomiting has been no greater than encountered during the anticubital injection of similar volumes of contrast material during excretory urography.

There has been approximately a 2 percent incidence of redness and tenderness at the site of the injection occurring within the first twenty-four hours after injection and presumably secondary to a superficial phlebitis in that area. On the other hand, there has been no recognized progression of the deep venous thrombosis nor the appearance of a new deep venous thrombosis following phlebography. Two patients have developed a localized area of sloughing where extravasation of the dye occurred during its injection.[19] A presumptive diagnosis of pulmonary embolization has been made on a few patients within the first twenty-four hours after phlebography but has never been proven. We know of three deaths occurring within twenty-four hours following the examination. All three of these were sudden deaths and massive pulmonary emboli were suspected. All three patients had complete autopsies and the cause of death was found to be myocardial infarction and there was no evidence of recent pulmonary embolism.

Phlebography has proven to be a safe, accurate and exceedingly useful tool which is helpful in the diagnosis and management of thromboembolism.

REFERENCES

1. Adams, James T. and DeWeese, James A.: Comparative evaluation of ligation and partial interruption of the femoral vein in the treatment of thromboembolic disease. *Ann Surg, 172*:795-803, 1970.
2. Adams, James T., Feingold, Bertram E. and DeWeese, James A.: Comparative evaluation of ligation and partial interruption of the inferior vena cava. *Arch Surg, 103*:272-276, 1971.
3. Bauer, G.: Venographic study of thromboembolic problems. *Acta Chir Scand, Suppl, 84*: 61:1-75, 1940.
4. _____: Roentgenological and clinical study of sequels of thrombosis. *Acta Chir Scand, 86 Suppl, 74*:1-115, 1942.
5. Berberich, J. and Hirsch, S.: Die Roentgenographische Darstellung der Arterieri und Venen am Lebenden Menschen. *Klin Wochenschr, 2*:2228, 1923.
6. DeWeese, James A. and Rogoff, Stanley M.: Clinical uses of functional ascending phlebography of the lower extremity. *Angiology, 9*:268-278, 1958.
7. _____: Functional ascending phlebography of the lower extremity by serial long film technique. *Am J Roentgenol Radium Ther Nucl Med, 81*:841-854, 1959.
8. _____: Phlebographic patterns of acute deep venous thrombosis of the leg. *Surgery, 53*:99-108, 1963.
9. DeWeese, James A.: Thrombectomy for acute iliofemoral venous thrombosis. *J Cardiovasc Surg, 5*:703-712, 1964.
10. DeWeese, James A., Adams, James T. and Rogoff, Stanley M.: Restoration and maintenance of venous patency in venous thrombosis: Anticoagulation, thrombectomy, and partial venous interruption. *Pacific Med Surg, 75*:77-82, 1967.
11. Daugherty, J. and Homans, J.: Venography. Clinical study. *Surg Gynecol Obstet, 71*:697-702, 1940.
12. Felder, D. A. and Murphy, T. O.: Evaluation of method of phlebography of lower extremities. *Surgery, 37*:198-205, 1955.

13. Greitz, T.: Technique of ascending phlebography of lower extremity. *Acta Radiol,* 42:1-20, 1955.
14. Kakkar, V.: The diagnosis of deep vein thrombosis using the ^{125}I-fibrinogen test. *Arch Surg,* 104:152-159, 1972.
15. Lea, Thomas M.: Phlebography. *Arch Surg,* 104:145-151, 1972.
16. LeVeen, Harry H.: Thromboembolic phenomena: A symposium. *Contemp Surg,* 1:68-108, 1972.
17. Nicolaides, A. N., Kakkar, V. V., Field, E. S. and Renney, J. T. G.: The origin of deep venous thrombosis: A venographic study. *Br J Radiol,* 44:653-663, 1971.
18. Rabinov, Keith and Paulin, Sven: Roentgen diagnosis of venous thrombosis in the leg. *Arch Surg,* 104:134-144, 1972.
19. Rogoff, Stanley N. and DeWeese, James A.: Phlebography of the lower extremity. *JAMA,* 172:1599-1606, 1960.
20. Scott, H. W., Jr. and Roach, J. F.: Phlebography of leg in erect position. *Ann Surg,* 134:104-109, 1951.
21. Sigel, Bernard, Felix, W. Robert, Jr., Popley, George L. and Ipsen, Johannes: Diagnosis of lower limb venous thrombosis by Doppler ultrasound technique. *Arch Surg,* 104:174-179, 1972.
22. Wheeler, H. Brownell, Pearson, Daniel, O'Connell, Daniel and Mullick, Subhas C.: Impedance phlebography. *Arch Surg,* 104:164-169, 1972.

DISCUSSION

Dr. Zimmerman (Rockfort): Dr. DeWeese, you presented two cases of embolization from calf vein, and the previous speaker commented that he felt calf veins high I^{131} counts were not dangerous. Is there a discrepancy here or is this based on techniques or have you found evidence of disease that already have embolized, or how can we reconcile these two points of view?

Dr. DeWeese: I think probably in both of these instances the clot had progressed into the popliteal vein and the previous speaker did specify that with thrombi in the popliteal and femoral veins they would use anticoagulants.

Dr. Hume (Boston): Some years ago we corresponded about a patient who had been on the pill and wanted to sue the company that made the pill, because the thrombosis that was said to have occurred after she had been on the pill for awhile was due to the oral contraceptive. When a phlebogram was done it was entirely normal, but of course the phlebogram wasn't done for several months. She had had proper treatment on Heparin and Coumadin. The question was, does the phlebogram ever return to normal if venous thrombosis has been present and he showed a nice slide today. Do you think then that the likelihood of the phlebogram becoming normal after proper treatment is to be expected or is it frequent, or can you judge after a properly treated episode?

Dr. DeWeese: I'm continually surprised at how complete a return to normal you can see. A patient was seen last week that had extensive thrombosis, nonobstructing, of the femoral vein six months ago. He now has a normal appearing vein with valves in it and he has not had a thrombectomy. Looking at the new films, I would not have been able to say that he had deep venous thrombosis in the past, although I have the phlebogram that shows that he did.

Dr. Oliver (St. Louis): Would you care to comment on the technique of transosseous or intraosseous venography?

Dr. DeWeese: Only to say that we have not used it. I cannot fairly evaluate it. I know it is even more painful than our technique, which is less painful if you use angioconray and it has not been necessary to go to the extra bother of injecting into the bone.

Dr. Mobin-Uddin: Let me ask Dr. DeWeese, how often our clinical diagnosis of thrombophlebitis is correct. What is the clinical correlation with phlebography and thrombophlebitis?

Dr. DeWeese: It is very poor. It was pointed out in studies by McLaughlin and also studies we did a few years ago, that the best objective sign of venous thrombosis is swelling and many other things cause swelling of the leg. In addition, if there is only calf vein thrombosis, the swelling that is present is only minimal. Tenderness was only present in 80 percent of patients with calf vein thrombosis, 90 percent in those with femoral vein thrombosis and, of course, always in iliofemoral venous thrombosis. So it is easy to make a diagnosis of iliofemoral and femoral but difficult to make that of calf vein thrombosis.

Dr. Pearlman (Boston): How often have you had to do a cut-down in order to do a phlebogram?

Dr. DeWeese: Very rarely, but again in a massively swollen leg, you may have to do it. With increasing experience of the person doing it, the need for cut-downs decreases. You can almost always find a small vein, even if it is that good dorsal vein on the big toe.

Dr. Cacera (Delray): Are you still doing venous thrombectomy for iliofemoral phlebitis?

Dr. DeWeese: Yes.

Dr. Silver (Durham): These are beautiful phlebograms. I wonder if you have a pattern that you look for before you do a thrombectomy. Do you use your phlebograms to help you decide who to operate on?

Dr. DeWeese: The answer is yes, the more localized and proximal it is, the more apt we are to do it.

Chapter 6

THE EFFECT OF COMPRESSION UPON THE DEEP VENOUS SYSTEM OF THE LOWER EXTREMITIES DURING INACTIVE RECUMBENCY

Bernard Sigel, Annette L. Edelstein,

W. Robert Felix, Jr., and Charles R. Memhardt

COMPRESSION HAS BEEN a time-honored method for preventing stasis in the lower extremities. Elastic bandages, and more recently elastic stockings, have been employed to prevent venous thrombosis in patients who for various reasons are felt to be at risk for thromboembolism. In an effort to determine the efficacy of elastic compression for preventing venous thrombosis, we undertook a study of venous flow in inactive recumbent subjects. Our plan of study was to employ a noninvasive Doppler ultrasound blood flow technique to measure femoral vein blood flow velocity. The details of this study* have been reported previously and only a summary of our findings will be presented.[1]

METHOD

Ten volunteers, fully informed as to the purposes of examination, were studied. Each subject was placed in a supine position on the examining table and three transducers were applied as follows: (1) a Doppler ultrasound transducer was applied over one femoral vein at the inguinal ligament; (2) a similar transducer was applied over the opposite groin to fit over the femoral artery; and (3) a mercury-in-rubber strain gauge was fixed to the chest to time the respiratory movements. The transducer over the vein was connected to a bidirectional Doppler ultrasound flow detector (Parks Model 806). The arterial transducer was connected to a non-directional Doppler ultrasound detector and the mercury-in-rubber strain gauge

*Supported by a grant (HL-11774) from the National Institutes of Health, Veterans Administration, and The John A. Hartford Foundation.

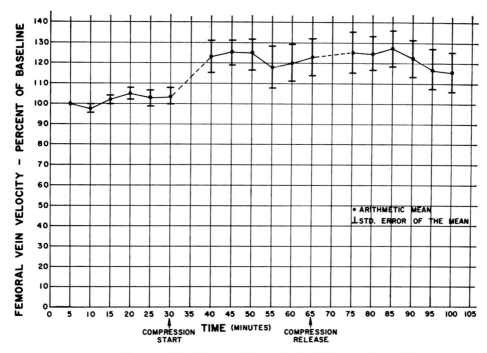

FEMORAL VEIN VELOCITY DURING ELASTIC STOCKING COMPRESSION
IN NINE LOWER EXTREMITIES

THIRTY MINUTE COMPRESSION STUDY

Figure 6-1. The effect of 30-minute elastic stocking compression on femoral vein flow. Compression produces an increase of about 20 percent in femoral flow velocity. This increase persists for up to 30 minutes after release of compression.

was coupled to an electrical impedance plethysmograph. Signals from these three sources were recorded on an instrumentation tape recorder and subsequently analyzed by simultaneously displaying the data on a multichannel pen recorder.

We first tested inactive supine subjects for up to three hours to determine the stability of our recording system. This was performed at first without compression and revealed that flow velocity baselines were constant for up to three hours of continuous measurement. After this time, either a change in the transducer position, restlessness of the subject, or both, precluded continued monitoring. Thus, we limited our experiments to three hours or less.

Prior to the study, measurements were made of the circumferences of the lower extremity of each subjcet at various locations. Thigh-length knitted nylon/spandex stockings similar to those used in hospitals to prevent venous thrombosis were then prepared for each subject according to the dimen-

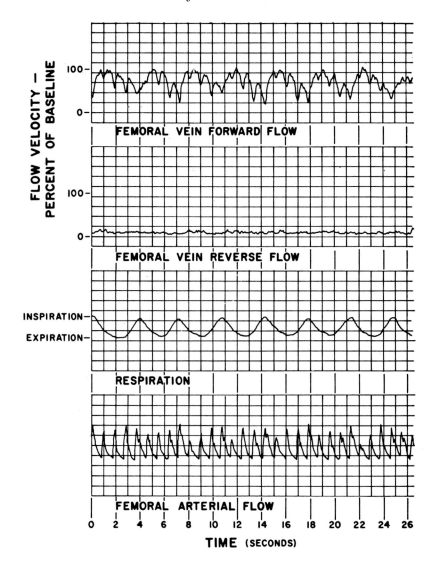

CYCLICAL PATTERN OF VENOUS VELOCITY SIGNAL

Figure 6-2. The dual cyclical pattern of the venous velocity signal is shown in the forward flow tracing compared to respiration and cardiac pulsations represented by a femoral artery velocity tracing.

sions of his lower extremity. These stockings were fitted to provide pressure at the ankle of eighteen mm Hg and pressure at the upper thigh of 6.5 mm Hg. In addition, each stocking was fitted with a full-length zipper along its anterior aspect to permit rapid application and decompression during the study periods.

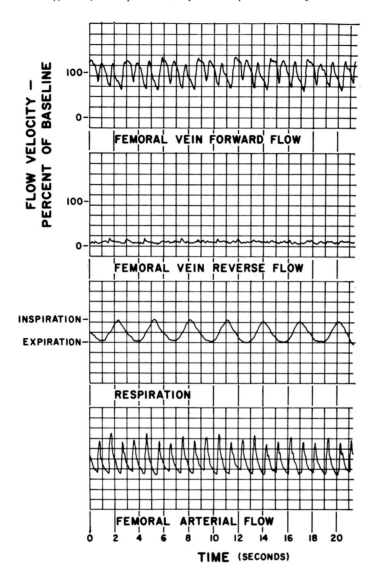

EFFECT OF COMPRESSION ON CYCLICAL PATTERN
OF VENOUS VELOCITY

Figure 6-3. Elastic compression reduces the amplitude of the respiratory cycle effect. The venous velocity pulses in cadence with the cardiac pulses are relatively enhanced by this maneuver.

INTERPRETATION OF RESULTS

Figure 6-1 shows the summary results obtained in nine lower extremities before, during and after thirty-minute stocking compression. The baseline of femoral blood flow velocity has been set at 100 percent. With compression, the average femoral blood flow velocity increased to about 120 per-

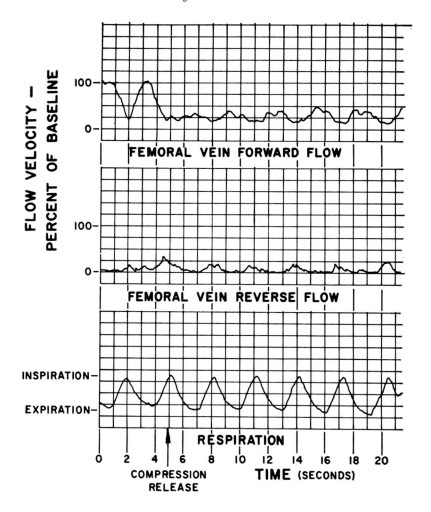

RELEASE OF COMPRESSION IN SUBJECT WITH
COMPETENT VALVES

Figure 6-4. With rapid decompression, there is a marked decrease of forward flow velocity. In this subject with competent valves, the transient increase in reverse flow velocity did not occur as in the subject with incompetent valves.

cent of baseline. Following release of compression, the increase in blood velocity persisted for approximately thirty minutes after decompression.

Figure 6-2 shows recordings from the extremity without compression. Note the fluctuations of the femoral vein velocity tracing. These fluctuations are in phase with the respiratory excursions. There is a decrease in femoral vein flow velocity with inspiration and an increase in flow velocity with expiration. In addition, the femoral vein velocity tracing shows a more rapid pulsatile component which is in cadence with the heart rate when

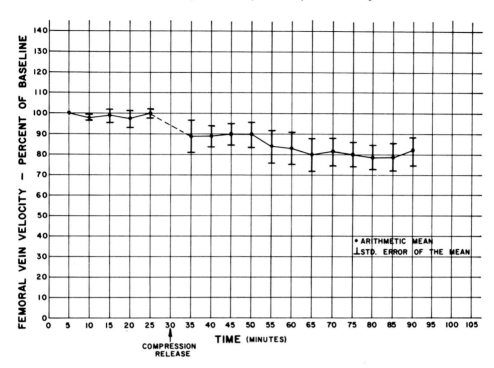

FEMORAL VEIN VELOCITY DURING AND AFTER ELASTIC COMPRESSION
OF THREE HOURS DURATION
STUDY OF EIGHT LOWER EXTREMITIES

Figure 6-5. The effect of compression lasting three hours is measured in the last thirty minutes of compression and for sixty minutes following release of compression. Following decompression, flow velocity decreased over a period of thirty minutes to reach a baseline which was about eighty percent of the average flow velocity during the latter part of the three-hour compression period. (*All figures in this chapter by permission of Archives of Surgery.*)

compared to the arterial velocity pulse seen in the lower part of the figure.

Figure 6-3 shows the effect of elastic stocking compression on the femoral vein velocity tracing. Note that compression greatly diminishes the effect of respirations and accentuates the pulsatile component which is in cadence with the heart rate. Thus, there is a qualitative effect in the venous flow tracing produced by elastic compression consisting of a more constant flow of venous blood toward the heart.

Figure 6-4 shows what happens to femoral vein flow immediately after rapid removal of elastic compression. Femoral vein blood velocity transiently diminishes. We regard this as being due to an expansion of the venous bed following decompression with an increased filling of the bed with blood resulting in a brief reduction in femoral vein flow. We interpret this event, therefore, as indirect evidence that elastic stockings reduce the capacitance of the venous bed thereby decreasing stasis.

Figure 6-5 is a summary of the study performed in eight lower extremities to determine the length of persistence of increased flow following removal of elastic stockings. In this experiment, all the subjects wore elastic stockings for at least three hours. Following removal of the stockings, there was a gradual reduction in flow lasting approximately thirty minutes. This experiment shows that elastic compression still exerts an effect at the end of three hours and that this effect persists for up to thirty minutes following removal of the elastic stockings.

DISCUSSION

Initially, we employed plastic inflatable air splints as well as elastic stockings on the same subjects. We found the effect of air splints to be quite different from elastic stockings exerting the same average pressure. Air splints, with pressure levels comparable to elastic stockings, produced less consistent increases in flow velocity. As the splint pressure was increased, there was an actual decrease in femoral vein flow velocity. We believe that the different effects are due to at least two causes. First, the splints exert a uniform pressure throughout the region being compressed. In contrast, the stockings used in this study (as is the practice with elastic stockings used in hospitals) exert a graduated pressure which is greatest at the ankle and least at the thigh. Second, the inflatable plastic splints which we employed fully extend the leg when inflated. Full extension of the knee will diminish popliteal vein blood flow. Consequently, the decrease in femoral vein flow velocity seen with the use of splints may result from decreased venous flow produced by extension.

In addition to showing that elastic stocking compression increases femoral vein blood flow velocity, our study has revealed other relevant findings. First, there is a persistence of increased flow velocity for up to thirty minutes after removal of the stockings. Second, there was a qualitative change in the femoral vein velocity during compression. The fluctuations caused by respirations became markedly decreased indicating that venous flow with compression is more constant. Third, there appears to be indirect evidence that there is a reduction in the capacitance of the venous bed with elastic stocking compression suggesting that such compression reduces venous stasis. Finally, this study shows that the effects of elastic stocking compression persist for at least three hours of continuous wear. All the changes produced by elastic compression would appear to reduce conditions which are regarded as predisposing to the development of venous thrombosis. Thus, the results support the efficacy of employing elastic compression stockings to prevent lower extremity venous thrombosis in subjects at risk for venous thromboembolism.

Conclusions

1. Elastic compression of the lower extremities by elastic stockings will increase blood flow velocity in the femoral vein. This effect persists at the end of three hours of compression indicating that elastic stocking compression does maintain an increase in venous flow velocity under conditions resembling those used in hospitalized patients.

2. Compression reduces the effects of the respiratory excursions on flow velocity. Venous flow with compression, therefore, is more constant.

3. There is indirect evidence that elastic compression reduces the capacitance of the venous bed resulting in decreased stasis in the veins of the lower extremities.

4. The effect of compression in inactive recumbent subjects appears to lessen factors which predispose to the occurrence of deep venous thrombosis.

REFERENCE

1. Sigel, B., Edelstein, A. L., Felix, Jr., W. R. and Memhardt, C. R.: Compression of the deep venous system of the lower leg during inactive recumbency. *Arch Surg 106*:38-43, 1973.

DISCUSSION

Dr. Ochsner (New Orleans): Concerning your observations on the use of elastic stockings, I wonder if there may not be another factor, because we made an observation on our orthopedic service that individuals with femoral fractures which are ideal candidates for phlebothrombosis, that those treated by traction developed a high incidence whereas those treated by plaster encasement in which the mobility is even more complete than by traction had a very low incidence. I'm wondering if it isn't the retention of heat in the extremity and the increase of the arterial flow and the increased vis-a-tergo through the capillary system, because of the insulating effect of the stockings.

Dr. Sigel: This is a possibility.

Dr. Powell (Fort Knox): I was just wondering, do these increased flow effects still obtain after the patient has been wearing the stocking for seven days or so like we do have when we have very sick patients we keep the stocking on?

Dr. Sigel: No, the longest we did was three hours.

Dr. Powell: If I could just briefly say, I've been somewhat involved with the NASA Apollo Project and Commander Evans, the last time out, wore a lower body negative pressure suit to control his venous stasis that we worried about, the other two men did not. We found after twelve days of this situation, Commander Evans showed absolutely no difference in venous tone when we measured them when we brought him down. I was wondering if it reaches a point at which the effect diminishes.

Dr. Sigel: I'm sure this will happen, that with time the pressure effect is diminished and finally disappears, but I can only say that it at least lasts for three hours.

Chapter 7

ILIOFEMORAL THROMBECTOMY—
PRESENT STATUS

ALLAN M. LANSING

DESPITE THE USE of elevation of the legs and vigorous heparin therapy, the late morbidity of the post-phlebitic syndrome has created great interest in a better type of treatment of iliofemoral venous thrombosis. Surgical thrombectomy has been recommended to obtain immediate relief of the comprised venous drainage, to decrease early morbidity, to preserve the venous valves, and to prevent the later post-phlebitic syndrome. The operative procedure was described by Leriche in 1948[11] and became known in America through the work of Mahorner et al in 1957.[12] A series of forty-five cases was reported from the University of Louisville in 1963 by Haller and Abrams[8] with early good results. However, when these were reviewed five years later, the end results were not nearly as satisfactory.[10]

The morbidity and mortality in thirty-nine of these patients is shown in the first slides. Ten patients died, five while still in the hospital. Three of the hospital deaths resulted from other diseases (heart disease, cancer, and stroke) and two from pulmonary embolism that occurred one and two days after operation. The other five patients died later of other diseases or from unknown causes. Thus, two deaths were directly attributable to the operation (5%).

Of the patients who left the hospital, the average duration of stay following operation was thirty days, ranging from six to 240 days. The median hospital stay of twelve days, however, gives a more accurate picture, since the average was distorted by one chronic disease patient who stayed 240 days. Blood transfusion was required in all but three patients, ranging from 100 cc in a thirteen-pound child to 3,500 cc, with an average of 1,000 cc. Local wound infection or hematoma that had to be drained occurred in twelve of the thirty-nine patients (30%), and nonfatal pulmonary embolus in one.

73

The evidence of stasis disease five years after early operative intervention, that is clinical disease present for one week or less, was identified in twenty-five of the thirty-four patients in whom this situation existed. Nine of the patients died and eight others could not be located. Of the seventeen survivors, all except one had significant edema and wore an elastic support five years after operation, and one had a stasis ulcer that first appeared three months after operation. The only patient free of edema was a six-year-old boy who underwent thrombectomy when he was one year old for the treatment of an infected long saphenous phlebitis resulting from an ankle vein cut-down.

Venograms were performed on fifteen of the patients who underwent early operation. The involved area of the deep venous system was found to be incompetent in all cases and there were no functioning valves. Two of these are demonstrated in the next two slides, each of which shows a normal right leg ninety seconds after injection of contrast material with venous valves present, whereas the operated left side was patent but showed no valve. Evidence of the previous thrombosis and recanalization on the left side can be seen easily.

The immediate reduction in swelling and the disappearance of numbness and cyanosis reported after operative removal of the thrombus are not necessarily due to the operation itself. We have observed the same dramatic response after a few hours of marked elevation of the limbs combined with intravenous heparin therapy, two elements that form part of the operative treatment of the disease, and it is difficult to separate the benefits of thrombectomy from those of the other two measures. Karp and Wylie[2] reported ten patients, all of whom were clinically improved within a few hours after thrombectomy, but in eight of these who underwent postoperative venograms recurrent occlusion was present. They concluded that some factor other than continuing patency of the veins was responsible for the clinical improvement. We observed eight patients in whom bilateral iliofemoral thrombosis was treated on one side by operative intervention and on the second by conservative, nonoperative measures. The clinical results and the venograms were indistinguishable on the two sides, so that it was impossible to separate the effects of the thrombectomy from those of the concomitant elevation and heparin therapy. The next slide shows one of these cases in whom iliofemoral thrombectomy was performed on the right leg five years before, while left iliofemoral thrombosis was treated medically on the other side one month later. You can see the dilated superficial femoral vein and the absence of the valves on the operated right side and the thrombosed common femoral vein with collateral channels around it. On the left, the superficial femoral vein is thrombosed, but the saphenous, common femoral and iliac veins are patent. Edema was present in both legs.

Patency of the veins, as demonstrated in the postoperative venogram, cannot in itself be an aim of the operation or proof of its success. For one thing, an equally acceptable early clinical result has been achieved even in the absence of such patency. In addition, Dale[4] demonstrated that the time in the postoperative period when the venogram was performed must also be considered. His experimental study of venous suture techniques and vein graft showed that at least one half of the patent veins had in fact undergone thrombosis and recanalization in the postoperative period.

It is evident, therefore, that the key factor in prevention of the post-phlebitic syndrome is not patency of the veins, but preservation of the venous valves. The experience at the University of Louisville showed that the vein in which thrombectomy has been performed was frequently patent when studied at a later date, but functioning venous valves in the involved segment have not been demonstrated in any of the cases. Edwards and Edwards[6] reviewed both experimental and clinical data and showed very clearly that destruction of the venous valves occurred despite recovery of venous patency after thrombosis. Fontaine[7] also showed that recanalization was common, but the veins involved were valveless and poorly functioning if the follow-up period was long enough. In spite of this, a satisfactory end result will likely be obtained if the popliteal and calf veins have not been involved in the original process or if therapy has prevented extension of the thrombus to these areas. Even though the femoral and iliac channels are occluded or recanalized with no functioning valves, the patient may have little or no edema if the popliteal and calf veins and their valves have not been damaged. The only good result in our series is shown in this slide, that of the six-year-old child who underwent operation at the age of ten months. Note that most of the superficial femoral vein is occluded and the deep femoral channels are dilated. However, there are valves in the distal femoral and popliteal veins, and no edema was present. Other films showed recanalized iliac veins and an occluded distal inferior vena cava with lumbar collaterals, further indicating the important benefits that result when the popliteal and calf veins are not involved in the process.

As a result of these studies and other experiences, American surgeons have tempered their enthusiasm for performing thrombectomy in all cases of iliofemoral venous thrombosis. In fact, most of the more recent literature on the subject has come from British authors. Cranley et al.[3] reported on the immediate and late results in fifty-six patients who were followed up for five to fourteen years after thrombectomy (16 cases), caval ligation (13 cases), and conservative treatment (37 cases). They compared the incidence of swelling, varicose veins, pigmentation, and ulceration. While there were no patients with uncontrolled edema among the sixteen who underwent thrombectomy and ligation, only 15 percent of those who had either conservative treatment or caval ligation alone had uncontrolled edema. There was no difference in the incidence of varicose veins, pigmentation, or ulceration between the group that underwent thrombectomy and those who had conservative treatment alone. The only really significant difference was that the patients who had caval ligation alone had a much higher incidence of all three of these complications: 61 percent had varicose veins, 46 percent had pigmentation, and 14 percent had ulcers. As a result of these studies Cranley now recommends that bed rest, elevation, and heparin therapy should be the standard procedure for treatment of iliofemoral venous thrombosis.

Another British author who has investigated the surgical management of deep vein thrombosis is Mavor.[15, 16] He divided deep vein thrombosis into the peripheral types that rarely extend to the iliac system or cause pulmonary embolism, and the proximal or iliofemoral types that usually extend distally, are associated with pulmonary embolism in about one half of the cases, and may be nonocclusive or totally occlusive. If total occlusion has occurred, subsequent venous insufficiency usually follows. He is still a proponent of the surgical treatment, but considers contraindications to surgical intervention to include poor general condition of the patient such as malignancy, generalized disease, or obesity; local conditions such as infection or a useless leg in a hemiplegic patient; or the lapse of over seventy-two hours after the occurrence of complete occlusion, except in patients with threatening gangrene or involvement of the inferior vena cava. He recommends that before operation is undertaken bilateral phlebography must be undertaken and the thrombectomy should be done with radiographic control. In a series of 257 patients he had a mortality of only four percent, three of these during operation and six later of pulmonary embolism, and two of unrelated causes. Rethrombosis occurred in less than fourteen days in twenty-one patients, including seven of sixty-one in whom complete clearance of the vein had been considered to have been accomplished at the time of operation and in fourteen of thirty-four in whom some residual clot remained at the time of operation. A further eight patients were found to have rethrombosed between three months and five years including four of eighteen with complete clearance at the time of the first operation and four of twelve with incomplete clearance. In spite of his extensive surgical experience, he now recommends treatment with Streptokinase, Heparin, and Coumadin as the first line of treatment, especially if over seventy-two hours have occurred from the onset of symptoms. Immediate operation is undertaken only for threatened gangrene or for involvement of the inferior vena cava.

Mansfield and his colleagues have also been investigating the surgical treatment of venous thrombosis.[13, 14] He reported upon his experiences in thirty-two patients operated upon less than ten days after the onset of the disease. If the procedure is to be undertaken he recommends the following prerequisites. A bilateral venogram must be performed preoperatively and this is usually done both through the ankle veins and by the pertrochanteric route using general anesthesia. A mobile image intensifier is employed in the operating room to give accurate radiographic control during the procedure and the inferior vena cava is occluded through the saphenous vein of the good leg at the level of the second lumbar vertebra. A thrombectomy catheter employing an eight-ml or ten-ml balloon is used after control of the inferior vena cava has been achieved, and operative venography is performed at the end of the procedure. Both the vena cava catheter and the thrombectomy catheter balloons are inflated with a radio-opaque material to facilitate these steps. He states that the advantages of these measures include exact positioning of the inferior vena cava catheter, demonstration of occlusion of the inferior vena cava by the balloon, observation of the sites of venous compression, and close observation of the course of the thrombectomy catheter. However, he does not have any long-term follow-up studies to support his conclusions.

It is evident from these studies that neither the early clinical result nor patency of the involved veins is a reliable criterion of the final result, and the critical factor in evaluating the benefit of any therapy is the passage of enough time so that the late sequelae can be documented. Hojensgard[9] demonstrated that treatment by elevation alone without anticoagulation will give a high percentage of limbs that look satisfactory for one or two years, but in the period between two and five years edema begins to appear, and between six and ten years ulceration becomes increasingly frequent. As Bauer[1] so aptly expressed the situation in his monograph on venography: "... if thrombotic patients are followed-up, not for one or a couple of years, but for decennia, it will be found that the late complications, contrary to what might be supposed, increase in commonness and severity as the years pass by ...." Other authors, including DeWeese et al.[5] and Fontaine,[7] have reported similar results when patients who had undergone thrombectomy were followed for several years, and they concluded that thrombectomy offered little benefit as far as the long-term results were concerned. Although the early results of thrombectomy appear satisfactory, the situation is much like that of an aortic valve that has been damaged by rheumatic fever: the leak may appear to be fairly minimal and cause little hemodynamic disturbance for many years, but its effect gradually becomes progressively more severe and devastating.

In summary, the present status of surgical treatment is indicated in the final slide. The initial mainstays of treatment include complete bed rest, marked elevation of the legs, and intravenous heparin therapy. Operation is undertaken for threatened gangrene that does not immediately respond to these measures or if the disease has been present for less than forty-eight hours. It should be preceded by bilateral phlebography to rule out the presence of disease on the other side or inferior vena cava involvement, and operation should be performed with radiographic control through an image intensifier, balloon catheter occlusion of the inferior vena cava, and operative venography, and venous interruption is not part of the procedure. On the other hand, if over seventy-two hours have occurred since the onset of the symptoms, we must concentrate first on local therapy with Streptokinase followed by Heparin and Coumadin to prevent recurrence of the thrombosis.

REFERENCES

1. Bauer, G.: Roentogenological and clinical study of the sequels of thrombosis. *Acta Chir Scand, 86*: Supplement 74, 1942.
2. Karp, R. B. and Wylie, E. J.: Recurrent thrombosis after iliofemoral venous thrombectomy. *Surg Forum, 17*:147, 1966.
3. Cranley, J. J., Krause, R. J., Strasser, E. S. and Hafner, C. D.: Femoroiliac thrombophlebitis: Immediate and late results after thrombectomy, caval ligation, and conservative treatment. *J Cardiovasc Surg, 10*:463, 1969.
4. Dale, W. A.: Thrombosis and recanalization of veins used as venous grafts. *Angiology, 12*:603, 1961.
5. DeWeese, J. A., Jones, T. I., Lyon, J. and Dale, W. A.: Evaluation of thrombectomy in the management of iliofemoral venous thrombosis. *Surgery, 47*:140, 1960.
6. Edwards, E. A. and Edwards, J. E.: The effects of thrombophlebitis on the venous valves. *Surg Gynecol Obstet, 65*:310, 1937.
7. Fontaine, R.: Remarks concerning venous thrombosis and its sequelae. *Surgery, 41*:6, 1957.
8. Haller, J. A., Jr. and Abrams, B. L.: Use of thrombectomy in the treatment of acute iliofemoral venous thrombosis in forty-five patients. *Ann Surg, 158*:561, 1963.
9. Hojensgard, I. C.: Sequelae of deep thrombosis in the lower limbs. *Angiology, 3*:42, 1952.
10. Lansing, A. M. and Davis, W. M.: Five-year follow-up study of iliofemoral venous thrombectomy. *Ann Surg, 168*:620, 1968.
11. Leriche, R.: Y-a-t-il des thrombosis primitives localisees a l'Embouchure de la Veine Cave? A propos de la thrombectomie dans les phlebites, thrombose, et stase. *Presse Med, 56*:825, 1948.
12. Mahorner, H., Castleberry, J. W. and Coleman, W. O.: Attempts to restore function in major veins which are the site of massive thrombosis. *Ann Surg, 146*:510, 1957.
13. Mansfield, A. O.: Thrombectomy employing continuous radiological control. *Ann Roy Coll Surg Eng, 48*:3-4, 1971.
14. Mansfield, A. O., Carmichael, J. H. and Parry, E. W.: Thrombectomy employing continuous radiological control. *Br J Surg, 58*:119, 1971.

15. Mavor, G. E.: Deep vein thrombosis: Surgical management. *Br Med J*, 4:680-682, 1969.

16. Mavor, G. E., Galloway, J. M. D. and Karmody, A. M.: The surgical aspects of deep vein thrombosis. *Proc Roy Soc Med*, 63:126-130, 1970.

DISCUSSION

Dr. McCranie (California): Dr. Lansing, do you have any phlebograms demonstrating long-term patency with presence of functioning valves on the cases you just mentioned?

Dr. Lansing: No, in fact the opposite was true. In no case was there patency with a functioning valve in the involved area. The veins were patent, but there were no valves.

Dr. Lansing: Could I have time just to emphasize one more point? Could I see those last three slides? I always have to keep something up my sleeve. This is to show what we would like to obtain and to emphasize again the difference between a normal and the operative side. Here is a normal leg with venous filling and the beautiful valves present. Next slide—When you re-X-ray the patient, three minutes later the normal side is empty with only a few little pockets of dye in the cusps, the place that the venous thrombosis is believed to start, but on the operative side, the dye is still present in the vein illustrating the venous insufficiency, stasis and the absence of any valves. Next slide please—This is what we would like to see, but have not seen in any of the patients in the involved segments of the vein. We would like to see nice valves like this with cusps like this. When we see that, we will know that we have found the proper treatment of iliofemoral venous thrombosis.

Dr. Wheeler (Wooster): I'd just like to leave with one slightly positive note. I'm not an enthusiast for this operation, we rarely do it, but I have had a couple of patients who have not responded to conservative treatment within forty-eight hours who have had an ileofemoral thrombectomy. At least one of them had good functioning valves on venogram about three years later. The other had good function by Doppler and impedance studies.

SECTION II

PULMONARY
THROMBOEMBOLISM —
PATHOPHYSIOLOGY

Chapter 8

HYPERCOAGULABLE STATES

JOHN A. SPITTELL, JR.

I F A hypercoagulable state is defined as a state in which one can demonstrate an increased concentration of a normal or abnormal procoagulant, or a decrease in a normal inhibitor, or an acceleration of the coagulation mechanism of the blood, then hypercoagulable states are common. Numerous studies have demonstrated such changes and their occurrence in conditions and disease states predisposing to or characterized by thrombosis.[1]

There is much controversy and much resistance to the concept of hypercoagulability and its role in thrombosis. This ignores the fact that in the converse and well-accepted concept of hypocoagulability causing bleeding, changes in vascular integrity are necessary before bleeding takes place. By analogy, the hypercoagulable state is best considered as a condition of the blood favorable or predisposing to thrombosis, given the proper set of circumstances (changes in blood flow or in the blood vessels or in both) in which thrombosis can occur. Such a concept is well supported by studies showing, in experimental hypercoagulable states induced by the injection of serum[2] or ellagic acid,[3] that thrombosis does not occur without accompanying stasis of blood flow.

Studies of the blood cells have included not only the cells themselves but also their behavior in the liquid medium of blood. Myeloproliferative disorders have long been known to be associated with an increased incidence of thrombosis. However, the exact mechanism by which the increased numbers of erythrocytes (in polycythemia) or of platelets (in thrombocytosis) contribute to thrombosis is not clear. In polycythemia the phenomenon of "sludging," so well documented in the experiments of Knisely and associates,[4] may be the mechanism. In the case of the platelets and their relationship to thrombosis several possible mechanisms exist. Not only can increased numbers of platelets be implicated, but the characteristics of platelet adhesiveness and the phenomenon of platelet aggregation also have been shown to be increased in conditions associated with an increased incidence of thromboembolism. The constituents of platelets may also be important in thrombosis.[5]

Before proceeding to studies of the coagulation factors, the dysprotein-emic states—cryoglobulinemia, macroglobulinemia, and cryfibrinogenemia —should be mentioned as possible hypercoagulable states. Whether by "sludging," by altering the characteristics of the cellular elements of the blood, or by some other mechanism, diseases with these abnormal proteins may be complicated by thrombosis.

Most of the established tests of coagulation are not well suited—by their design for detecting deficiencies of coagulation—for detecting hypercoagu-lability. Even so, numerous studies using standard tests lend support to the concept of hypercoagulability.[1]

An example from our own laboratory is the suggestive evidence provided by comparing the whole-blood coagulation times of patients who have arterial thrombosis with those of a group of normal persons (Fig. 8-1). The mean coagulation time of the patients with thrombosis was six minutes while that of the normal persons was seven and one half minutes. Several modifications of this rather crude test have also shown a shortening of the clotting time in some patients with arterial and venous thromboses.

By various types of tests of coagulation, increased concentrations of most

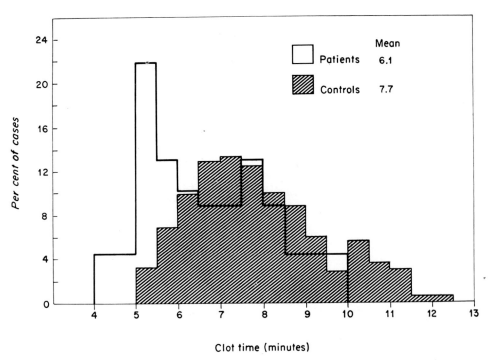

Figure 8-1. Whole-blood coagulation times in normal persons with thrombosis.

of the plasmatic coagulation factors have been observed in patients with thrombotic disorders. Likewise, deficiency of antithrombin and inhibition of fibrinolysis have also been reported to occur in persons who have a predisposition to thrombosis. Rather remarkable increases in some coagulation factors (Factor VII, Factor VIII, Factor IX, and Factor X as well as fibrinogen) have been reported in pregnant women,[6,7] but despite these changes thromboembolism did not occur. However, the possible role of such coagulation-factor changes in thrombosis gained support by the occurrence of arterial and venous thromboses in some women taking anovulatory drugs. In these women, coagulation changes mimicking those seen in pregnancy, though less pronounced, have been reported.[8]

In our laboratory we have been particularly interested in the earliest phases of the clotting mechanism, since from *in vitro* tests, at least, it appears that the limiting factor in normal clotting is the rate of formation and amount of available thromboplastin. With modification of the thromboplastin generation test we have been able to demonstrate accelerated thromboplastin generation in persons with various thrombotic disorders.[9]

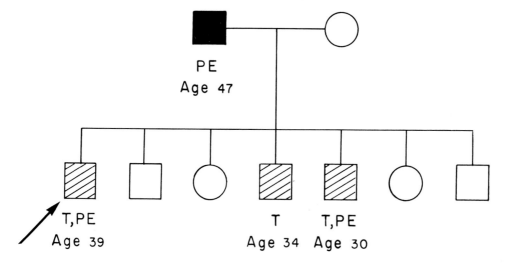

T-thrombophlebitis
PE-pulmonary embolism

Figure 8-2. Familial idiopathic thrombophlebitis: proband is a man whose recurring idiopathic thrombophlebitis began at age 39; his father died of pulmonary embolism of indeterminate cause at age 47. Two younger brothers developed idiopathic recurrent thrombophlebitis in their early 30's. (From Spittell, J. A. Jr.: Coagulation, thrombosis, anticoagulants, and fibrinolysis. In Fairbairn, J. F. II, Juergens, J. L., Spittell, J. A., Jr. (Eds.): *Peripheral Vascular Diseases*, 4th ed. Philadelphia, W. B. Saunders, Company, 1972, pp. 79-109. By permission.)

Of particular interest is the occurrence of thrombosis in certain families. Egeberg[10] found heparin resistance and low levels of antithrombin, apparently inherited as an autosomal dominant, in members of a family predisposed to venous thrombosis. In a young woman who had recurrent venous thrombosis, perhaps familial, Penick[11] also found reduced levels of antithrombin. We have observed several families with multiple members affected by recurring venous thromboembolism. One such family is illustrated in Figure 8-2. It thus appears that some hypercoagulable states, the result of abnormalities of coagulation, may be inheritable.

Recent years have witnessed more attention to the possible role of activated clotting factors, rather than excessive amounts of normal coagulation factors, as the stimulus for thrombosis. Wessler and Yin[12] have found in their experimental studies of thrombosis in animals that activated Factor X is immensely more thrombogenic than nonactivated Factor X.

Further supporting the concept that intravascular thrombosis can be triggered by activation of the clotting mechanism, is the now well-accepted clinical syndrome of disseminated intravascular coagulation.[13] Complicating numerous and diverse diseases, this syndrome is characterized by abnormal hemostasis that, depending on the relative degrees of activation of the clotting and fibrinolytic mechanism, may result in thrombosis or overt bleeding.[14] The clinical syndrome can be reproduced in animals by infusing precoagulant materials such as thromboplastin and thrombin.

The complexity of the problem of thrombosis and its mechanism(s) is evident. The diversity and the large number of clinical conditions in which it occurs suggest that multiple factors effect its genesis. There is little doubt, from the data presented, that changes in the blood which accelerate *in vitro* tests of clotting do occur. Such alternations in clotting can also be induced experimentally. If these changes can be defined as hypercoagulable states, just as defects in clotting are hypercoagulable states, then the concept that hypercoagulability favors thrombosis seems as tenable as the well-accepted association of hypocoagulability and bleeding.

REFERENCES

1. Spittell, J. A., Jr.: Coagulation, thrombosis, anticoagulants, and fibrinolysis. In Fairbairn, J. F., Juergens, J. L., and Spittell, J. A., Jr. (Eds.): *Peripheral Vascular Diseases*, 4th ed. Philadelphia, W. B. Saunders Company, 1972, pp. 79-109.
2. Wessler, S.: Studies in intravascular coagulation. III. The pathogenesis of serum-induced venous thrombosis. *J Clin Invest*, 34:647-651, 1955.
3. Ratnoff, O. D.: The role of the blood-clotting mechanism in the pathogenesis of thrombosis. In Sherry, S., Brinkhous, K. M. and Genton, E., et al. (Eds.): *Thrombosis*. Washington, D. C., National Academy of Sciences, 1969, pp. 339-344.

4. Knisely, M. H., Warner, L. and Harding, F.: Ante-mortem settling: microscopic observations and analyses of the settling of agglutinated blood-cell masses to the lower sides of vessels during life: A contribution to the biophysics of disease. *Angiology, 11*:535-588, 1960.
5. Zucker, S. and Mielke, C. H.: Classification of thrombocytosis based on platelet function tests: Correlation with hemorrhagic and thrombotic complications. *J Lab Clin Med, 80*:385-394, 1972.
6. Pechet, L. and Alexander, B.: Increased clotting factors in pregnancy. *N Engl J Med, 265*:1093-1097, 1961.
7. Todd, M. E., Thompson, J. H., Jr., Bowie, E. J. W., et al.: Changes in blood coagulation during pregnancy. *Mayo Clin Proc, 40*:370-383, 1965.
8. Owen, C. A., Jr., Thompson, J. H., Jr., Bowie, E. J. W., et al.: Coagulation studies during pregnancy and hormone treatment. In Astrup, T. and Wright, I. S. (Eds.): *Blood Coagulation, Thrombosis, and Female Hormones.* Washington, D. C., James F. Mitchell Foundation, 1968, pp. 24-26.
9. Spittell, J. A., Jr., Thompson, J. H., Jr. and Owen, C. A., Jr.: Mechanism and management of intravascular thrombosis. *Minn Med, 49*:331-334, 1966.
10. Egeberg, O.: Inherited antithrombin deficiency causing thrombophilia. *Thromb Diath Haemorrh, 13*:516-530, 1965.
11. Penick, G. D.: Blood states that predispose to thrombosis. In Sherry, S., Brinkhous, K. M., Genton, E., et al. (Eds.): *Thrombosis.* Washington, D. C., National Academy of Sciences, 1969, pp. 553-565.
12. Wessler, S., Yin, E. T.: Experimental hypercoagulable state induced by Factor X: Comparison of the nonactivated and activated forms. *J Lab Clin Med, 72*:256-260, 1968.
13. Deykin, D.: The clinical challenge of disseminated intravascular coagulation. *N Engl J Med, 283*:636-644, 1970.
14. Cooper, H. A., Bowie, E. J. W., Didisheim, P., et al.: Paradoxic changes in platelets and fibrinogen in chronically induced intravascular coagulation. *Mayo Clin Proc, 46*:521-523, 1971.

DISCUSSION

Question: What does the last letter in the ICF syndrome stand for?

Dr. Spittell: Intravascular coagulation fibrinolysis syndrome.

Question: Have you had any luck at predicting patients who are about to develop clinical clotting from laboratory tests?

Dr. Spittell: I have been reluctant to try to do that. I don't have that much confidence in our laboratory tests at this point. I think we need better tests than we now have before we can try to do that, and I still follow clinical criteria.

Question: Dr. Spittell, in the thirty-four-year-old patient with the ICF you initially treated him with heparin and EACA and then subsequently with heparin alone. When did you decide and why did you decide to use EACA as well as heparin?

Dr. Spittell: In the first instance, the man was on heparin in our usual clinical doses when he developed pulmonary embolism, so we went up in the dose of heparin and felt that this man was in such dire shape that we needed to add EACA to stop lytic mechanisms. We don't use EACA by itself and we only use it in situations where we don't feel that we are able to get on top of things with heparin alone. We didn't feel that we were in that man. Subsequently, we were in the situation where we recognized it early and felt that we would be able to handle it with heparin alone. We use EACA very infrequently.

Question: One syndrome associated with spontaneous thrombosis is polycythemia vera. I wonder if any of your studies show anything in this condition.

Dr. Spittell: Consistently we haven't been able to show acceleration of the clotting mechanism in these people, and I myself have wondered for a long time whether it isn't related to the platelets in polycythemia. I have no data on that. Once in a while, you will see people who have digital thrombosis and markedly elevated platelet levels, and I have never been able to do any more than associate the two.

Question: In the slide of familiar idiopathic thrombophlebitis, just how many of those offspring have varied?

Dr. Spittell: I think it is very important to rigidly define this group of people. If we don't, then we really lose our clinical model. If they do not have any cause for the thromboembolism I won't classify them as idiopathic until I have followed them through for at least three years. Whether this is really a syndrome or not, I don't know, but it is an interesting group of people and I think that when you see them and you inquire of family histories, you will be surprised how often you will encounter familiar occurrences.

Question: Dr. Spittell, have you done the blood viscosity studies on these patients?

Dr. Spittell: No, I haven't.

Question: What is the usual dose of heparin that you use in these patients in initiating therapy?

Dr. Spittell: We usually start with 5,000 units every four hours intravenously. I think when our platelet Factor IV studies get better, I will have a better method of identifying those patients who need more than 5,000 units every four hours. There is a problem in large practices in monitoring heparin therapy. We used the PTT like everyone else but we would like to try to identify the patient who at the very outset needs more than 5,000 units.

Question: Another syndrome that occasionally is associated with spontaneous thrombosis is the idiopathic thrombosis associated with malignancy. Do you have any insight on the cause of thrombosis in these folks?

Dr. Spittell: First of all, if you will pardon me, that's not idiopathic. There is a cause for that. I am going to hang tough on that because otherwise I lose the purity of the idiopathic group of people that interests me. In people with malignancy, one can frequently demonstrate accelerated thromboplastin generation and it is due to excessive levels of Factor VIII. Today we would feel that this may represent an overcompensation for occult intravascular thrombotic process. We would look at the diffuse intravascular thrombosis levels of the factors consumed may fall to zero. Some people may have a high fibrinogen because they are not only using it but their mechanism of production has responded and actually overshot and sometimes in diffuse intravascular coagulation we have observed elevated platelets, elevated fibrinogen, and elevated Factor VIII.

Question: Within the initial group of patients that you followed with idiopathic hypercoagulability or idiopathic recurrent thromboembolism, you said that one half of them had, on initial examination, hypercoagulability demonstrable by your laboratory examinations, then I understand that you followed the other thirteen that were normal to begin with and half of those again had acceleration.

Dr. Spittell: No, when we saw abnormal clotting in only half of the patients, we wondered what was wrong with our test; was it insensitive and we were only measuring the top of a disorder? We didn't know what the problem was, so it seems logical that what we should do, is to follow a group of these people and if indeed as we suspected, the clotting mechanism can change, that it is a dynamic thing, then it may be that over a period of time you can observe them at times when clotting is abnormal and at others normal. This we think is what has happened; that the clotting mechanism can change from time-to-time and that any given time these people may be relatively more prone to thrombose, given the right set of circumstances; i.e. that their clotting mechanism may be just right for thromboembolism to occur. The clotting change may be a permissive thing.

Question: Did you pick up any additional acceleration in the group that was previously normal?

Dr. Spittell: Yes. We observed normal to go accelerated and accelerated to go normal and we have seen this many many times.

Question: I know that your group of ulcerative colitis patients are not idiopathic but, I know that you have published on that group particularly. Do they have a longitudinal continuing hypercoagulability?

Dr. Spittell: In that little red slide box there are four slides.

Question: Could you answer another question while you are waiting on that? Do you have comments on the role of platelet inhibitors in the management of idiopathic hypercoagulability?

Dr. Spittell: No. We haven't tried that yet. We are still using oral anticoagulant therapy which works in our hands in the idiopathic group, if they are truly idiopathic. Are the slides ready?

Dr. Spittell: Chronic ulcerative colitis is an intriguing disease. There are some that say that one shouldn't give anticoagulants to these people. I don't happen to agree to that. This is an interesting case and one that got me interested in this disorder. This is a man thirty-four, who had chronic ulcerative colitis develop in 1953 and with almost each of his flares he had thrombophlebitis and during the course of these many episodes, he had two pulmonary emboli. In 1960, we did a retarded TGT on him. We noted that he was moderately accelerated about two times to three times, and because of his severe disease on gastrointestinal indications, a total colectomy was performed. The next slide happens to be his colon which shows diffuse involvement with multiple areas of neoplastic development. The next slide shows where he was moderately accelerated preoperatively. His acceleration remained postoperatively, and by the time that he was dismissed, it was still present. Nine months later he had only a questionable acceleration and he was asymptomatic, having gained twenty-five to thirty pounds and looked like a picture of health. I haven't heard from this man since, and I specifically requested that both the patient and his wife contact me if he had any more thrombophlebitis or any more pulmonary embolism. After this intriguing patient, we went on to study other series of patients. The next slide is on ulcerative colitis both with and without thromboembolism. Here is a group of people, the first man, of course, was the patient you have seen in detail, five more patients with thrombosis, one lady, patient number six, with brachial artery thrombosis who lost her arm. If you practice cardiovascular disease and see many people lose an upper extremity from thrombosis, it's unusual. In CUC when thrombosis occurs, it is severe, and she is just an illustration of it. It is interesting to us that the acceleration was present whether or not these patients had clinical evidence of thrombosis and that it could vary in degrees. Of course, patient number 2 being followed serially showed you that with recrudesence of the disease the coagulation abnormality that we were able to demonstrate can change also.

Question: Dr. Spittell, could I ask you just one comment? Knowing how difficult the TGT test is and most people do not have the expertise of the Mayo Clinic at their hand, is there some other laboratory tests that may be a little more simpler to do, that we could, kind of out in the field that would give us a handle on this disease?

Dr. Spittell: A well done plasma recalcification time or PTT may, but you will have a great deal more overlap and it is more difficult to demonstrate the abnormality. I don't think that the retarded TGT or modified TGT is necessarily the answer to thromboembolism. We've used it and continued to use it, because it gives us an opportunity to identify people whom we want to follow and study further. I really think that we are looking at what may be a manifestation of some other abnormality in the clotting mechanism, but it's a good handle on the disease and we haven't found a better test in our hands, difficult though it is.

Question: Dr. Spittell, have you noticed in your experience among very young women, a genetic group that is fair skinned, either blonde or red head with rhumatoid like complaints and chronic recurrent phlebitis?

Dr. Spittell: Yes, and they usually have lupus and a circulating anticoagulant.

Chapter 9

CLINICOMORPHOLOGIC CONSIDERATIONS
OF PULMONARY THROMBOEMBOLISM*

Joseph C. Parker, Jr.

THROMBOSIS occurs when there is a decrease in blood flow, damaged vessel walls and altered blood clotting mechanism. Since these abnormalities may be difficult to appreciate clinically, many thrombi are recognized only at autopsy. With extensive necropsy dissections of the venous system in the legs,[1] thromboses were found in eighty-one of 125 autopsies on patients without pulmonary embolism (65%). Venous thrombi were found most frequently in the calf veins, next in the thigh or pelvic veins and less frequently in the popliteal veins. Prolonged bed rest was associated with increased thigh thrombi. In ninety-three unselected autopsies, Beckering and Titus[2] found thigh vein thrombi in 26.9 percent which included thrombi within the femoral-popliteal venous sinuses in almost half these cases. Forty percent of these leg thrombi were bilateral, and inflammation was infrequent. Their patients with femoral-popliteal venous thrombi often had long confinements in bed and were usually women. Although pulmonary embolism was present in 22.6 percent of this total series, it was fatal in only 3.2 percent. In their patients with thigh vein thrombi, 60 percent had pulmonary emboli, but in individuals without these thrombi, pulmonary emboli were found in 9 percent.

THE PROBLEM

Pulmonary thromboembolism has been observed in 3 percent of autopsied patients and over 60 percent in a more detailed necropsy series.[4] Its frequency at autopsy depends obviously on the thoroughness of the prosecutor, but seems to have remained around 10 percent over the past forty years (Table 9-I). Emboli to the lung account for about 47,000 deaths a year in the United States.[9] Even though patients with pulmonary emboli may be totally asymptomatic or die suddenly, characteristically

*Technical assistance of N. F. Gerard, R. F. Heineman, and T. Watts is greatly appreciated.

they develop varying degrees of dyspnea and tachypnea. The condition has been associated with childbirth, obesity, severe trauma and thrombophlebitis, including continuous intravenous therapy.[10] Smith and colleagues[11] in 1965 found pulmonary embolism to be the single most common cause of death in 370 autopsies. Sevitt[12] found that thromboemboli in the lungs were frequent after injury in patients over forty years of age who were confined to bed for more than a few days. In his experience pulmonary embolism was the most common single cause of death in elderly injured subjects and tended to occur in patients over fifty years of age who usually had experienced prolonged bed rest and injury.

TABLE 9-I

AUTOPSY FREQUENCY OF PULMONARY THROMBOEMBOLISM

Year reported	Total autopsies	Pulmonary emboli
1934 (Belt[5])	567	10%
1940 (Hampton & Castleman[6])	3,500	9%
1951 (Raeburn[7])	130	15%
1964 (Smith et al.[8])	225	15%
1973 (Parker)	472	12%

The postmortem frequency of pulmonary thromboembolism.

Thromboembolism in the lung is not synonymous with pulmonary infarction,[13] which may be seen in only half the cases. The source for these blood clots are usually the deep veins of the lower extremities and pelvic veins. Less common sources include the right heart, inferior vena cava and veins of the neck and upper extremities.[10] Frequently, at postmortem examination the embolus represents the entire thrombus, and there is no apparent source for it. Although the vast majority of blood clots in the lung are metastatic from other sites, primary pulmonary thrombosis has been described rarely in patients with pulmonary tuberculosis, emphysema, pneumoconioses, and severe cardiac failure.[3] Primary thrombosis in smaller pulmonary muscular arteries and veins is usually associated with decreased blood flow.[3] In fifty-four autopsied patients with pulmonary emboli, eleven multiple blood clots were found in every instance and usually within muscular pulmonary arteries. Variable aged emboli in the lung were common, and less than 10 percent were associated with infarcts.

PATHOLOGIC FEATURES

Pulmonary thromboembolism is an impaction of a thrombus formed within the vascular system and transported by the systemic veins to the pulmonary artery. Emboli also include a multiple of other intrinsic and extrinsic substances capable of being transported to pulmonary vessels, such as fat, air, bone marrow, liver, fatty tissue, amniotic fluid trophoblastic tissue, brain, cotton fibers, parasites, vegetables, and other foreign particles.

Most patients with pulmonary thrombolism have multiple thrombi which tend to lodge in their lower lobes, apparently due to the character of blood flow.[3] They appear more common on the right than the left side and usually are small thrombi in the peripheral lung near the pleura. Larger thromboemboli are often coiled clots wedged in one or both main pulmonary arteries (Fig. 9-1), and when blood flow decreases suddenly over 60 percent, they tend to produce death.[3] With postmortem removal of the thrombus, casts of the parent vein with venous valve impressions may be discerned. Smaller emboli usually produce no symptoms and can be found protruding above the cut lung parenchyma. When recurrent, these thromboemboli may lead to pulmonary hypertension and often precede a fatal larger embolus.

Grossly, antemortem blood clots may be confused with postmortem blood clots, but possess certain distinguishing features including a coiled

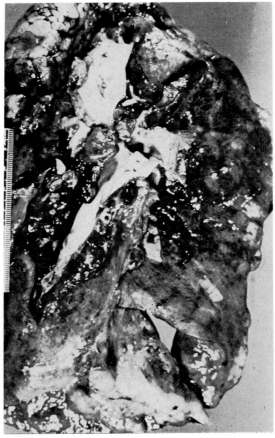

Figure 9-1. A large thrombus originating in the leg almost totally occludes a major pulmonary artery in the left lung.

friable firm dry laminated appearance. Thromboemboli may distend the involved vessel. More recent antemortem clots have gross characteristics similar to some postmortem blood clots; however, older organized thrombi are firmly adherent to the vessel wall. Inadequate sampling of a blood clot at autopsy may lead to confusion since an antemortem thrombus may be associated with adjacent postmortem clots. Microscopic evidence of early degeneration and/or organization within the blood clot may be the only convincing feature for an antemortem origin. A recent antemortem thrombus has a laminated pattern with degenerated polymorphonuclear neutrophils (Fig. 9-2). Later, spindle-shaped mononuclear cells appear within the clot, and epithelioid cells grow over the surface of the blood clot and into spaces formed by retraction of the fibrin. Eventually, new thin-walled sinusoidal channels completely recanalize the thrombus (Fig. 9-3).

In view of both pulmonary and bronchial blood supply with variable perfusion to the lung, an infarct is often not found with a thromboembolus.[3, 10] When passive congestion of the lung compromises blood flow, the patient develops an infarct with his embolus. The pulmonary infarct is typically sterile and varies in size and configuration depending upon the occluded vessel.[13] Some infarcts are irregular or quadrilateral. Their base often rests upon the pleural surface, and the occluded vessel may be found

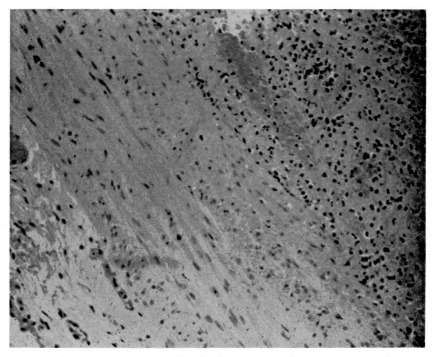

Figure 9-2. Recent antemortem blood clot in a pulmonary artery demonstrates scattered degenerated leucocytes and erythrocytes with focal spindle-shaped mononuclear cells (right upper area). H&E X 250.

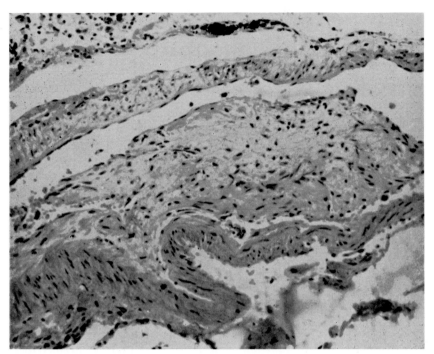

Figure 9-3.   Later, the pulmonary thromboembolus becomes recanalized and fibrotic. H&E X 125.

in the lung proximal to the infarct. When a pulmonary infarct occurs, there is initially an acute fibrinous pleuritis overlying the lesion, and the infarcted lung parenchyma swells. Within the first few days, induration and hemorrhage are evident in the lesion which possesses a somewhat ill-defined, moist, dark purple cut surface. Several days later, the adjacent pleura becomes depressed, and the pulmonary infarct appears drier, granular, and pale red. Eventually, the necrotic tissue becomes brown due to accumulated hemosiderin and its margins become more distinct. Organization and retraction of the involved lung parenchyma leave a well-concealed thin scar at right angles to the pleural surface which also undergoes focal thickening. The thrombus during this period of organization is transformed into a recanalized fibrous mass (Fig. 9-3). Within the first two days a pulmonary infarct possesses intense alveolar capillary congestion and hemorrhage (Fig. 9-4A). After this period, the intraalveolar septa develop coagulative necrotic changes with loss of nuclear detail (Fig. 9-4B). Erythrocytes degenerate, and hemoglobin is converted into hemosiderin and deposited within phagocytes. During the second week the pulmonary infarct develops ingrowths of fibroblasts from its periphery, and organization progresses over a period of weeks to months varying with the size of the lesion. Septic thromboemboli produce infarcts with focal abscesses.

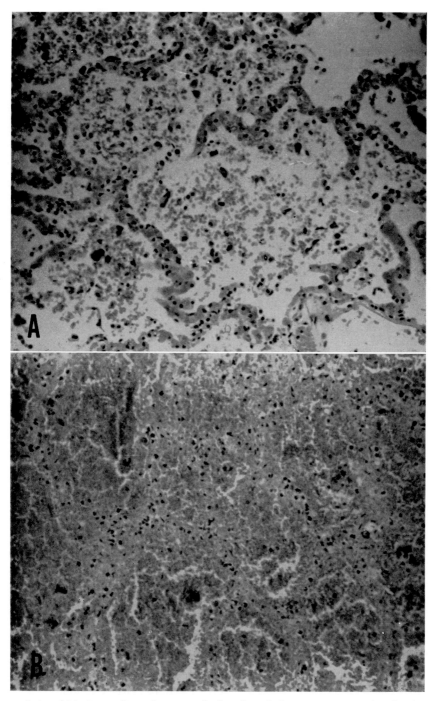

Figure 9-4. (A) An early pulmonary "infarct" includes severe intraalveolar hemorrhage and congestion. H&E X 125 (B) Coagulative necrosis with indistinct alveolar septa and prominent hemorrhage is consistent with an early hemorrhagic infarct. H&E X 125.

POSTMORTEM STUDY

TABLE 9-II

POSTMORTEM PULMONARY THROMBOEMBOLI

(472 autopsies)

Abnormality	Study group (56)	Control group (416)
Heart disease	41 (73%)	132 (32%)
Malignancy	21 (38%)	71 (17%)
Tissue damage	56 (100%)	259 (62%)
Two or more abnormalities	56 (100%)	46 (11%)

Autopsy study of pulmonary thromboemboli at the University of Kentucky Medical Center (1970-1971).

At the University of Kentucky Medical Center, 472 consecutive autopsies were done during 1970 and 1971 and revealed fifty-six patients (12%) with significant pulmonary thromboemboli (Table 9-II) that contributed to the patient's demise. This series included eighteen females and thirty-eight males varying from six months to eighty years with an average age of fifty-two years. Five of the fifty-six patients (9%) were considered to be obese. Thirty-one (55%) were admitted to a medical service, and the remaining twenty-five patients (45%) were on a surgical service. Hospitalization for this population varied from less than one day to over 180 days with an average confinement of seventeen days. Pulmonary infarcts were associated with thromboembolism in twenty-eight of the fifty-six cases (50%). Prominent associated disorders in this study group (Table 9-II) included heart disease in forty-one (73%) and malignant lesions in twenty-one (38%). In all autopsied patients with significant pulmonary thromboembolism, focally prominent tissue damage tended to involve the liver and brain primarily. In patients with any significant cardiac disease, focal necrosis in the liver was associated with acute and chronic passive congestion and fatty change. Brain damage manifested by recent hemorrhagic infarcts, brain injury, abscesses and metastatic carcinoma was found in twenty-five out of forty-nine autopsies with central nervous system examinations (55%). In patients with pulmonary thromboemboli who failed to demonstrate recent liver or brain damage, other significant tissue damage included metastatic necrotic neoplasm (25%), infections (20%), and trauma related to recent surgery (43%). Malignant lesions were found primarily in the lung (7) and gastrointestinal tract (6) including the pancreas (2), stomach (1), esophagus (1), duodenum (1) and liver (1). Other locations included the breast (2), ovary (2), blood (2), bladder (1), prostate (1), and skin (1). In the remaining

416 autopsies without recognizable pulmonary thromboemboli, heart disease was found in only 32 percent, malignancy in 17 percent, and significant tissue damage in 62 percent (Table 9-II). Unlike the study group in which the combination of tissue damage with heart disease and/or malignancy was observed consistently, the control patients demonstrated this association in only 11 percent. In the present retrospective autopsy study no other abnormalities were apparent.

Comment

Thrombosis of peripheral veins and pulmonary thromboembolism are more common than clinically appreciated. The 12 percent postmortem incidence of significant pulmonary thromboembolism at the University of Kentucky Medical Center is consistent with previous studies (Table 9-I). Significant tissue damage when associated with heart disease and/or malignancy seem to predispose patients in this series to the development of peripheral venous thrombi and subsequent pulmonary embolism. In order to create venous thrombi, alterations of Virchow's triad (blood flow, vessel wall integrity and clotting mechanisms) are required and can be precipitated apparently by many different conditions. In the current postmortem study, heart disease was a major factor that appeared to produce congestion (blood stasis) with intimal hypoxia. When blood clotting was altered possibly by the addition of thromboplastin from necrotic tissue, this catalyst seemed to create thrombi in dependent veins with the subsequent risk of pulmonary thromboembolism. The phenotype for a patient with potential pulmonary thromboembolism as revealed by this study included a middle-aged man with some cardiovascular disease, moderate inactivity (prolonged hospitalization), a likely malignant lesion, and a possible source for thromboplastin as manifested by tissue damage especially in the liver and central nervous system.

Even though the morphologic features of pulmonary thromboembolism with or without pulmonary infarction are well defined; postmortem examinations have demonstrated a broad kaleidoscopic somewhat confusing spectrum of patients and disorders that are associated with pulmonary embolism. Possible sources for thromboplastin from tissue damage in almost any site, especially the liver and brain, and from almost any cause, particularly malignancy, seem to be major considerations in precipitating thrombi in patients already compromised by cardiovascular disease, obesity and/or prolonged bed rest. Hopefully, postmortem characterization of patients with significant pulmonary thromboemboli will enable clinicians to maintain a high index of suspicion for this potentially lethal disorder in any patient with possible tissue damage from any cause.

REFERENCES

1. Sevitt, S. and Gallagher, N. G.: Venous thrombosis and pulmonary embolism. A clinico-pathological study in injured and burned patients. *Br J Surg, 48*:475-489, 1961.
2. Beckering, R. E., Jr. and Titus, J. L.: Femoral-popliteal venous thrombosis and pulmonary embolism. *Am J Clin Pathol, 52*:530-537, 1969.
3. Spencer, H.: *Pathology of the Lung.* New York, MacMillan Co., 1962, pp. 435-464.
4. Freiman, D. G.: Pathologic observations on experimental and human thromboembolism. In Sasahara, A. A. and Stein, M. (Eds.): *Pulmonary Embolic Disease.* New York, Greene and Stratton, 1965, pp. 81-85.
5. Belt, T. H.: Thrombosis and pulmonary embolism. *Am J Pathol, 10*:129-144, 1934.
6. Hampton, A. O. and Castleman, B.: Correlation of postmortem teleroentgenograms with autopsy findings, with special reference to pulmonary embolism and infarction. *Am J Roentgenol Radiation Ther, 43*:305-326, 1940.
7. Raeburn, C.: The natural history of venous thrombosis. *Br Med J, 2*:517-520, 1951.
8. Smith, G. T., Dammin, G. J. and Dexter, L.: Postmortem arteriographic studies on the human lung in pulmonary embolization. *JAMA, 188*:143-151, 1964.
9. Hodgson, C. H. and Good, C. A.: Pulmonary embolism and infarction. *Med Clin North Am, 48*:977-992, 1964.
10. Millard, M.: Lung, pleura and mediastinum. In Anderson, W. A. D. (Eds.): *Pathology,* 6th ed. St. Louis, C. V. Mosby Co., 1971, pp. 888-892.
11. Smith, G. T., Dexter, L. and Dammin, G. J.: Postmortem quantitative studies in pulmonary embolism. In Sasahara, A. A. and Stein, M. (Eds.): *Pulmonary Embolic Disease.* New York, Greene and Stratton, 1965, pp. 120-130.
12. Sevitt, S.: Anticoagulant prophylaxis against venous thrombosis and pulmonary embolism. In Sasahara, A. A. and Stein, M. (Eds.): *Pulmonary Embolic Disease.* New York, Greene and Stratton, 1965, pp. 265-276.
13. Heitzman, E. R., Markarian, B. and Dailey, E. T.: Pulmonary thromboemboli disease—a lobular concept. *Radiology, 103*:529-537, 1972.

DISCUSSION

Question: I'd like to ask two questions raised by some of the earlier pathology literature. Dr. Belt from Toronto, whose paper you listed in 1934, had two conclusions, and I wonder if they are true today? (1) He believed that *in situ* thrombosis occurred in the pulmonary artery system and that all thrombi at autopsy were not emboli. (2) He said that at autopsy the antemortem thrombus is not always easy to distinguish from the postmortem thrombus and that even in experienced hands, this was a commonly overlooked diagnosis. Will you comment on these two statements?

Dr. Parker: I will comment on the last statement first. Dr. Belt's experience is identical to mine. It is at times difficult to recognize a fresh recent thromboembolus in any artery. In surgical specimens, fresh unorganized blood clots are seen commonly in patients with clinically significant occlusive clots. Histologically, these fresh antemortem clots lack features we use to recognize organized antemortem thrombi, possibly due to the freshness of the clot as well as inadequate sampling. Recently propagated clot often occurs both proximal and distal to the original embolus, making sampling important in accurately evaluating the material. The clinical information is most helpful in interpreting these specimens. To answer the second question, I think most people consider that primary pulmonary thrombosis is an exceedingly uncommon condition which is almost impossible to prove. I would be happy to hear experiences from the audience about documented cases of primary pulmonary thrombosis. I have never seen a well-documented case.

Question: Are your patients embalmed before you autopsy them?

Dr. Parker: Our patients are not embalmed before autopsy.

Question: Have you isolated to your satisfaction the factors that lead to pulmonary infarction in the event of embolization?

Dr. Parker: Some compromise to the pulmonary blood flow appears significant in patients at autopsy with pulmonary infarcts. This is usually manifested by severe pulmonary congestion. I have not seen an otherwise healthy person with a pulmonary embolus develop a pulmonary infarct that was documented at autopsy. Characteristically, the postmortem pulmonary infarct is associated with some element of heart failure.

Question: (1) Why doesn't bone trauma play a more important part in your list? It was not mentioned. (2) Can you tell us about the features of a clot undergoing lysis? If it takes seven to ten days for fibrovascular formation to occur, what does the clot look like before and during that time if thrombolytic agents are used?

Dr. Parker: In answer to the first question, the absence of trauma in this autopsy series is due to the nature of our postmortem material. A great deal of trauma occurs in young otherwise healthy people, who often survive. In older patients with trauma, pulmonary thromboemboli are common, but unlike young healthy individuals with extensive trauma, the elderly are compromised often by heart failure, malignancy, or both and frequently die. These latter factors which stood out in our postmortem study at the University of Kentucky Medical Center appeared to be major compromising factors. In other words, if someone with trauma has other superimposed compromising factors such as heart disease or malignancy, there is an increased likelihood that this patient will develop spontaneous thromboses with a subsequent pulmonary thromboembolus. The second question about the lysis of a clot is difficult to answer in view of generally inadequate data. If the clot breaks up, it should occur early during the first few days of its formation. The early organized clot with fibroblasts and a few delicate capillaries may be lysed, but once the thrombus develops dense fibrosis, it cannot be lysed effectively. There are no morphologic characteristics of a resolving lysed clot of which I am aware.

Question: Dr. Parker, I appreciated your comments about organ damage, but I wasn't sure whether you were referring to this as a cause, effect or neither in relation to pulmonary embolism.

Dr. Parker: I wish I could be specific about this, but unfortunately I cannot. The association of heart disease, malignancy and tissue damage appear more frequent in the postmortem population with pulmonary thromboemboli than in the postmortem population without them. There are obviously gradations here, and I think Dr. Spittell implied this. Not everyone who is hypercoagulable develops spontaneous venous thrombosis. In some people, without recognizable hypercoagulability, pulmonary emboli occur. Exacerbations and remissions of this hypercoagulable state may be important. The same phenomena exist in my retrospective study, for not everyone with tissue damage has thromboemboli at autopsy.

Question: Dr. Parker, would you comment about the stage in the formation of pulmonary infarction which would be visible on X-ray?

Dr. Parker: The pulmonary infarct should be visible within twenty-four hours if it is large enough. What you see is consolidation manifested by tremendous extravasation of blood. The earliest stage of a pulmonary infarct before coagulation necrosis is similar to congested lung. After a few hours, coagulation necrosis is evident and more extravasated blood is seen. At this time you should be able to recognize the infarct on a chest X-ray if it is large enough. In patients who have a massive pulmonary embolus, with careful postmortem studies we can demonstrate commonly many small multiple pulmonary emboli that are usually not associated with any infarcted tissue and are not suspected clinically.

Question: In view of the ability of the lung to lyse clots, do you have any ideas about why some cases will go on to cor pulmonale with multiple emboli? What are the limiting factors for recovery or progressive disease?

Dr. Parker: I really don't have any good answers. Some of the small pulmonary thromboemboli tend to resolve into the involved vessel wall. This can create increased arterial resistance and subsequent pulmonary hypertension. The problem histologically is trying to separate a vessel with a thickened wall due to idiopathic or primary pulmonary hypertension, whatever that entity means, from multiple small pulmonary thromboemboli organizing into the vessel wall. Damage to the vessel wall is a helpful finding. If the vessel wall appears damaged and possesses medial fibrosis and hemosiderin deposits as illustrated in a venous thrombus on an earlier slide, this supports an organized area of an ancient thrombus. On the other hand, if the media is diffusely hyperplastic, as illustrated again on a previous slide, medial hypertrophy due to pulmonary hypertension from almost any cause including multiple pulmonary thromboemboli may be involved. I have difficulty morphologically distinguishing primary from secondary pulmonary hypertension. All available clinical and morphological data are required for accurate titration and even then there are some unresolved cases.

Chapter 10

PHYSIOLOGY OF ACUTE PULMONARY EMBOLISM

Donald Silver

Pulmonary embolism remains a significant contributor to most morbidity and mortality statistics. The ubiquitousness and the potential seriousness of pulmonary embolism indicate the need for symposia, such as this one, to evaluate new concepts of underlying mechanisms, new methods for recognition, and new modes of therapy.

My colleagues and I have attempted to gain additional information about the mechanisms responsible for the cardiopulmonary changes that occur during acute pulmonary embolism in order to treat the disorder more effectively. This report will review some of our studies of these mechanisms.

Historical

Although Laennec clearly described the findings of pulmonary embolism ("pulmonary apoplexy") in 1819,[1] and Rudolph Virchow established the principles of pulmonary thromboembolism in 1846,[2] meaningful studies of the mechanisms that alter the cardiopulmonary physiology during pulmonary embolism have been accomplished primarily in the past three to four decades. There have been numerous studies of the cardiopulmonary responses to foreign body emboli (e.g., barium sulfate, starch granules, fungus spores, etc.), to balloon occlusion of one or more pulmonary arteries, and to fresh and aged autologous and homologous thromboemboli produced *in vivo* and *in vitro*. In recent years emphasis has been placed upon utilizing thromboemboli that more closely correspond to those which occur clinically.[3]

In general, previous investigators have demonstrated that the cardiovascular changes (i.e., increase in pulmonary artery pressure, right ventricular dilatation, decreased cardiac output, and decreased blood pressure) and the pulmonary changes (i.e., decrease of lung compliance and increase of

Supported by U.S.P.H.S. Grant HL-08929.

airway resistance) could be caused by neural reflexes,[4-5] by the release of humoral substances from/by the thromboembolus,[6-9] or by mechanical blockade of the pulmonary circulation by the thromboembolus.[10-13] Most investigators seem to agree that reflex changes are secondary and of minor importance. The relative importance of the humoral and mechanical factors remains controversial.

Many recent studies have added strong support for a humoral etiology of the acute cardiopulmonary changes associated with pulmonary embolism and have indicated that serotonin and possibly other bioactive amines released from the platelets within or adherent to the thromboembolus are the humoral agents responsible.[14-19] It has also been suggested that serotonin antagonists will alleviate some of the acute changes that occur during pulmonary embolism.[8, 9, 15] If serotonin or other humoral agents are primarily responsible for the acute cardiopulmonary changes that occur with pulmonary embolism, then clinical trials of specific antagonists are indicated.

If the cardiopulmonary changes are secondary to the mechanical blockage which occurs with acute pulmonary embolism, then major efforts should be directed to the development of effective, safe thrombolytic agents and, as will be discussed in this symposium, to ways for detecting and treating venous thrombosis before pulmonary embolism occurs.

Experiences obtained while treating patients with pulmonary embolism, in which clinical improvement, reductions of right heart pressures and increased pulmonary artery flow paralleled dissolution of the emboli,[20] suggested that mechanical blockage of the pulmonary circulation by the thromboembolus could be primarily responsible for initiating the cardiopulmonary changes which occur. These observations have prompted my colleagues and me to perform several experimental studies that were designed to determine the relative contributions of the mechanical or humoral factors to the cardiopulmonary pathophysiology which occurs in acute pulmonary embolism.

EXPERIMENTAL STUDIES

The first study was designed to evaluate the effect of a variety of volume standardized emboli upon the cardiopulmonary parameters. It was elected to use large rather than small or miliary emboli because significant clinical changes usually occur only after embolization with large emboli and because miliary embolization is not often recognized in the clinical situation. Furthermore, the possible vasomotor reflexes thought to be associated with miliary embolism[21] could be avoided.

Adult mongrel dogs, 15 to 22 kg in weight and free of Dirofilaria immitus, were utilized in all of the studies.[22] The animals were anesthetized with pentothal and respirated at sixteen cycles per minute. Tidal volumes were selected by using a tidal volume which fell on the linear portion of the pulmonary pressure-volume curve for each dog. Endotracheal air flow and pressures, and pulmonary artery and left atrial pressures were monitored for an hour. Pulmonary blood flow was measured by placing an electromagnetic flow probe around the main pulmonary artery. Compliance and total lung resistance were calculated by a modification of the method of Mead and Whittenberger.[23] All emboli were 0.75 ml/kg and were volumetrically standardized by correcting for the hematocrit.

The emboli were prepared *in vitro* and injected as a single bolus into the right jugular vein. The four types of emboli included: (1) Fresh emboli. The calculated amount of blood was clotted with one ml autologous serum and incubated for ten minutes at 37°C. (2) Aged emboli. These emboli were prepared in a similar manner but were incubated for ninety minutes. (3) Serum 0.75 ml of serum/kg were obtained from ninety-minute-old clot and were injected into the pulmonary artery through the catheter used for measuring pulmonary artery pressures. (4) Agarose emboli. 0.5 percent agarose gels (0.75 ml/kg) form "clots" of similar density and consistency as whole blood clots. The agarose "jelled" in polyethylene tubes and was embolized in a manner similar to that used for the whole blood clot.

There was no mortality in the serum or fresh clot emboli groups. The agarose emboli group experienced a 40 percent mortality and the aged clot group a 65 percent mortality. The difference in mortality between the dogs embolized with fresh clot emboli and dogs receiving older emboli may have been related to the relative friability of the fresh clot and the susceptibility of the fresh clot to compression and rapid lysis. Some of the fresh clot emboli demonstrated up to 50 percent reductions in volume when studied at autopsy at the end of the experiments. The smaller increase in pulmonary artery pressure by the fresh clot (Table 10-I) may also be explained by this mechanism.

Serum produced minimal, probably physiologically insignificant, changes in pulmonary artery pressure, compliance and total lung resistance (Table 10-I). The fresh clot emboli produced the greatest changes in compliance and total lung resistance. The changes that occurred after agarose emboli-

TABLE 10-I

AVERAGE MAXIMUM CHANGES AFTER EMBOLIZATION

	Pul. Artery Pressure *mm Hg*	*Compliance* *ml/cm H2O*	*Total Lung Resistance* *cm H2O/L/sec.*
Serum	+ 1.4	− 0.7	+0.3
"Fresh" Clot	+18.2	−11.6	+2.4
"Aged" Clot	+20.2	− 5.2	+1.0
Agarose	+24.5	− 4.1	+1.75

zation were slightly more pronounced than those produced by the aged clot.

The minimal changes that followed the serum infusion indicate that "stable" humoral substances which are exuded from a thrombus are not responsible for the cardiopulmonary changes observed in acute pulmonary embolism. However, the maximum changes in compliance and total lung resistance which were noted after embolization with fresh clot suggest that humoral substances released from/by fresh clot may augment the changes produced by mechanical obstruction of the pulmonary circulation. These observations of the effect of fresh clot upon the cardiopulmonary changes of acute pulmonary embolism are supported by the work of Marshall and associates,[24] who did not note significant changes in airway resistance or compliance in dogs embolized with six- to fourteen-day-old autologous emboli, and by Thomas and associates,[7] who noted striking changes in resistance and lung compliance when animals received fresh clot emboli. Furthermore, significant support for the humoral contributions to the cardiopulmonary changes of acute pulmonary embolism have come from the notable reports of Thomas and Gurewich and their associates.[7, 16, 17, 19, 25, 26] These reports have emphasized the role of humoral agents, especially serotonin and other bioactive amines transported by platelets, in initiating the cardiopulmonary changes which occur during acute pulmonary embolism. However, the similar alterations in pulmonary arterial flow and pressure and in airway resistance and lung compliance produced by aged clot and agarose emboli, which contain lesser amounts of the humoral agents, suggest that mechanical obstruction is probably the major factor in initiating the cardiopulmonary changes.

Although platelet accretions were not found to be adherent to the aged or agarose clot emboli, the possible contributions of serotonin or other bioactive amines transported by platelets to the acute changes could not be eliminated. Consequently, another study was done in which platelets and serotonin were varied in dogs undergoing embolization.[27]

Adult mongrel dogs free of heart worms were also used in this study. The preparation was the same as that used in the earlier experiments and similar parameters were monitored. The dogs were divided into six groups. All dogs received a 0.75 ml/kg embolus which was volumetrically standardized by correcting for the hematocrit. The first group received an aged embolus which had been incubated for ninety minutes at 37°C. Group 2 was similar to the first but received 400 u/kg of aqueous heparin immediately prior to embolization. Group 3 received 0.05 mgm/kg of reserpine per day for three days before embolization with an aged clot. Blood serotonin levels were immeasurable at the time of embolization. Platelets were removed from the Group 4 dogs by a blood cell separator (Celltrifuge®). The average platelet count at the time of embolization with an agarose clot (0.75 ml/kg of a

0.5 percent agarose gel) was 8,000 ml³. Group 5 dogs received a fresh clot embolus. The serotonin content in the fresh clot was two to three times that found in the aged clots. Group 6 dogs also received fresh clot emboli but, like the Group 3 dogs, had received reserpine for three to five days before embolization and had immeasurable levels of blood serotonin at the time of embolization.

Tracheal air flow, left atrial pressure, and the electrocardiogram did not change significantly during the experiments. Increases of pulmonary artery pressures and decreases of pulmonary artery flow, increased resistance to air flow and decreases of compliance occurred after embolization in all animals. The changes are summarized in Table 10-II. The fresh clot emboli again produced a smaller increase in pulmonary artery pressure, a greater increase in lung resistance (except Group 3), and a larger decrease in compliance than did the other types of emboli. Pretreatment with heparin reduced the magnitude of all the changes.

TABLE 10-II

MAXIMAL CHANGES AFTER EMBOLIZATION IN SECOND GROUP OF DOGS

Type Embolus	Tracheal Pressure % Increase	Lung Resistance Increase cm H2O/L/sec.	Compliance % Decrease	PA Pressure % Increase
Aged Clot (AC)	40.02	2.17	26.3	238.74
Heparin—AC	15.06	1.90	13.75	219.64
Reserpine—AC	31.08	3.59	24.00	109.89
Platelet depletion—Agarose	27.01	2.49	21.60	138.46
Fresh Clot (FC)	38.57	3.22	27.19	95.74
Reserpine—FC	41.95	3.14	23.14	146.66

The effect of serotonin depletion prior to embolization was assayed in dogs embolized with aged and fresh autologous clot. Except for the notable increase in lung resistance, pretreatment with reserpine seemed to protect the animals from the effects of an aged clot, i.e., lesser changes in tracheal pressure, compliance and pulmonary artery pressure. On the contrary, pretreatment with reserpine did not offer the fresh clot emboli group any significant protection, as demonstrated by the increase in tracheal pressure, fall in compliance, and increased pulmonary artery pressure. If serotonin were responsible for the acute changes in pulmonary embolism, one would expect a greater effect of reserpine in the fresh clot group than in the aged clot group.

The platelet depleted dogs were embolized with agarose in an attempt to limit the incorporation of any bioactive amines into the embolus. The cardiopulmonary changes in these platelet depleted dogs were similar in time course and only slightly less in magnitude than those seen in the other groups of dogs. The response of the platelet depleted agarose embolized dogs to embolization offers strong evidence that mechanical obstruction is the primary initiator of the cardiopulmonary changes that occur after pulmonary embolization.

Statistical comparisons (paired Student t-test) revealed that the heparin protected dogs (Group 2) were the only ones that were significantly different from the others in their cardiopulmonary responses to pulmonary embolism. All of the changes occurred very quickly, were maximal in thirty to 120 seconds, and usually resolved within fifteen to sixty minutes.

The similarity of responses in all groups, despite the absence of any measurable blood serotonin in two groups and the embolization of a bland protein clot in a third group of platelet depleted dogs, suggests that the cardiopulmonary changes which occur during acute pulmonary embolism are not dependent upon the presence of serotonin or other platelet transported bioactive amines as has been suggested by others.[15, 18, 28] Our data clearly are in conflict with the observations of Stein and Thomas that airway constriction after pulmonary embolism does not occur unless at least 50,000 platelets per ml^3 are present.[29] The differences in cardiopulmonary effects between fresh and aged clot are minor and probably relate to the differences of consistency and tensile strength of the emboli.

The beneficial effects of pretreatment with heparin were significant. Additional studies are needed to better define the mechanism of action of heparin. Heparin may be beneficial by reducing the propagation of the embolus after it lodges in the pulmonary artery, or may augment thrombolysis.[30]

The data from these studies add additional support to the theory that mechanical blockage is primarily responsible for the changes which occur during pulmonary embolism. The changes may be augmented by humoral substances released from (by) the embolus.

We have initiated an additional series of experiments to evaluate the effects of humoral agents on lung compliance, air flow resistance, and on bronchoconstriction. These studies are designed to compare the effects of infusions of physiological and pharmacological amounts of serotonin on these parameters. Although the studies are incomplete, they do indicate that the responses to the infusion of serotonin into the right ventricle are dose dependent. In this study, mongrel dogs are initially infused with concentrations of serotonin that approach that found in a 0.75 ml/kg fresh clot embolus. At appropriate intervals, after baseline conditions are obtained, the concentration of serotonin is doubled, and later doubled again. A final infusion of serotonin is given which approximates the total amount of circulating serotonin for the animal being studied. Tracheal air flow and pressure are monitored and compliance and lung resistance are calculated.

Bronchoconstriction is monitored by performing tantalum bronchograms and using videotape cinemicroradiography.

In the four dogs studied thus far, there were no changes in compliance, lung resistance or bronchial diameters when serotonin concentrations equal to that found in a 0.75 blood/kg body weight fresh clot embolus were infused. When the amount of serotonin infused was doubled the parameters remained unchanged and continued unchanged when four times the amount of serotonin in a standard fresh clot embolus was infused. Only when the massive amounts of serotonin were infused were changes in compliance, lung resistance and bronchoconstriction noted. A review of the literature reveals that most of the investigations upon the cardiopulmonary effects of serotonin describe the effects of infusions of massive amounts of serotonin[7, 14, 31, 32, 33] and not the effects of amounts comparable to that found in the standard experimental embolus. These preliminary studies and the available reports indicate once again that while humoral agents, especially serotonin, may augment the cardiopulmonary responses found in pulmonary embolism, they probably are not responsible for initiating the responses.

Summary

The increasing frequency and sequelae of clinical pulmonary embolism make it mandatory that pulmonary embolism be prevented whenever possible, or treated properly when it occurs. Proper therapy bespeaks an understanding of the cardiopulmonary alterations which accompany pulmonary embolism and of the mechanisms responsible for producing these alterations. While the alterations have been clearly documented, controversy still exists about the mechanisms, especially about the relative contributions of the mechanical and humoral factors to the cardiopulmonary changes.

A series of studies of experimental pulmonary embolism have been done in an attempt to learn more about the mechanisms responsible for the cardiopulmonary changes. Data have been obtained from normal dogs, serotonin depleted dogs, and platelet depleted dogs embolized with autologous emboli of different ages and with inert protein emboli. Data have also been obtained from serotonin infusions in dogs. The data add strong support to the concept that mechanical obstruction of the pulmonary artery is primarily responsible for the cardiopulmonary changes that occur during acute pulmonary embolism. Although the data suggest that humoral agents, especially serotonin or other agents released from/by platelets, are not primarily responsible for the acute cardiopulmonary changes, an augmentative role for these substances cannot be denied.

Since mechanical obstruction of the pulmonary circulation appears to be primarily responsible for the cardiopulmonary changes of pulmonary embolism, major investigational efforts should be directed toward preventing deep venous thrombosis, detecting deep venous thrombosis early before embolization occurs, preventing migration of the embolus and lysing the embolus. It seems appropriate that this symposium on "Pulmonary Thromboembolism—New Concepts" is oriented toward developing information about preventing, detecting, lysing, and preventing the migration of venous thromboemboli.

REFERENCES

1. Laennec, R. T. H.: Mediate Auscultation on Traite du Diagnostic des Maladies des Poumons et du Coeur. Paris, 1819.
2. Virchow, R.: Die Verstopfung der Lungenarterie und ihre Folgen. *Beitr Z Exp Pathol Physiol*, 2:1, 1846.
3. Wessler, S., Reiner, L., Freiman, D. G., Reimer, S. M. and Lertzman, M.: Serum-induced thrombosis. Studies of its induction and evolution under controlled conditions *in vivo. Circulation*, 20:864, 1959.
4. Cahill, J. M., Attinger, E. O. and Byrne, J. J.: Ventilatory responses to embolization of lung. *J Appl Physiol*, 16:469, 1961.
5. Griffin, G. D. J. and Essex, H. E.: Experimental embolism of the pulmonary arterioles and capillaries. *Surgery*, 26:707, 1949.
6. Halmagyi, D. F. J., Starzecki, B. and Horner, G. J.: Humoral transmission of cardiorespiratory changes in experimental lung embolism. *Circ Res*, 14:546, 1964.
7. Thomas, D., Stein, M., Tanabe, G., Rege, V. and Wessler, S.: Mechanisms of bronchoconstriction produced by thromboemboli in dogs. *Am J Physiol*, 206:1207, 1964.
8. Gurewich, V., Cohen, M. and Thomas, D.: Humoral factors in massive pulmonary embolism. *Am Heart J*, 76:784, 1968.
9. Hamilton, W. M. and Nemir, P., Jr.: The humoral factor in pulmonary embolism. *Arch Surg*, 105:593, 1972.
10. Daley, R., Wade, J. D., Maraist, F. and Bing, R. J.: Pulmonary hypertension in dogs induced by injection of Lycopodium spores into the pulmonary artery, with special reference to the absence of vasomotor reflexes. *Am J Physiol*, 164:380, 1951.
11. Hyland, J. W., Smith, G. T., McGuire, L. B., Harrison, D. C., Haynes, F. W. and Dexter, L.: Effect of selective embolism of various sized vessels of the pulmonary arterial circulation in dogs. *Am J Physiol*, 204:619, 1963.
12. Knisely, W. H., Wallace, J. M., Mahaley, M. S. and Satterwhite, W. M., Jr.: Evidence including *in vivo* observations suggesting mechanical blockage rather than reflex vasospasm as the cause of death in pulmonary embolism. *Am Heart J*, 54:483, 1957.
13. Dexter, L. and Smith, G. T.: Quantitative studies of pulmonary embolism. *Am J Med Sci*, 247:641, 1964.
14. Cobb, B. and Nanson, E. M.: Further studies with serotonin and experimental pulmonary embolism. *Ann Surg*, 151:501, 1960.
15. Daicoff, G. R., Chavez, F. R., Anton, A. H. and Swenson, E. W.: Serotonin-induced pulmonary venous hypertension in pulmonary embolism. *J Thorac Cardiovasc Surg*, 56:810, 1968.

16. Gurewich, V., Sasahara, A. A. and Stein, M.: Pulmonary embolism, bronchoconstriction and response to heparin. In Sasahara, A. A. and Stein, M. (Eds.): *Pulmonary Embolic Disease*. New York, Grune & Stratton, 1965, p. 162.

17. Gurewich, V., Thomas, D., Stein, M. and Wessler, S.: Bronchoconstriction in the presence of pulmonary embolism. *Circulation, 27*:339, 1963.

18. Jacobsen, D. C., Soden, K. J., Allen, P. D. and Daicoff, G. R.: Humoral blockade on lethal pulmonary embolism in the awake dog. *Surg Forum, 22*:209, 1971.

19. Rosoff, C. B., Salzman, E. W., Gurewich, V. and Schroeder, H. K.: Reduction of platelet serotonin and the response to pulmonary emboli. *Surgery, 70*:12, 1971.

20. Urokinase pulmonary embolism trial: Phase I results—A cooperative study. *JAMA, 214*:2163, 1970.

21. Price, K. C., Hata, D. and Smith, J. R.: Pulmonary vasomotion resulting from miliary embolism of the lungs. *Am J Physiol, 182*:183, 1955.

22. Silver, D., Rhodes, G. R., Oates, T. K. and Puckett, C. L.: Unpublished data.

23. Mead, J. and Whittenberger, J. L.: Physical properties of human lungs measured during spontaneous respiration. *J Appl Physiol, 5*:779, 1953.

24. Marshall, R., Sabiston, D. C., Allison, P. R., Bosman, A. R. and Dunnill, M. S.: Immediate and late effects of pulmonary embolism by large thrombi in dogs. *Thorax, 18*:1, 1963.

25. Thomas, D. P. and Gurewich, V.: Role of platelets in sudden death induced by experimental pulmonary emboli. *Circulation* (Suppl. II): 207, 1965.

26. Thomas, D. P., Tanabe, G., Khan, M. and Stein, M.: Humoral factors mediated by platelets in experimental pulmonary embolism. In Sasahara, A. A. and Stein, M. (Eds.): *Pulmonary Embolic Disease*. New York, Grune & Stratton, 1965, p. 59.

27. Puckett, C. L., Gervin, A. S., Rhodes, G. R. and Silver, D.: The role of platelets and blood serotonin in acute massive pulmonary embolism. *Circulation, 46* (Suppl. II): 57, 1972.

28. Thomas, D. P., Gurewich, V. and Ashford, T. P.: Platelet adherence of thromboemboli in relation to the pathogenesis and treatment of pulmonary embolism. *N Eng J Med, 274*:953, 1966.

29. Stein, M. and Thomas, D. P.: Role of platelets in the acute pulmonary response to endotoxin. *J Appl Physiol, 23*:47, 1967.

30. Silver, D. and Hall, J. H.: Effect of heparin on the fibrinolytic system. *Surg Forum, 17*:11, 1966.

31. Comroe, J. H., Jr., Van Linge, B., Stroud, R. C. and Roncoroni, A.: Reflex and direct cardiopulmonary effects of 5-OH-tryptamine (serotonin); their possible role in pulmonary embolism and coronary thrombosis. *Am J Physiol, 173*:379, 1953.

32. Sackner, M. A., Will, D. H. and DuBois, A. B.: The site of pulmonary vasomotor activity during hypoxia or serotonin administration. *J Clin Invest, 45*:112, 1966.

33. Ozdemir, I. A., Katsuyuki, K., Wax, S. D. and Webb, W. R.: Effects of serotonin on pulmonary vascular resistance and microcirculation. *Circulation, 46* (Suppl. II): 56, 1972.

DISCUSSION

Dr. Sasahara: I think these are gorgeous studies, Dr. Silver, and some concepts are, I think, new to us who have been working in the field. As you well know, we felt that serotonin was an important agent, although in the human we could not demonstrate pulmonary vasoconstriction. However, we could demonstrate bronchoconstriction in patients, analogous to the animal study that you quoted from Thomas. If this response is due only to the mechanical act of blockade, it would be difficult to explain the sudden rise in airway resistance and the drop in compliance for that short period of time. It could, however, be explained by the biologic half-life of serotonin which is very short.

Dr. Silver: Art, we were aware of the importance that your Boston colleagues have assigned to the role of humoral factors in initiating the cardiopulmonary changes that occur during acute pulmonary embolism. However, we felt that the humoral factors weren't primarily responsible for the changes. The studies were done to test our thesis that mechanical factors were the most important.

Serotonin is the humoral agent most widely acclaimed as being responsible for initiating the cardiopulmonary changes of acute pulmonary embolism. One must be critical in his evaluation of the cardiopulmonary effects of serotonin infusions. Most reports on the similarity of the cardiopulmonary changes after serotonin infusions and pulmonary embolism describe the effects of infusions of massive amounts of serotonin and not amounts that might accompany pulmonary thromboembolism. We have an ongoing study in which the amount of serotonin contained in an LD_{50} embolus is infused into the pulmonary artery—no changes occur in the cardiopulmonary parameters. Double and quadruple this amount of serotonin may be infused without producing alterations of these parameters. Changes in the cardiopulmonary parameters similar to those seen in pulmonary embolism occur only when a quantity of serotonin equal to the total circulating serotonin is infused.

Agarose emboli and the use of serotonin and platelet depleted dogs were additional attempts to evaluate the role of humoral agents in pulmonary embolism. These studies also suggested that the humoral agents have a secondary role in initiating the cardiopulmonary responses.

Question: Dr. Silver, was there any difference in the serotonin level of those dogs who were treated with heparin and who were not treated with heparin?

Dr. Silver: I am not sure I understand your question. Do you mean before or after embolization, or are you referring to that amount in the thrombus?

Question: What I am leading to is, was there any demonstrable decrease in serotonin level of the dogs that were embolized with heparin and without heparin? Was there an antiserotonin effect of heparin?

Dr. Silver: I'm sorry, but I can't answer that question. We did not measure serotonin levels after the dogs received heparin. The embolus was made from autologous blood obtained before heparin was administered. Heparin will interfere with most enzyme reactions. This may have been one of the reasons for the "protective effect" of heparin.

Question: Dr. Silver, did you make any quantitative correlation between the effects that you have demonstrated and the volume of the clot that you put in?

Dr. Silver: No. However, the volume and size of the embolus is very important. We embolized large clots in order to approximate the acute situation which occurs clinically. We have chosen not to use starch granules, barium sulfate, fungus spores, microspheres, etc., which are much smaller than the usual clinical embolus, do not contain bioactive amines, and lodge in smaller branches of the pulmonary artery. We chose to produce emboli that would approximate the size of the jugular vein of the dog. Because of the marked variation in hematocrits of dogs, all of our emboli were volumetrically corrected for the hematocrits. We did not inject the embolus through a syringe (as is so often done) which tends to fragment the embolus.

When one reads papers on experimental pulmonary embolism, one ought to be curious about how the embolus was prepared, how it was injected, and where it lodged. These things greatly influence the effects of the embolus. Miliary emboli appear to behave, as Art Sasahara suggested, in a different fashion than larger emboli.

Dr. Hirsh: I would also like to congratulate you on your work. Dr. Cade, in our department, has done similar studies and our conclusions are very much the same as yours. The one thing that continues to puzzle us, and Dr. Sasahara has referred to this, is the explanation for the rise and fall in pulmonary artery pressure following massive sublethal embolus. There is a sudden rise in pulmonary artery pressure coincident with embolism, but this falls to normal limits within half an hour despite the fact that there is little change in the size of the embolus. We have used very accurate means of quantitating the embolus (radioactive embolus) and find that very little of the embolus has disappeared in thirty minutes. This suggests that it is not just the embolus which is causing the rise in pulmonary artery pressure but it is the embolus plus some other factor. This experimental observation is supported by some clinical studies that were published in the Japanese literature some years ago. In these studies, the investigators infused serotonin into normal subjects and into patients who had pulmonary embolism and found there was virtually no rise in pulmonary artery pressure in normal subjects but a very considerable rise in patients who had pulmonary embolic disease.

Dr. Silver: Thank you for your comments, Dr. Hirsh. Most of the acute changes observed in our studies were maximal in 30 to 120 seconds and usually resolved in 50 to 60 minutes. We did not correlate cardio-pulmonary measurements with the size of the embolus remaining at autopsy. I would guess that fragmentation, movement, and/or lysis of the embolus occurs early in the recovery phase. However, I do not have any data on this aspect of pulmonary embolism. Additional studies on the mechanism of the recovery phase are needed.

Chapter 11

THE HEMODYNAMIC RESPONSE TO
PULMONARY EMBOLISM

KEVIN M. McINTYRE AND ARTHUR A. SASAHARA

Introduction

A VARIETY of hemodynamic disturbances have been observed after pulmonary embolism. Some patients show no abnormality while others may have pulmonary hypertension of varying severity, venous pressure elevation, low cardiac output or shock. With few exceptions, however, the various hemodynamic disturbances after embolism have not been interpreted meaningfully. Despite extensive use of diagnostic selective pulmonary angiography which provides in turn, a method for estimating the extent of embolic involvement, the relationship between the hemodynamic disturbance and the extent of involvement has not been extensively explored. Because it appeared to us that the postembolic hemodynamic status had important therapeutic and prognostic implications, a complete profile of pressure and flow measurements were obtained, when possible, in patients with acute pulmonary embolism. In addition, perfusion lung scans and pulmonary angiograms were obtained to qualify the extent of pulmonary vascular obstruction.

RESULTS

The observed hemodynamic responses appeared to fall into two groups: those patients with no prior cardiopulmonary disease and those with underlying heart and lung disease.

Pulmonary Embolism in Patients With No Prior Heart and Lung Disease

The Hemodynamic Response

A depression of systemic arterial oxygen tension (PaO_2) was the most frequent disturbance observed after embolism in patients without prior heart and lung disease.[1,2] A depression in PaO_2 may be observed with as little as 5 to 15 percent embolic obstruction (estimated by lung scanning or angiography). With more extensive involvement, PaO_2 may fall to forty

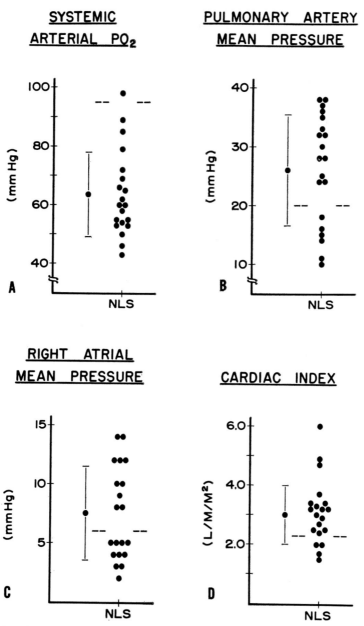

Figure 11-1. Systemic arterial partial pressure of oxygen, mean pulmonary arterial pressure, mean right atrial pressure and cardiac index are plotted for each of twenty patients. The mean and one SD is shown for each index. Horizontal broken lines indicate normal levels.

to fifty mm Hg. The range of values observed in twenty patients with no prior heart and lung disease who suffered pulmonary embolism is shown in Figure 11-1A.

The next most frequent abnormality after embolism in this population of patients was an elevation of the pulmonary arterial mean pressure (PAm) (Fig. 11-1B). Seventy percent with no preembolic heart or lung disease showed elevations in the PAm (normal less than 20 mm Hg). It is of particular interest to note that no patient had a PAm in excess of forty mm Hg, despite massive obstruction in some. It was concluded from this series[1-3] and affirmed in other series of comparable patients[4, 5] that

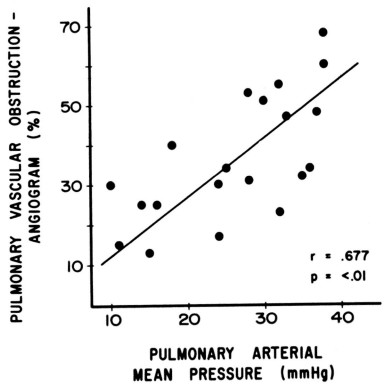

PERCENT ANGIOGRAPHIC OBSTRUCTION – PULMONARY ARTERIAL MEAN PRESSURE RELATIONSHIP

Figure 11-2. A highly significant relation existed between mean pulmonary arterial pressure (abscissa) and estimated angiographic obstruction (ordinate) in patients free of prior heart and lung disease.

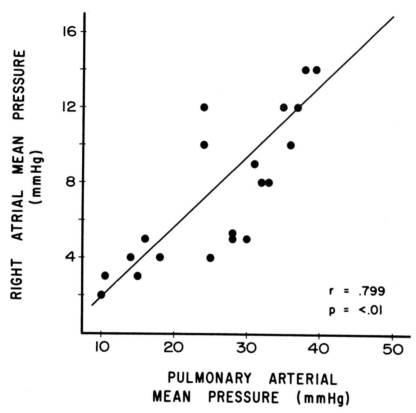

Figure 11-3. The mean right atrial pressure (ordinate) related to the mean pulmonary arterial pressure (abscissa) with a high degree of significance in patients free of preembolic cardiopulmonary disease.

forty mm Hg very likely approximates the maximum PAm pressure which the previously normal right ventricle can sustain acutely, so that a PAm between thirty and forty mm Hg after embolism is considered to represent *severe* pulmonary hypertension in these patients.

The right atrial mean pressure (RAm) was elevated above the normal in our laboratory (6 mm Hg) in roughly half of the patients studied (Fig. 11-1C). It is clear, therefore, that the absence of central venous or right atrial mean pressure elevation generally cannot be used to exclude the diagnosis of pulmonary embolism. On the other hand, as shown in Figure

11-10, an elevation of right atrial or central venous pressure after embolism in patients with no prior heart or lung disease is a clear indication that extensive embolic obstruction has occurred.

The cardiac index (CI) is usually not depressed after embolism in this population of patients, but is generally either normal or elevated (Fig. 11-1D). Despite extensive obstruction estimated by angiography in a number of patients, only 20 percent showed a depressed CI.

Relationship of Hemodynamic Status to Angiographic Obstruction

The magnitude of pulmonary embolic involvement was found to determine directly the type and severity of the hemodynamic abnormality in this group of patients with no prior heart or lung disease. When the level of pulmonary vascular obstruction was below 25 percent, PAm tended to remain normal (Fig. 11-2). Generally, when angiographic obstruction

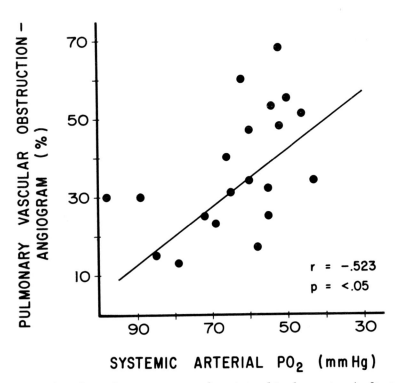

Figure 11-4. The relation between estimated angiographic obstruction (ordinate) and the degree of systemic arterial hypoxemia (abscissa) is shown in patients free of pre-embolic heart and lung disease.

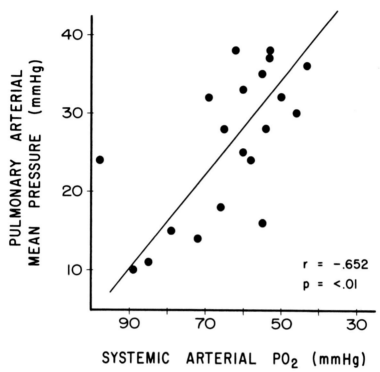

Figure 11-5. A high degree of correlation was observed between mean pulmonary arterial pressure (ordinate) and systemic arterial hypoxemia (abscissa) in patients without preembolic heart and lung disease.

exceeded 25 to 35 percent, PAm was elevated. With additional increases in pulmonary vascular obstruction, elevation of RAm was commonly observed. The RAm after embolism in patients free of prior cardiopulmonary disease appears to be directly related to both the extent of embolic obstruction and to the level of PAm.[1, 3] While PAm was below thirty mm Hg, which generally occurs with angiographic obstruction up to thirty-five percent, the RAm was generally normal (Fig. 11-3). Once pulmonary pressure exceeded this level, the RAm was usually elevated. One could presume from an elevated RAm, therefore, that PAm and vascular obstruction had reached these levels. Depression of PaO_2, also appeared to depend on the severity of embolic obstruction (Fig. 11-4) and PAm, in turn, was observed to bear a significant relationship to PaO_2, with increasingly severe pulmonary hypertension being observed as hypoxemia became more severe (Fig. 11-5). The CI is usually preserved until pulmonary angiographic obstruction exceeds 50 percent.

General Considerations and Conclusions

The observation that pulmonary hypertension may be observed with as little as 25 percent angiographic obstruction is not inconsistent with experimental studies and observations on unilateral pulmonary artery occlusion in man which have shown that 50 percent or more of the pulmonary vasculature must be obstructed before pulmonary hypertension occurs.[6, 7] Angiography generally underestimates total effective pulmonary vascular obstruction since it cannot entirely appreciate small vessel obstruction and

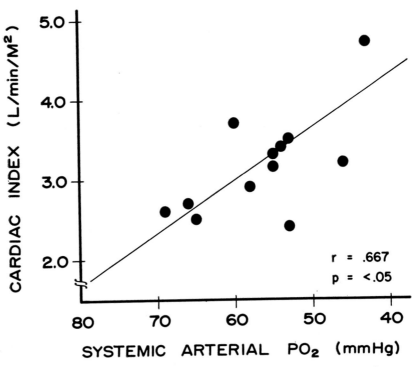

Figure 11-6. Cardiac index (ordinate) related to the severity of the hypoxemia (abscissa). There was a close relation in patients in whom systemic hypoxemia was well established (pO_2 less than 75 mm Hg) and cardiac failure, as manifested by a depression of cardiac index, was not present. See text.

is insensitive to vasoconstriction, both of which may contribute substantially to effective pulmonary vascular obstruction.

An elevation of right atrial or central venous pressure is generally considered to be a manifestation of right ventricular failure. The fact that the CI remained normal or increased in a number of patients in whom the RAm was elevated suggested that failure of the right ventricle in terms of its ability to maintain forward flow indeed had not occurred. It appeared instead that a compensatory adjustment had been provided by the Frank-Starling mechanism, allowing the right ventricle to maintain its output.[1-3] Furthermore, it has been shown in normal man that acute depressions

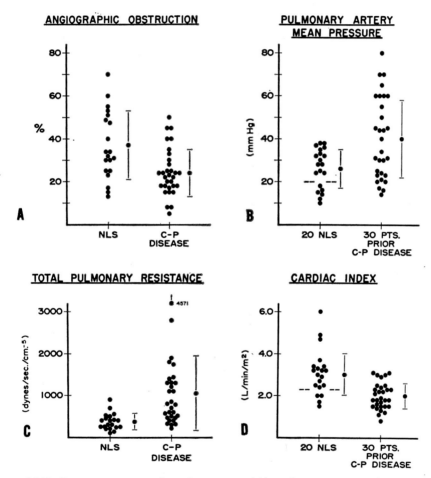

Figure 11-7. Percent angiographic obstruction (A) pulmonary arterial mean pressure (B) total pulmonary resistance (C) and cardiac index (D) in thirty patients with and twenty patients without prior cardiopulmonary disease. The mean and one standard deviation are shown to the right of each aggregate of values. Normal levels are indicated by the horizontal dashed lines.

of systemic arterial oxygen tension to a range of forty to sixty mm Hg were generally followed by an increase in cardiac output.[8] This observation was also made in our series (Fig. 11-6). Experimental evidence suggests that this high flow response to hypoxemia may be mediated by a marked increase in cardiac sympathetic discharge both in animals[9] and in man.[10] Another explanation for increased flow may be that the hypoxic stimulus to venoconstriction[11] may result in an increase in venous return with a resultant increase in stroke output, again by means of the Frank-Starling mechanism. It is likely that both enhancement of cardiosympathetic tone and the Frank-Starling mechanism are involved as compensatory phenomena after pulmonary embolism in patients with previously normal heart and lungs. Failure of these mechanisms to sustain stroke output may ultimately be expressed by a low-flow state with a high central venous pressure or RAm and a dominantly chronotropic expression of cardiosympathetic stimulation, which is the characteristic clinical syndrome after massive embolism in patients free of prior heart and lung disease.

While depressions in PaO$_2$ may not occur after embolism in some patients

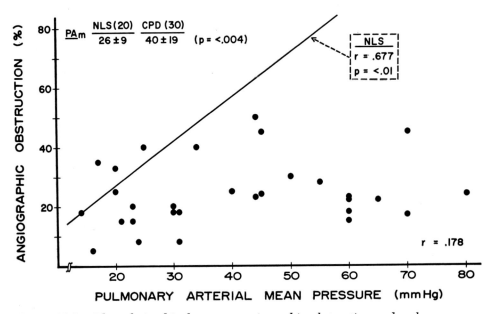

Figure 11-8. The relationship between angiographic obstruction and pulmonary arterial mean pressure for thirty patients with prior cardiopulmonary disease (dots). No significant relationship could be established. By contrast, a highly significant relationship was present in twenty patients without prior heart and lung disease (regression line).

they may be expected with sufficient frequency (approximately 85 percent) that this measurement continues to have value as a screening test for PE in patients free of prior cardiopulmonary disease.[12, 13] Furthermore, the relationship between PAm and PaO_2 observed in this study (Fig. 11-5) as well as previous observations on the role of hypoxemia in the production of pulmonary vasoconstriction[14] suggest that the administration of oxygen could have immediate therapeutic value by reducing, however slightly, (what might represent) a critical right ventricular load.

The Hemodynamic Response in Patients With Prior Heart or Lung Disease

Similar observations to those noted above were made in a series of thirty patients *with* prior heart or lung disease, including coronary heart disease,

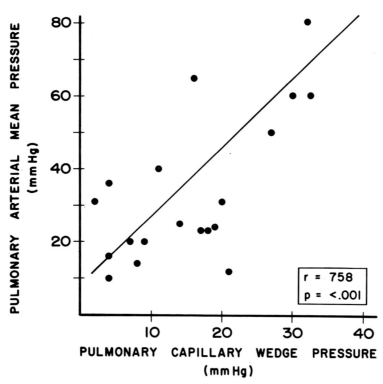

Figure 11-9. The pulmonary arterial mean pressure (ordinate) bore a highly significant relationship with the pulmonary capillary wedge pressure (abscissa) in the nineteen patients with preembolic heart or lung disease in whom it was measured.

aortic valve disease, mitral valve disease and chronic obstructive lung disease. Comparisons between this latter population and the population of patients with normal cardiopulmonary status before embolism were made. Angiographic obstruction averaged 34 percent in the population of patients with no prior heart or lung disease, but was significantly less in patients in whom heart or lung disease was present prior to embolism, averaging 23 percent (Fig. 11-7A). While angiographic obstruction was higher in patients with no prior heart or lung disease, the PAm (mean 26 mm Hg) was significantly lower than in the group with prior heart or lung disease (mean 40 mm Hg), as shown in Figure 11-7B. The PAm in the latter group ranged from normal levels, which were observed in only a few patients, to eighty mm Hg. A large number of patients in this group had pressures in excess of forty mm Hg. Total pulmonary resistance (TPR)

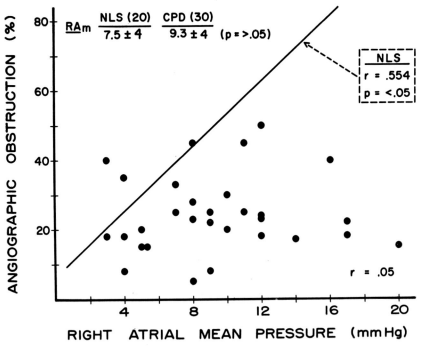

Figure 11-10. The severity of angiographic obstruction, plotted in percent on the ordinate, was found to bear no relationship to the level of right atrial mean pressure (abscissa) in the thirty patients with preembolic heart or lung disease (solid dots). The regression line for the relationship in twenty patients with no preembolic heart or lung disease indicates a significant relation. See text.

averaged approximately 400 dynes/sec/cm^{-5} in the previously normal group while the mean value exceeded 1000 dynes/sec/cm^{-5} in patients with prior heart or lung disease (Fig. 11-7C). It clearly appeared that factors other than the magnitude of embolic obstruction were important determinants of the postembolic PAm and the TPR in these patients. CI was generally depressed in this population, averaging two liters/min/M^2, in contrast to the normal or usually elevated postembolic CI in patients with no prior heart or lung disease (Fig. 11-7D). The PAm bore no relationship to angiographic obstruction in the population of patients with prior heart or lung disease (Fig. 8), as it had in the previously normal group (Fig. 11-2). On the other hand, the PAm could be directly related to the pulmonary capillary wedge pressure in patients with prior heart or

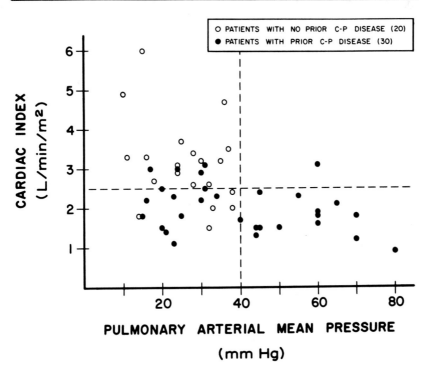

RELATIONSHIP OF CARDIAC INDEX TO PULMONARY ARTERIAL MEAN PRESSURE

Figure 11-11. The cardiac index and the pulmonary arterial mean pressure in twenty patients without preembolic cardiopulmonary disease (open circles) and in thirty patients with preembolic cardiopulmonary disease (solid dots). None of the first group displayed a pulmonary arterial mean pressure in excess of forty mm Hg (vertical broken line), despite extensive angiographic obstruction in some. The horizontal broken line, is the minimal normal (2.3 to 2.5 L/min) of cardiac index.

lung disease (Fig. 9). It appeared, therefore, that left atrial pressures or left ventricular diastolic pressures played a much more important role in the level of PAm in this population than did the severity of pulmonary vascular obstruction. Similarly, the PAm was unrelated to angiographic obstruction among patients with prior heart or lung diseases, while a significant relationship was noted in the previously normal patients (Fig. 11-10). The interpretation of RAm or central venous pressure in patients with preembolic heart or lung disease, therefore, must be quite different, since it may be due entirely to congestive heart failure which predated embolism, and therefore bore no relationship to the embolic event per se. When the CI was related to the PAm in the two groups, a rather distinct separation in the two groups was apparent. The CI was generally normal

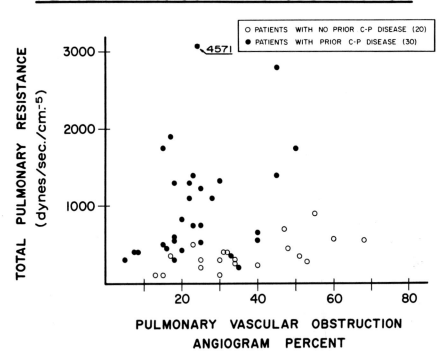

Figure 11-12. Total pulmonary resistance is plotted on the vertical axis, angiographic pulmonary vascular obstruction on the horizontal axis, for thirty patients with (solid dots) and twenty patients without (open circles) prior cardiopulmonary disease. A highly significant relationship between resistance and angiographic obstruction was observed in previously normal patients (p = less than .01). No relationship could be established in patients with preceding heart or lung disease.

or increased while the PAm was below forty mm Hg in the previously normal group while in the group of patients with prior heart or lung disease, the PAm exceeded forty mm Hg in half and the CI was depressed in more than 70 percent (Fig.11-11). The relationship of TPR and the percent of angiographic obstruction in the two groups was of particular interest. Whereas elevation of the TPR was found to be directly proportional to the extent of embolic obstruction in patients previously free of cardiopulmonary disease, TPR was elevated out of proportion to angiographic obstruction in patients with prior heart and lung disease (Fig. 11-12). The difference in the TPR between the two groups may represent an approximate measure of the extent to which the preembolic cardiopulmonary status contributes to the postembolic hemodynamic status. These observations indicate that an awareness of the preembolic cardiopulmonary status as well as the extent of pulmonary vascular involvement is of real importance in the interpretation of the hemodynamic status following pulmonary embolism.

Conclusions

It was concluded, based on the data presented above, that the hemodynamic status in patients after pulmonary embolism is determined by both the preembolic cardiopulmonary status and by the magnitude of pulmonary embolic obstruction. The hemodynamic abnormalities observed after pulmonary embolism in patients free of prior heart and lung disease are usually linearly related to the magnitude of embolic obstruction. Lesser degrees of obstruction result in relatively minor hemodynamic derangements. Massive degrees of obstruction are associated with serious or critical hemodynamic disturbances.

The hemodynamic status after embolism in patients with preembolic heart or lung disease, on the other hand, may be determined primarily by the nature and severity of the cardiopulmonary abnormality that existed prior to embolism. Small degrees of embolization, therefore, may be associated with very substantial hemodynamic abnormalities, since such hemodynamic derangements may have been present prior to and independent of the embolization. In patients with preembolic heart or lung disease, therefore, the postembolic hemodynamic status may be determined primarily by the embolic event per se, by the preembolic hemodynamic status or, as is the usual case, by a combination of the two processes.

REFERENCES

1. McIntyre, K. M. and Sasahara, A. A.: The hemodynamic response to pulmonary embolism in patients without prior cardiopulmonary disease. *Am J Cardiol,* 28:288, 1971.

2. McIntyre, K. M., Sasahara, A. A. and Sharma, G. V. R. K.: Pulmonary thromboembolism: Current concepts. In Stollerman, G. H. (Ed.): *Advances in Internal Medicine.* Year Book Medical Publishers, Inc. Vol. 18, 1972, p. 199.

3. McIntyre, K. M. and Sasahara, A. A.: Determinants of cardiovascular responses to pulmonary embolism. In Moser, K. M. and Stein, M. (Eds.): *Pulmonary Thromboembolism.* Chicago, Year Book Medical Publishers, Inc., 1973, p. 154.

4. Miller, G. A. and Sutton, G. C.: Acute massive pulmonary embolism. Clinical and haemodynamic findings in 23 patients studied by cardiac catheterization and pulmonary arteriography. *Br Heart J, 32*:518, 1970.

5. Dalen, J. E., Banas, J. J., Brooks, H. L., Evans, G. L., Paraskos, J. A. and Dexter, L.: Resolution rate of acute pulmonary embolism in man. *N Engl J Med, 280*:1194, 1969.

6. Brandfonbrener, M., Turino, G. M., Himmelstein, A., et al.: Effects of occlusion of one pulmonary artery on pulmonary circulation in man (Abstract). *Fed Proc, 17*:19, 1958.

7. Nelson, J. R. and Smith, J. R.: Pathologic physiology of pulmonary embolism. Physiologic discussion of the vascular reactions following pulmonary arterial obstruction by emboli of varying size. *Am Heart J, 58*:916, 1959.

8. Kontos, H. A., Jevasseur, J. E., Richardson, D. W., et al.: Comparative circulatory responses to systemic hypoxia in man and in unanesthetized dogs. *J Appl Physiol, 23*:381, 1967.

9. Downing, S. E. and Siegle, J. H.: Some factors concerned with the regulation of sympathetic discharge to the heart (Abstract). *Clin Res, 10*:171, 1962.

10. Richardson, D. W., Kontos, H. A., Raper, A. J., et al.: Modification by beta-adrenergic blockade of the circulatory responses to acute hypoxia in man. *J Clin Invest, 46*:77, 1967.

11. Eckstein, J. W. and Harsley, A. W.: Effects of hypoxia on peripheral venous tone in man. *J Lab Clin Med, 56*:847, 1960.

12. Szucs, M. M., Jr., Brooks, H. L., Grossman, W., Banas, J. S., Meister, S. G., Dexter, L., Dalen, J. E.: Diagnostic sensitivity of laboratory findings in acute pulmonary embolism. *Ann Int Med, 74*:161, 1971.

13. Urokinase Pulmonary Embolism Trial: A national cooperative study. *Circulation, Suppl II XLVII*(4):51, 1973.

14. Sasahara, A. A.: Pulmonary vascular responses to thromboembolism. *Mod Concepts Cardiovasc Dis, XXXVI*(10):55, 1967.

DISCUSSION

Question: Could you comment on the time interval between the pulmonary embolism and the findings presented?

Dr. Sasahara: The time interval between the embolism and study in these patients was within forty-eight hours.

Question: Dr. Hamilton: If a patient is seen with severe shortness of breath or hypotension and the jugular venous pressure is not elevated, would you say that this was not due to a pulmonary embolus?

Dr. Sasahara: That's correct. It's most likely due to massive myocardial infarction with primary pump failure on the left side. Perhaps Dr. Sautter, will discuss this on Saturday, but this relationship seems to hold. Looking for neck veins in the serious situation where the differential diagnosis could be massive embolism or myocardial infarction is a very good differentiating clinical observation.

Dr. Zimmerman (Rockford): It would sound then as though you wouldn't need such a tool as the Swan-Gans catheter in order to get wedge pressures on such people in emergency situations. Would you agree with this? We were evaluating whether under circumstances of shock we need to institute Swan-Gans catheters in a community hospital and looking for circumstances in which they are needed, one of which is the sudden appearance of shock. From this discussion, it would seem that differentiating pulmonary emboli from the other causes of shock does not require the use of wedge pressures or left atrial pressures to help make the differential since you can do this on simple central venous pressures.

Dr. Sasahara: Yes, that is basically correct. In differentiating the shock of massive pulmonary embolism from that of acute myocardial infarction the simple bedside observation of the neck veins is invaluable. It is a rough index of the state of the right ventricle. In massive pulmonary embolism, the severe pulmonary hypertension places a great load on the right ventricle and therefore the right atrial pressure rises, which is reflected in distention of the neck veins. In shock due to massive myocardial infarction, the failure of the left ventricle is reflected in the elevated wedge pressure which reflects left atrial pressure. Therefore, the neck veins in such an acute situation are not distended. The value of the Swan-Gans catheter measurement lies in the moment to moment measurement of the wedge pressure in a very unstable hemodynamic condition involving the left ventricle. The right atrial pressure in this situation is useless.

Dr. Hecker (Michigan): I think we're confused, because what you have measured is mean pressure and what that doctor was talking about was wedge pressure and wedge pressure is the reflection of left sided failure and it may be different than in the mean pressure in the pulmonary arteries.

Dr. Sasahara: No, he was talking about my use of the right atrial mean pressure in the diagnosis of pulmonary embolism. That's central venous pressure as opposed to the Swan-Gans wedge pressure which is left atrial mean pressure, isn't that correct?

Dr. Hecker: Yes.

Chapter 12

PULMONARY MICROEMBOLISM

RICHARD P. O'NEILL, ROBERT B. PENMAN AND A. J. MILLETT

PULMONARY EMBOLISM occurs when a thrombus on the venous side of the circulation is loosened and freed from its site and reaches the lungs.

The determinants of intravascular clotting are still not precisely known but several factors involved are well documented such as (1) local venous injury produced by trauma, infection or infiltration, (2) local stasis produced by inefficient arterial supply or venous outlet obstruction with resultant acidosis and (3) increased clotting tendency caused by platelet abnormality, polycythemia, increased tissue breakdown, abnormal humoral states and others.

Pulmonary embolism may be acute, subacute and chronic. All may produce acute and/or chronic pulmonary hypertension. Acute pulmonary embolism occurring in association with large thromboemboli is familiar enough and will not be dealt with here. Subacute and chronic pulmonary embolism can be divided into three main groups, as described by Oakley and Goodwin.[1]

1. Thromboembolic
   a. Major segmental branches
   b. Arterioles and muscular arteries
   c. Pulmonary venous occlusive disease

2. Other Emboli
   a. Fat
   b. Air
   c. Marrow
   d. Amniotic Fluid and trophoblast
   e. Tumor, e.g. chorion
   f. Ova-bilharzia
   g. Contrast Materials

3. Generalized disease
   a. Polyarteritis
   b. Scleroderma

4. Embolism associated with D.I.C. Syndrome
   a. Tissue Injury, obstetrical, surgical; neoplastic; associated with chemotherapy.
   b. Endothelial Injury: Gram positive and Gram negative Septicemia; viremia; prolonged hypotension
   c. Platelet or red cell injury
   d. Reticuloendothelial cell injury; liver injury; acute pyogenic hepatitis; cirrhosis; postsplenectomy

It has recently been suggested[2] that temporary clotting of the blood in the pulmonary microcirculation and elsewhere is relatively common. Such temporary clotting may be initiated by hemorrhage, trauma, or infection and is accompanied by arteriolar vasoconstriction. Arteriovenous shunts then open up, circumventing the occluded vessels, adding to the already slowed capillary circulation and causing local lactic acidosis. Capillary stasis and local acidosis produce local thrombosis.

The classical picture of subacute or chronic pulmonary embolism and/or pulmonary hypertension is seen in the woman of childbearing age. It is not known whether multiple, recurrent embolisations over many years and shed to the lung from peripheral thrombotic sites is the cause or whether the hypertension occurs from *in situ* thromboses in the smaller pulmonary vessels. It is reasonably certain that the disease is rarely caused by pulmonary venous thrombosis.

Early diagnosis of this "entity" depends on an alert and aroused clinical sense. The initial symptoms are frequently vague and ill-described. What appear to be psychosomatic and neurotic complaints in a fit-looking young woman, particularly after pregnancy, should spell at least caution. The symptoms are those of undue fatigability, light-headedness and dizziness, particularly on effort, hyperventilation syndrome or recurrent episodes of ill-defined "pneumonia" or "pleurisy." Abnormal physical findings are conspicuous by their absence. The chest X-ray is read as being normal. Spirometry is normal. Arterial blood gases, particularly when performed at rest, are normal. Later, generally within 3 to 4 years, the patient complains of severe dyspnea, particularly on exertion, exertional syncope and anterior chest pain suggestive of angina pectoris. There is evident marked tachypnea, tachycardia and not infrequently cyanosis. Even when significant pulmonary hypertension is present the diagnosis can be missed. There is often an increased presystolic "a" wave in the neck which may only be brought out on or after exertion. There may be present a right ventricular heave, appreciated in the parasternal or epigastric region, increased pulmonary artery pulsation, pulmonary ejection click and accentuated pulmonic valve closing sounds. A low cardiac output then develops with cold and cyanosed extremities, a narrowed systemic arterial blood pressure and the early diastolic murmur of pulmonary incompetence. Right ventricular hypertrophy is associated with a fourth and later a third heart sound and the second sound becomes widely split. Terminally, dancing jugular pulsations and a pulsatile liver are indicative of tricuspid insufficiency and congestive heart failure and death is not far round the corner. Death in syncope is not unusual secondary to low cardiac output, arrythmias and cerebral ischemia. The picture elaborated falls into the group of insidious, so-called idiopathic pulmonary hypertension. It is argued as to whether its cause is progressive obliteration of the small pulmonary vessels versus thromboembolism without apparent source of emboli.

Pulmonary microemboli have at least three possible sources and pathologically at least two varieties can be distinguished.[3, 4] Unfortunately, the same histological section may show more than one type and this may cause differential difficulty.

The largest arterial microemboli occur in pulmonary vessels of 0.25 to 1 mm in diameter. Most of these, when fresh, look like macroscopic emboli and microscopically are red thrombi, containing fibrin, platelets and leucocytes. Occasionally larger emboli in larger arteries are found in association with microemboli. Here deep vein thrombi are found in the peripheral venous system in the majority. It would seem then that microemboli are the microscopic counterpart of large thromboemboli, and that they have their origin as deep vein thrombi under conditions of venous stasis and injury. They become detached and are embolized to the pulmonary vessels in varying sizes and there further fragment into smaller sizes.

Microemboli also occur in the smaller than 0.25 to one mm diameter pulmonary vessels. They may occur in the prearteriolar capillaries and in the capillaries. It would appear that such microemboli are different. They are composed of compressed fibrin admixed with platelets. It is believed that such microemboli have two different sources: (1) they occur as a by-product of the circulation under special, stressful conditions, and (2) they derive from blood circulating expracorporeally or transfused, especially during various bypass procedures.

Microemboli have been seen in the small vessels of the pulmonary circulation in animals after experimental hemorrhage,[5, 6, 7] in patients dying following acute, generally extensive, trauma;[8] in rabbits subjected to endotoxic shock;[9] and in patients dying in shock following major vascular surgery, such as a repair on the aorta.[10]

It is thought that microemboli are emboli swept to the lung from the venous circulation during a change in coagulation or thrombogenesis. The process can be regarded, in general, as a stage of diffuse intravascular coagulopathy. The precipitating event seems to be a phase of sudden hypercoagulability associated with activated fibrinolysis. This later is presumably a protective mechanism. There is then a reduction in plasma-clotting factors and a fall in platelets. Consumptive coagulopathy is now recognized as an important factor in the complex coagulative and fibrio-lytic reactions in injury, burns, hemorrhage, and various shock-like states.[11, 12]

Accelerated clotting and activated fibrinolysis are the chief factors in the first few hours. They are followed by decreased clotting, inhibited fibrinolysis, and a fall in circulating platelets. Adrenaline has been impli-cated as a trigger mechanism and the accelerated clotting is likely the result of a thromboplastin or thrombolic accelerator. The spleen may well play a major role because it has been shown that the shortening of clotting time after severe hemorrhage in dogs[13] and rabbits[6] did not arise in pre-viously splenectomised animals.

These microemboli appear to be of real importance. Blaidsell et al.[10] reviewed deaths following major vascular surgery and found a group of patients with shock, respiratory disturbances and decreased arterial oxygen saturation. Fibrin thrombi were found in the small vessels of the lung of patients dying within the first three postoperative days. They concluded that microembolism is a frequent cause of morbidity and mortality follow-ing major vascular surgery.

The picture is probably more complex than this but it is certainly pos-sible that a seemingly minor insult to the pulmonary microcirculation may set off a chain reaction. Embolic trauma is succeeded by platelet disrup-tion, release of active amines, vasoconstriction, increased stasis and *in situ* thrombosis.

The third type of microembolism could perhaps be termed iatrogenic. It is seen in venovenous bypass operations with blood circulating through a pump oxygenator[14] and in patients dying after cardiac surgery with veno-aortic bypass and large blood transfusions.[15] In venovenous experiments Allardyce[14] found a picture of hypotension, raised right ventricular pres-sure, and decreased PaO₂ within minutes and on autopsy extensive micro-emboli in the small pulmonary vessels and capillaries. The cause was ascribed to blood damaged by the pump oxygenator (the debris acting as microemboli), because microembolism did not occur when the pump was excluded nor when a filter was introduced into the system.

Systemic microembolism has been found in the kidney and myocardium following transfusion in association with cardiopulmonary bypass and in the lungs of patients following large intravenous blood transfusions. These emboli were mainly fused, aggregated platelets.[16]

The clinical diagnosis of microembolism is difficult and confounding. It should be looked for in the setting of trauma, accidental or surgical and particularly so in association with vascular and bypass procedures; in shock syndromes; in association with large blood transfusions, burns, and in obstetrical accidents. The clinical picture found is essentially that of some degree of shock with hypotension, low cardiac output, peripheral vasoconstriction and dyspnea, this latter often being described by patients as, "I can get air in but it isn't doing me any good." Laboratory studies may reveal a low PaO_2 with hyperventilation; an EKG showing evidence of myocardial ischemia due to poor coronary perfusion and low cardiac output; occasionally pulmonary infiltrates on chest X-ray indicative of intra-alveolar hemorrhage, focal atelectasis, or pulmonary edema; thrombocytopenia and decreased plasma fibrinogen level.

The treatment is if possible, the avoidance of systemic shock or prolonged surgical clamping shock, the introduction of efficient filters into pump oxygenators, and measures to avoid unnecessarily large transfusions. Corrective treatment is with heparin, maintenance of blood pressure, appropriate oxygenation and measures to combat lactic acidosis.

REFERENCES

1. Oakley, C. and Goodwin, J. F.: *Prog Cardiovasc Dis, 9*:495, 1967.
2. Hardaway, R. M.: *Ann Surg, 155*:325, 1962.
3. Brenner, O.: *Arch Intern Med, 56*:1189, 1953.
4. Hayem, G.: In *Du Sang et des Alterations Anatomiques*. Paris, 1889.
5. Crowell, J. W. and Read, W. L.: *Am J Physiol, 183*:565, 1955.
6. Turpini, R. and Stefanini, M. J.: *J Clin Invest, 38*:53, 1959.
7. Robb, H. J.: *Ann Surg, 158*:685, 1963.
8. Sevitt, S.: *Lancet, 2*:1203, 1966.
9. Brimson, J. G., Gamble, C. V. and Thomas, L.: *Am J Pathol, 31*:489, 1955.
10. Blaidsell, F. W., Lin, R. C., Amberg, J. R., Choy, S. H., Hall, A. D. and Thomas, A. N.: *Arch Surg, 93*:776, 1966.
11. Bachmann, F.: *Hosp Pract, 113*:6, 1971.
12. Deykin, D.: *N Engl J Med, 636*:283, 1970.
13. McClintock, J. T. and Magers, E.: *Proc Soc Exp Biol Med, 24*:203, 1926.
14. Allardyce, D. B., Yoshida, S. H. and Ashmore, D. G.: *J Thorac Cardiovasc Surg, 52*:706, 1966.
15. Jenevin, E. P. and Weiss, D. L.: *Am J Pathol, 45*:313, 1964.
16. *Lancet* (Editorial), *764*:429, 1967.

Chapter 13

PULMONARY THROMBOEMBOLISM IN CHILDREN

Jacqueline A. Noonan

Pulmonary thromboembolism is considered a rare problem in infants and children. Of 508 cases of pulmonary embolism occurring among 10,000 consecutive autopsies from the University of Chicago reported by Haber and Bennington[1] only seven or 1.4 percent occurred in children under age ten years. Deep vein thromboses are particularly rare in children so that other predisposing factors should be considered.

Hypercoagulable States

Hypercoagulable states which may be common to both adults and children is one important factor. Early reports in the literature of multiple platelet or fibrin thrombosis in small pulmonary vessels of infants dying with a variety of overwhelming acute illnesses were considered by pathologists as a possible Schwartzman reaction. Today the term disseminated intravascular coagulation, or DIC, is recognized as a complication of shock from a variety of causes, particularly septicemia. Autopsy findings in such patients frequently show fibrin or platelet thrombi in a variety of organs especially the pulmonary vessels.[2] (Fig. 13-1) An infant who died following head trauma with shock had the clinical picture of disseminated intravascular clotting with low platelets, low fibrinogen and a bleeding tendency. Multiple thrombi were present in the small pulmonary vessels including a bone marrow embolus seen in Figure 13-2.

Sickle cell anemia is another cause of intravascular thrombosis.[3, 4] Although pulmonary infarction from pulmonary thrombosis and sickle cell anemia is rare in children it does occur. Figures 13-3 and 13-4 are of a four-year-old girl who presented with signs of a cerebral vascular accident attributed to thrombosis of the right middle cerebral artery. Her chest X-ray suggested pulmonary infarction with a wedge shaped infiltrate. One and one-half years later at the age of five and one-half years, she returned with dyspnea, cough, and an infiltrate with a pleural effusion. Pulmonary infarction was again suspected.

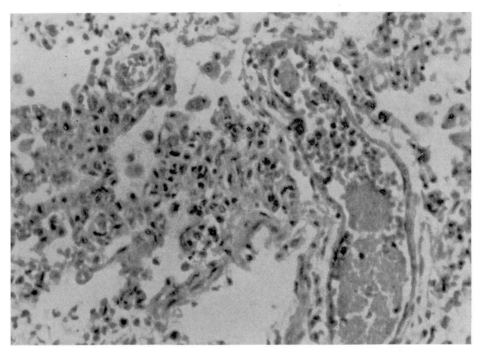

Figure 13-1.   Pulmonary vessel with fibrin thrombosis in a child dying with sepsis.

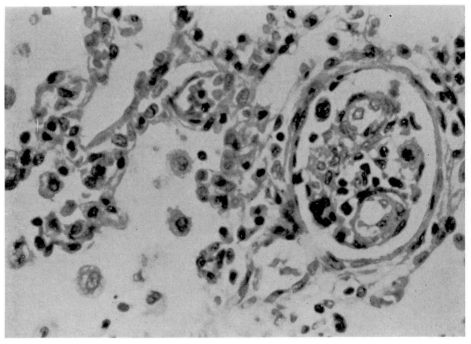

Figure 13-2.   Bone marrow embolus in pulmonary vessel following head trauma in an infant.

Fatal pulmonary thrombosis as well as peripheral venous and arterial thrombosis have been reported as a complication of the nephrotic syndrome.[5, 6] In all of the reported cases, the thrombosis occurred following diuresis. Treatment with steroids and diuretics almost always preceded

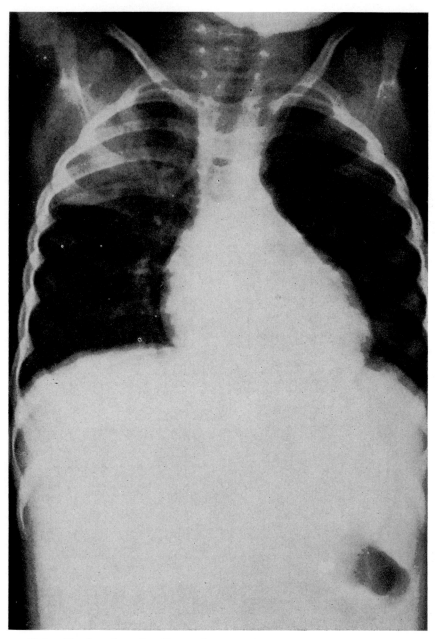

Figure 13-3. Wedge shaped infiltrate due to pulmonary infarction in a four-year-old girl in sickle cell crisis.

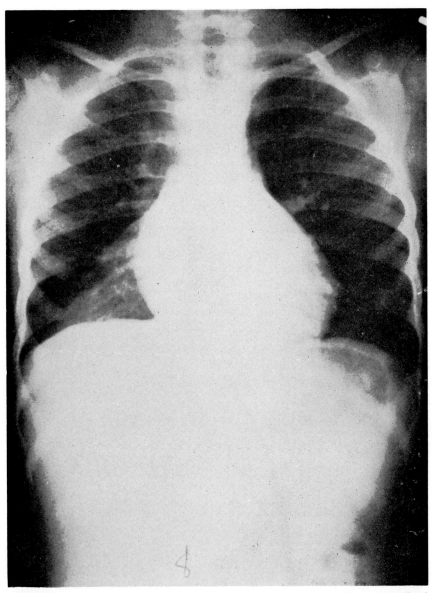

Figure 13-4.   Same patient as in Figure 13-3 in another crisis eighteen months later with clinical evidence of another pulmonary infarction.

this complication and it is postulated that an altered state of coagulation resulted secondary to the use of the diuretic or steroids. Severe dehydration from any cause may rarely be complicated by pulmonary thrombosis in children. Homocystinuria,[7] a rare metabolic defect, may also be complicated by vascular thrombosis. As in adults thromboembolism may become a problem in infants or children whenever a hypercoagulable state is present.

Septic Thromboemboli

Some of our recent medical advances have actually increased the over-all incidence of pulmonary thromboembolism in children. Septic emboli in the pulmonary vessels are frequently seen when infection occurs follow-ing prolonged deep intravenous therapy. The use of umbilical catheters, long-term deep intravenous therapy for alimentation and the presence of a foreign body in the vascular system are frequently complicated by in-fection, thrombosis and emboli. The organism is often of an indolent nature and frequently difficult to erradicate. Figure 13-5 shows the hyphae of monilia which was found in a pulmonary vessel at autopsy. Strict sepsis is essential and the prompt removal of a foreign body should infection occur is necessary to prevent this dreaded complication. The thrombus frequently involves the superior vena cava and tricuspid valve, and then, of course, may easily embolize to the lung.

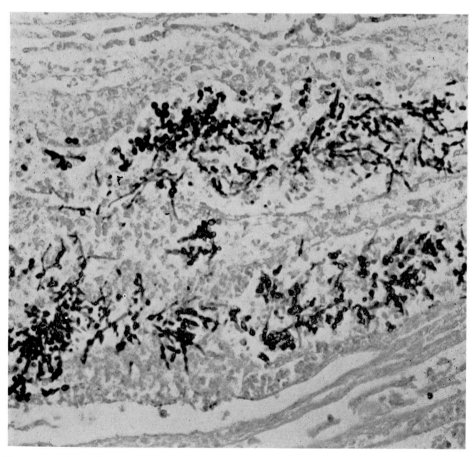

Figure 13-5. Pulmonary blood vessel showing monilia hyphae in an infant dying of sepsis following prolonged deep intravenous alimentation.

Ventriculovenous Shunts

We personally[8] have been interested in the problem of pulmonary emboli in children with ventriculovenous shunts to control hydrocephalus. A catheter is placed in the cerebral ventricle attached to a one-way valve which drains cerebral spinal fluid via another catheter directly into the cardiovascular system. The distal end of the catheter may be placed in the superior vena cava or right atrium. Acute cor pulmonale from massive pulmonary emboli has been reported as a complication particularly when acute infection occurs on the cardiac end of the catheter.[9] In addition, we have seen several children who developed insidious cardiac failure from cor pulmonale which could be attributed to multiple recurrent pulmonary emboli. This complication may occur with or without chronic infection.[10-12] The clinical picture resembles that of primary pulmonary hypertension. Both our patients developed chronic heart failure with evidence of tricuspid insufficiency and severe pulmonary artery hypertension which could be demonstrated at cardiac catheterization. There was a low cardiac output and death occurred a few months following diagnosis.

The exact mechanism of this interesting complication of ventricular venous shunts is unknown. The foreign body catheter in the vascular system frequently becomes plugged with small fibrin clots and results in so-called "shunt failure" which requires reoperation. It is possible that the repeated emboli of these small fibrin clots result in severe pulmonary hypertension. In many of the cases coming to autopsy, there is thrombosis of the superior vena cava around the catheter and often large thrombi are present in the right atrium so that repeated blood clots to the pulmonary artery is a more likely explanation. The possibility of an autoimmune reaction of the pulmonary vessels to cerebral spinal fluid has also been postulated.[13] The exact incidence of this complication is unknown but appears to be relatively uncommon. *Schistosomiasis*, a problem in some tropical countries, is also a recognized cause of cor pulmonale.[14-16] The schistosoma ova apparently embolize to the lungs and result eventually in an endarteritis, thrombosis, and intimal thickening of the pulmonary vessels. Granuloma in the lung tissue and identification of the ova permits differentiation from primary pulmonary hypertension.

Primary Pulmonary Hypertension

Primary pulmonary hypertension is a rare but recognized cause of cor pulmonale in children[17, 18] and it may be difficult to differentiate from repeated small pulmonary emboli. In the classic report by Wagenvoort[19] he found that of 156 cases diagnosed originally as primary hypertension, thirty-one on closer examination were due to chronic thromboembolism.

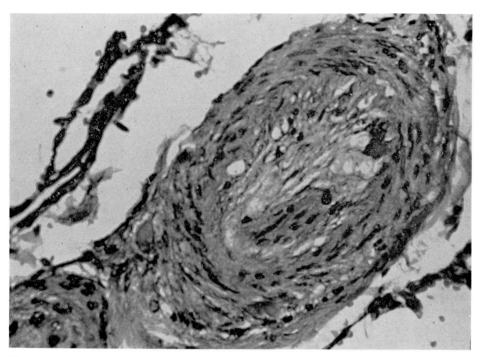

Figure 13-6. Marked intimal changes in a pulmonary vessel of an eleven-month-old infant with primary pulmonary hypertension.

Although primary pulmonary hypertension is usually considered a disease of young females, in Wagenvoort's report of 110 patients, thirty-nine were fifteen years of age or less, including eleven patients under one year of age. The etiology of primary pulmonary artery hypertension remains unknown although a genetic factor is suspected because in some cases there is a positive family history. The symptoms develop insidiously and include fatigue, dyspnea on exertion, syncope, convulsions and sometimes congestive cardiac failure. Figure 13-6 shows a small pulmonary vessel in an eleven-year-old child who died from primary pulmonary hypertension. She had frequent spells of hypernea resembling, in a striking fashion, the hypoxic spells seen in patients with tetralogy of fallot.

Tumor Thromboemboli

We recently saw an interesting patient who developed acute cor pulmonale during surgery. This was a two-year-old boy who presented with an abdominal mass. His initial chest X-ray was normal and no heart murmur was heard on physical examination. An intravenous pyelogram revealed displacement of the kidney and a diagnosis of Wilms' tumor was made. At operation there was involvement of the inferior vena cava so that

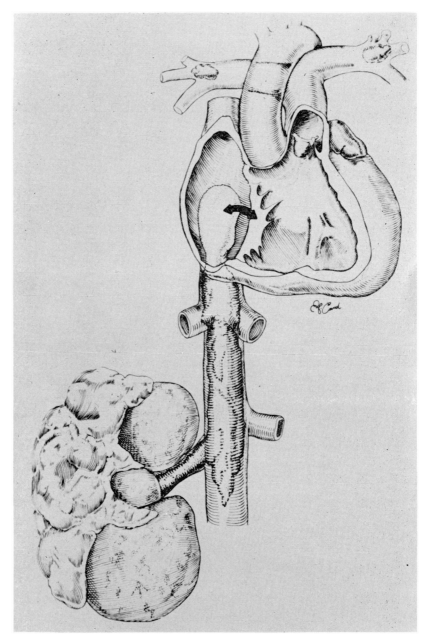

Figure 13-7.   Drawing of Wilms' tumor showing extension up the inferior vena cava into the right atrium with emboli to the pulmonary vessels.

complete resection was not possible. A diagnostic biopsy was obtained. At the conclusion of surgery, when the patient's position was changed, a sudden cardiac arrest occurred. Tumor embolization was suspected and under deep hypothermia cardiac exploration was performed. When the right atrium was opened, the tumor was seen to extend from the inferior vena cava into the right atrium through the tricuspid valve (Fig. 13-7). Tumor was also found in both pulmonary artery branches and this apparently accounted for the sudden acute cardiac arrest. After removal of the tumor from the heart and pulmonary arteries, the child made a good recovery. He awakened promptly and suffered no apparent neurological deficit.

An inferior vena cavagram was performed following surgery which showed complete obstruction of the inferior vena cava with all blood flow from the lower extremities occurring by a collateral flow through the azygous system. In retrospect, an inferior vena cavagram should have been performed prior to surgery and if inferior vena cava involvement were evident, cardiac exploration could have been planned. There are now a number of reports of tumors in children with extension from the inferior vena cava into the heart complicated by pulmonary emboli.[20, 21] With vigorous, aggressive treatment some of these children have had apparent cure.

Pulmonary Thromboemboli Complicating Cardiac Disease

As in adults, chronic congestive cardiac failure, particularly when associated with low cardiac output and stasis, may be complicated by pulmonary emboli and infarction. This may also occur when right-sided bacterial endocarditis complicates a cardiac defect. In my experience, children with primary myocardial disease are especially likely to have the complication of pulmonary emboli with infarction. The dreaded complication of pulmonary vascular disease as a complication of long-term severe pulmonary hypertension accompanying large left to right shunts in children is certainly another cause of pulmonary thrombosis. Microscopic findings in a child with advanced pulmonary vascular disease resembles that of primary pulmonary vascular disease which is felt to represent thrombosis of the pulmonary vessels with secondary recanalization. These lesions were first described by Rich[22] in patients dying with tetralogy of Fallot. The exact pathogenesis of these lesions is unknown.

Thrombosis of the pulmonary arteries may occur secondary to surgical procedures. The Glenn operation, in which the superior vena cava is anastamosed to the right pulmonary artery, may be complicated by thrombosis of the superior vena cava and the entire right pulmonary artery. Sometimes a shunt between the subclavian artery and the pulmonary artery may clot and a pulmonary thrombosis may result.

Congenital abnormalities of the pulmonary artery itself may predispose to thrombosis. A patient with multiple pulmonary artery branch stenoses was noted at his original study to have a main pulmonary artery pressure

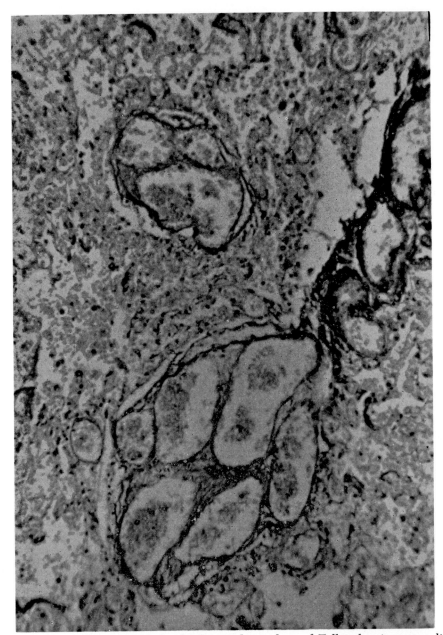

Figure 13-8.　Pulmonary vessels of infant with tetralogy of Fallot showing recanalization. (Rich lesions.)

of 80/6 mm Hg while that in the right pulmonary artery was 22/7 mm Hg. An angiogram made at that time showed a discrete narrowing at the origin of the right main pulmonary artery. There were also several areas of stenoses present in the left pulmonary artery. On follow-up the murmur previously present over the right chest disappeared. Repeat study showed the

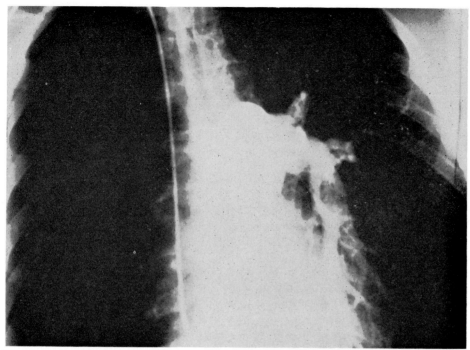

Figure 13-9.   Pulmonary arteriogram showing no filling of the right pulmonary artery. Patient had congenital stenosis of the right pulmonary artery on a previous study which progressed to complete obstruction on a follow-up study.

main pulmonary artery pressure to be 50/10 and in the left pulmonary artery 28/12. The right pulmonary artery could not be entered. An angiogram was performed and Figure 13-9 shows the lack of filling of the right pulmonary artery. The left pulmonary artery filled well and although the discrete areas of stenoses are not well seen there were pressure gradients apparent at several branches of the left pulmonary artery. Occlusion of the right pulmonary artery apparently occurred at the site of the congenital stenoses. Congenital absence of a pulmonary artery is a relatively uncommon cardiac defect and in a patient living at normal altitude, it is usually quite well tolerated.[23] Figure 13-10 shows the chest X-ray of another child who at first glance might suggest absence of the left pulmonary artery; however, in this case there was diffuse sacular bronchiectasis of the left lung with an entirely destroyed left lung. At cardiac catheterization, a catheter easily entered the left pulmonary artery although by angiogram no dye entered the pulmonary artery. The blood flow to the left pulmonary artery was from extensive bronchial collaterals. By angiography alone, such an entity could simulate thrombosis or absence of the left pulmonary artery. In this particular child, a left pneumonectomy was carried out and the child has done well since.

Figure 13-11 is of a rather interesting and unfortunate patient who had

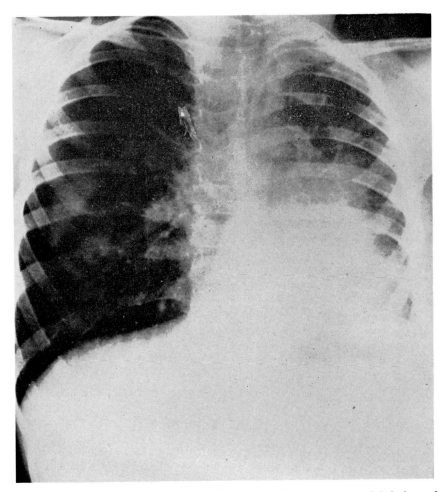

Figure 13-10.   Chest roentgenogram of three-year-old with destroyed left lung from bronchiectasis.

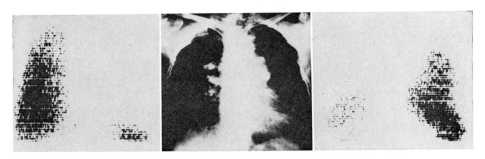

Figure 13-11.   Patient with "accidental" division of left pulmonary artery in place of a patent ductus arteriosis. Lung scan on right shows prompt filling of the right lung with no flow to the left lung. Aortic root injection on the left shows blood flow to the left lung is via collateral systemic circulation.

his left pulmonary artery accidently divided at the time of surgery instead of a patent ductus arteriosus. Injection of I-131 macroaggragate albumin showed prompt filling of the right lung and almost no flow to the left lung. An aortic root injection, on the other hand, showed the blood flow to the left lung was via collateral circulation from the aorta. Accidental division of a pulmonary artery is fortunately an uncommon cause of pulmonary artery occlusion.

In summary, pulmonary thromboembolism in children, while less frequent than in adults, does present a real challenge. We must be alert to the possibility of this complication whenever certain predisposing factors are present. The etiologic factors are varied and often extremely interesting.

REFERENCES

1. Haber, S. L. and Bennington, J. L.: Pulmonary embolism in an infant. *J Pediatr,* *61*:759, 1962.
2. Groniowski, J.: Thrombotic arteriolar lesions in the lungs of newborn. *Arch Path,* 75:144, 1963.
3. Diggs, L. W.: Sickle cell crises. *Am J Clin Pathol, 44*:1, 1965.
4. Yater, W. M. and Hansmann, G. H.: Sickle cell anemia: A new cause of cor pulmonale. Report of two cases with numerous disseminated occlusions of the small pulmonary arteries. *Am J Med Sci, 191*:474, 1936.
5. Gottman, N., Gross, J. and Mensch, A.: Pulmonary artery thrombosis; a complication occurring with prednisone and chlorothiazide therapy in two nephrotic patients. *Pediatrics, 34*:861, 1964.
6. Symchych, P. S. and Perrin, E. V.: Thrombosis of the main pulmonary artery in nephrosis. *Am J Dis Child, 110*:636, 1965.
7. McKusick, V.: *Heritable Disorders of Connective Tissue,* 3rd ed. St. Louis, C. V. Mosby Co., 1966, p. 150.
8. Noonan, M. A. and Ehmke, D. A.: Complications of ventriculovenous shunts for control of hydrocephalus. Report of 3 cases with thromboemboli to the lungs. *N Engl J Med, 269*:70, 1963.
9. Emery, J. L. and Hilton, H. B.: Lung and heart complications of treatment of hydrocephalus by ventriculoauriculostomy. *Surgery, 50*:309, 1961.
10. Nugent, G. R., Lucas, R., Judy, M., Bloor, B. M. and Warden, J.: Thromboembolic complications of ventriculoatrial shunts—Angiocardiographic and pathologic correlations. *J Neurosurg, 24*:34, 1966.
11. Sperling, D. R., Patrick, J. R., Anderson, F. M. and Fyler, D. C.: Cor pulmonale secondary to ventriculoauriculostomy. *Am J Dis Child, 107*:308, 1964.
12. Talner, M. S., Liu, H. Y., Oberman, H. A. and Schmidt, R. W.: Thromboembolism complicating holter valve shunt. A clinicopathologic study of four patients treated with this procedure for hydrocephalus. *Am J Dis Child, 101*:602, 1961.
13. Favara, B. E. and Paul, R. N.: Thromboembolism and cor pulmonale complicating ventriculovenous shunts. *JAMA, 199*:668, 1967.
14. De Faria, J. L.: Cor pulmonale in Manson's schistosomiasis. *Am J Pathol, 30*:167, 1954.
15. Kenaway, M. R.: The syndrome of cardiopulmonary schistosomiasis (cor pulmonale). *Am Heart J, 39*:678, 1950.

16. Naeye, R. L.: Advanced pulmonary vascular changes in schistosomal cor pulmonale. *Am J Trop Med, 10*:191, 1961.

17. Husson, G. S. and Wyatt, T. C.: Primary pulmonary vascular obstruction in children. *Pediatrics, 36*:75, 1965.

18. Thilenius, O. G., Nadas, A. S. and Jockin, H.: Primary pulmonary vascular obstruction in children. *Pediatrics, 36*:75, 1965.

19. Wagenvoort, C. A. and Wagenvoort, N.: Primary pulmonary hypertension: A pathologic study of the lung vessels in 156 clinically diagnosed cases. *Circulation, 42*:1163, 1970.

20. Anselmi, G., Suarez, J. A., Machado, L., Moleiro, F. and Blanco, P.: Wilms' tumor propagated through the inferior vena cava into the right heart cavities. *Br Heart J, 32*:575, 1970.

21. Murphy, D. A., Rabinovitch, H., Chevalier, L. and Virmani, S.: Propagation of Wilms' tumor into the right atrium. *Am J Dis Child, 126*:210, 1973.

22. Rick, A. R.: A hitherto unrecognized tendency to the development of widespread pulmonary vascular obstruction in patients with pulmonary stenosis (tetralogy of Fallot). *Bull Johns Hopkins Hosp, 82*:389, 1948.

23. Pool, P. E., Vogel, J. H. K. and Blount, S. G., Jr.: Congenital unilateral absence of a pulmonary artery. *Am J Cardiol, 10*:706, 1962.

Chapter 14

PULMONARY THROMBOEMBOLISM—
PATHOPHYSIOLOGY

Joseph C. Parker, Jr. (Moderator), Arthur A. Sasahara,

Donald Silver, John Spittel

D R. DIXON (Utah): I would like to ask Dr. Spittell if he had documented a hypercoagulable state in women taking birth control pills?

Dr. Spittell: In the third trimester of pregnancy, one sees all sorts of clotting changes and there are remarkable elevations of Factor VII and Factor IX and several other plasmatic coagulation activities. In women taking the oral contraceptive, it's like a mini-pregnancy and one sees coagulation changes in the same direction. One of the problems we had with the concept of hypercoagulability in the early days was a rather nice study by Dr. Ben Alexander in Boston of a series of pregnant women showing these remarkable changes in the clotting factors and yet, none of those women had thromboembolism. Consequently our detectors at the time felt that we were looking at what amounted to a myth in terms of a possible cause of thrombosis. Why some women have thromboembolism when they take oral contraceptives, I'm not sure. The fact that some do, and the clotting changes that one can demonstrate in these patients are not different one from the other, which leads me to feel that hypercoagulability in some situations may be more of a permissive thing or a potentiating factor rather than the true initiating factor. I think this is important because you know the hemophiliac doesn't bleed all the time. He has a low level of Factor VIII all the time, but he doesn't bleed all the time. It takes something to initiate this bleeding and I think when we were having difficulty with the concept of hypercoagulability, those who were pressing us were insisting that we demonstrate cause and effect, so to speak. I am not at all sure that maybe the same situation in reverse doesn't happen in the hypercoagulable state that with some initiating factor, whatever it is, certain people are

151

more prone to thromboses than others. That's a long-winded answer to the pill.

Dr. Hanway (New York): Dr. Parker, I wonder if you would talk to us about the problems that you have had in the autopsy room deciding what part the emboli played in the patient's demise?

Dr. Parker: This can be a problem. Certain morphologic features at autopsy may not apply to an operative blood clot just freshly removed from an arteriotomy site in a recently occluded femoral vessel or an embolectomy specimen from a major pulmonary artery. It is very important to correlate morphologic features with the clinical situation, because there are changes in some postmortem clots—the so-called chicken fat and current jelly types —that mimic a real antemortem thrombus. Even lamination may be found in postmortem clots. Recent thrombi at autopsy cannot be accurately evaluated morphologically and must be correlated with the complete clinical picture. The same problems in the postmortem room occur in clinical settings; for when a thrombus forms, additional thrombotic material can be deposited on it. The latter may be exceedingly difficult to interpret morphologically. I am not aware of a reliable method to separate recent antemortem clots from postmortem clots.

Dr. Murphy (Lexington): Dr. Sasahara, your study showed us the cardiovascular responses to pulmonary embolism in a group of patients; however, I'm sure there were other patients that died before you could study them and I imagine some of these folks that you studied did succumb to their pulmonary emboli. I wonder if you could tell us the relationship between your studies and the survival of these patients?

Dr. Sasahara: I'm not quite sure what you're asking.

Dr. Murphy: Did all the folks that you catheterized survive their pulmonary embolism, or did some of them die?

Dr. Sasahara: No, some of them died.

Dr. Murphy: Was there any relationship between the cardiovascular changes and death or survival?

Dr. Sasahara: Yes, I think the remarkable thing is, if the patients were previously normal, they do remarkably well despite extensive degrees of vascular obstruction. The ones who die are primarily those with prior serious cardiopulmonary disease, as I will show you this afternoon. From our experience, as well as the NIH combined Urokinase Study, the high mortality is found in those patients who have moderate amounts of embolism superimposed on bad heart and lung disease.

Dr. Murphy: Just the second part of that question then, how many folks had sudden deaths and died of pulmonary embolism before you could get them down to the cath lab during this period of time?

Dr. Sasahara: I can quote you some data from the Tufts New England Medical Center where my colleague Dr. McIntyre made a survey. In that hospital, during the survey period, 50 percent of sudden deaths were due to pulmonary emboli.

Dr. Hirsh (Hamilton): Dr. Parker, it is not uncommon to see patients with pleurisy but no radiological changes and one is left uncertain as to whether the pleurisy is due to pulmonary embolism or not. Do you think from your experience with clinicopathological correlations that it is possible to get a pulmonary infarct producing pleurisy with no radiological changes?

Dr. Parker: I do not have any significant experience to help solve this problem. Occasional autopsied patients have small recurrent pulmonary emboli that are associated with localized areas of chronic fibrosing pleuritis. These lesions may represent small, well orgnized infarcts, but unfortunately, these are end stage changes of nonspecific scarring. An experimental model like Dr. Silver's dog studies should add some light to this matter. At autopsy occasional small recurrent pulmonary emboli are associated with focal chronic pleuritis but whether the latter represents a well organized infarct is not apparent. Maybe Dr. Silver has some information on this from his experimental models.

Dr. Silver: Our dog experiments were all acute and do not contain answers to the question. However, I do think, Dr. Hirsh, that patients have emboli and infarcts that don't appear roentgenographically. Dr. Sasahara, what do you think?

Dr. Sasahara: I think it's also a function of size, don't you?

Dr. Silver: Yes, there are patients that have pain and pleuritic symptoms with abnormal lung scans or pulmonary angiograms which never have abnormal chest films. I am confident that some of these patients have had an embolus and infarction in spite of the "normal" chest X-ray.

Dr. Hirsh: We would perform a venogram and a lung scan and if the venogram was negative and the chest X-ray and lung scan were negative, we would not treat this patient as a pulmonary embolus.

Dr. Parker: I would agree with Dr. Hirsh. A lung scan does not seem capable of defining the small peripheral pulmonary emboli found at autopsy. In most debilitated necropsied patients, small peripherally located organized and recent pulmonary thromboemboli are observed and are probably too small to be recognized in the lung scan.

Dr. Hirsh: I entirely agree. To elaborate on the answer to this question, we would do a venogram, and if the patient were ambulant, had a normal venogram including patent iliacs, and a negative lung scan, we would not treat this patient. If the patient were in the hospital we would perform ^{125}I-fibrinogen scanning.

Question: Supposing your hospitalized patient is postoperative with pleuritic chest pain yet a negative venogram and negative leg scan.

Dr. Hirsh: Before we had leg scanning available, we used to treat these patients. Now that we have leg scanning we would scan those patients who are at high risk from bleeding; for example, those patients in the first few postoperative days, and not treat them if the leg scan, venogram and lung scan were negative but if there were no contraindication to anticoagulants and the patient were in bed and immobile we would treat with anticoagulants. As so often happens in medicine, one has to weigh the risks associated with the various approaches.

Dr. Webber (Illinois): Dr. Spittell, in the pure form of idiopathic recurrent thromboembolism, do all of these people have an abnormal thromboplastin generation test and is it a completely accurate screening test?

Dr. Spittell: No, I can't say that 100 percent do. By the same token, I can't say that I have studied them all at the right time. I suspect that at some time, most of them do. Percentagewise, I can't give you a figure that I could document. If you look at a large series with just one study done on each patient, about half of them will show it, but with a limited number of serial studies over a long period, the percentage goes up over 70 percent, and perhaps if you studied them every week in bigger numbers, you might kick it higher. I don't know whether idiopathic recurrent thrombophlebitis and pulmonary embolism is a pure syndrome or not. I suspect that it isn't. There may be a familial type and there may be a nonfamilial or acquired type or several, I don't really know. At the moment, I prefer to lump them until I know more about them. There may be multiple mechanisms involved.

Dr. Webber: You do restudy them everytime they have another thrombotic episode if you can.

Dr. Spittell: Not anymore, unless they are a patient of particular interest to our study, because I think we've done enough to know what's going on. At the moment I am more interested in the familial type.

Dr. Zimmerman (Rockford): Dr. Sasahara, do you have any clues in the physiology of pulmonary emboli in chronic obstructive lung disease that would help you detect its occurrence in patients who already have cardiovascular changes secondary to their chronic lung disease, say such as responsiveness to oxygen.

Dr. Sasahara: We have looked at that and I am not sure that it really helps, because in hypoxemic patients, secondary to lung disease, if one does a catheter study with pulmonary pressure measurements, giving oxygen will probably drop the pulmonary artery pressure. I don't think that helps you. I thought you were referring to the fact that if one does a Xenon perfusion and ventilation scan in the acute state, it might help differentiate between pulmonary embolism and chronic lung disease. Pulmonary embolism would have no perfusion or bad perfusion, but good ventilation, whereas in chronic lung disease, there would be bad perfusion and bad ventilation. That's not absolute either, because there is a time interval in which this holds true. It must be done in the acute stage. I hope Dr. Wagner will cover that tomorrow, it appears to be a useful test, and it's not invasive, relative speaking.

Question: Dr. Spittell, I am sure you use Coumadin long-term on your patients with idiopathic thrombophlebitis. One question is, when do you decide on how long to treat them and if you do decide to stop therapy, what criteria do you use?

Dr. Spittell: We use Warfarin. I don't have any real good objective way to tell you when to use long-term anticoagulant therapy in recurrent thrombophlebitis and it is difficult after the first episode to know which patients should you manage long-term and what do you mean by long-term. After the first episode, if it is significant, I generally keep the patient on long-term anticoagulant therapy for about a year and discuss with him the fact that I don't have any way of telling if and when he will ever have another episode nor of what magnitude it will be. My therapy carries some risks as well, and he and I mutually decide whether we should try it with or without indefinite long-term anticoagulant therapy. I think a good rule of thumb about indefinite long-term anticoagulant therapy is that if the patient's episodes of thromboembolism are sufficiently frequent to warrant the expense and risk of long-term anticoagulant therapy, then it ought to be used. Once in a while you encounter a patient with this problem who lives in a community where he doesn't have access to good management of long-term anticoagulant therapy. In some of those situations, after a period of time, when we found a way to do it that was not really practical indefinitely, we took the patient off of anticoagulant therapy, and I have been surprised that some of them haven't had recurrences. I don't know any way to tell.

Question: Have you found that any unusual factors in these people with idiopathic thrombophlebitis, such as infection in the feet, ingrown toenail, or some psychic trauma, produce recurrent thrombi?

Dr. Spittell: No.

Dr. Sasahara: Could I just comment on that before the next question. I think the availability of the noninvasive tests for deep vein thrombosis which you will hear discussed, the Doppler or the electrical impedance, has really given us a nice handle on how long to continue anticoagulation. For the past year and a half we have tried to answer the question of how long to maintain Warfarin by assessing deep vein patency by impedance (IPG) and lung reperfusion by serial scanning. We continue oral anti-coagulation until the lung scan either becomes normal or stabilizes and the deep veins by IPG become patent. Once the IPG comes back to normal, indicating that the deep venous system is not patent, and the patient is ambulatory and the lung scan is stabilized or normalized, we stop the anti-coagulant. It's difficult to maintain effective long-term anticoagulation. When you really get right down to it, how long you continue anticoagulation depends upon patient reliability—how often he is going to get pro-thrombin time. Therefore, the duration depends on his lungs and legs and ambulation.

Dr. Spittell: Someone who's had a family history of pulmonary embolism, fatal perhaps and there are several families in the literature like that now. I'm more inclined to be aggressive and stay long-term if the patient under-stands the problem we're faced with and the risk we are assuming. I guess I really haven't got enough faith in our laboratory tests as yet to try to place my clinical judgments on them exclusively. I try to look at the situa-tion and the risk these patients take and discuss it with them. I may have a particular course I'd like to follow, but I think the patient, as Art men-tioned, if you are going on long-term anticoagulant therapy indefinitely, you have to have a cooperative patient. In the situation where the family history is bad and the patient has had one episode of thromboembolism or several, I'm inclined without laboratory studies to go long-term. Inciden-tally, with that particular disease, I often hear people talk about idiopathic thrombophlebitis that isn't controlled with oral anticoagulants and my experience with good effective long-term anticoagulant therapy is that I haven't had any problems with idiopathic thrombophlebitis breaking through. When it breaks through, there is something behind the thrombo-embolism. It is no longer idiopathic.

Dr. Alton Oschner (New Orleans): Dr. DeCamp of our institution who has been very much interested in idiopathic thrombembolism, is convinced that tobacco plays a very definite role. What is your experience?

Dr. Spittell: In our series, we haven't been able to document that, Dr. Oschner.

SECTION III

PULMONARY
THROMBOLISM—
DIAGNOSIS

Chapter 15

CHEST X-RAY, PREINFARCTION AND POSTINFARCTION

ALLAN L. SIMON

THE PLAIN CHEST radiographic findings in pulmonary embolism are non-specific; therefore, one can never diagnose pulmonary embolism but only infer the existence of this disease from the combination of clinical signs and radiographic findings.

The explanation for the nonspecificity of the plain film findings in pulmonary embolism is that the films reflect the effect of the embolus on the lungs rather than visualizing the embolus itself.

The sudden occlusion of a pulmonary vessel results in the following pulmonary events, not necessarily in sequence. There is oligemia and ischemia of the affected area of lung. Pleuritic pain causes splinting of respiration. There are marked intrapulmonary shifts in ventilation and circulation secondary to the effects of the embolus and the mechanical splinting.

Table 15-I lists the plain film findings from four relatively large series of patients with proven pulmonary embolism.

When one eliminates the very high incidence of local oligemia in the study by Kerr, the most common radiographic findings of pulmonary embolism are a triad of elevated diaphragm, pleural effusion, and an infiltrate or atelectasis.

TABLE 15-I

Signs	Stein series	Kerr	Szucs	McDonald	Total	
Normal chest	12/72	0/25	14/50	2/23	28/165	17%
Local oligemia		25/25		10/23	35/48	73%
Local hyperemia		10/25			10/25	40%
Plump PA/Hilum		17/25			17/25	68%
Atelectasis	19/72				19/72	26%
Infiltrate	39/72	14/25	25/50	9/23	78/148	53%
Elevated diaphragm	21/72	8/25	13/50		42/148	28%
Pleural effusion	33/72		17/50		50/122	41%

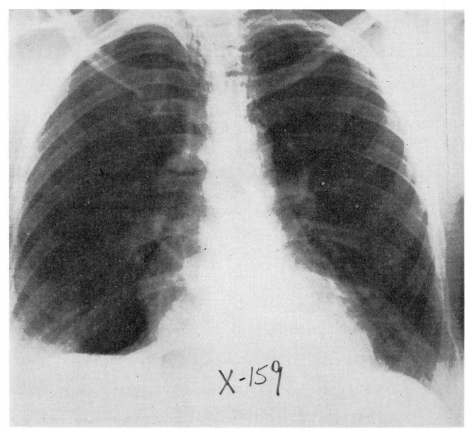

Figure 15-1A.   Plain chest radiograph in a patient with proven pulmonary embolism shows slightly plump right hilum as well as slight oligemia of the right lower lung field.

The combination of oligemia and a plump hilum, the so-called Wester-mark sign occurred in less than 3 percent of the series. (Fig. 15-1)

Infiltrates can be either of two types in this disease. The most commonly mentioned infiltrate is that seen when pulmonary infarction occurs. The characteristic radiographic appearance of an infarct has been described by Fleischner. The infarct presents as a hump-shaped consolidation with the base applied to a pleural surface and the apex pointing toward the hilum. This shadow is caused by edema and/or hemorrhagic necrosis of lung secondary to the ischemia. The incidence of infarction has been reported in various series to be from ten to forty percent of patients with pulmonary embolism and usually occurs only when there is embarrassed circulation along with the embolism.

The second type of infiltrate seen in pulmonary embolism is not the well-defined hump-shaped infiltrate of an infarction but is rather larger, less

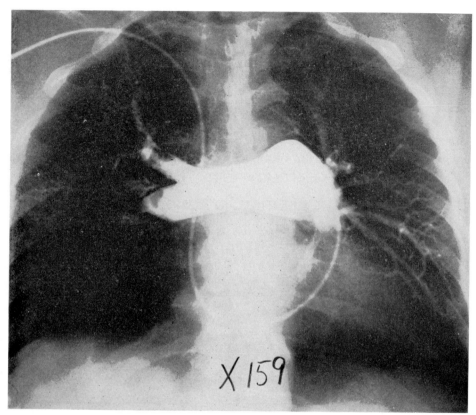

Figure 15-1B.   Is the angiogram made within hours of the chest X-ray. There is indeed a mass of pulmonary embolism occluding the right lower lobe pulmonary artery, causing a bulging hilum as well as oligemia to the right lower lobe. However, there is also a marked restriction of blood flow to the left lower lobe and considerable restriction of blood flow to both upper lobes.

dense, and less defined. This type is much more common, occurring in about three of four patients with embolism; it is most likely a small area of localized pulmonary edema rather than hemorrhage. This is the infiltrate which tends to disappear rapidly over three to five days and its method of resolution has been termed melting.

Oligemia is probably the first radiographic sign of pulmonary embolism, preceding the appearance of an infiltrate by up to 24 hours. The localization of the oligemia is not very helpful in localizing the site of pulmonary embolism. Generally, oligemia is quite focal in spite of diffuse embolism.

Atelectasis is the most commonly encountered plain film finding in pulmonary embolism in my experience. This phenomenon, however, is so nonspecific that one cannot determine whether it is secondary to the embolus or secondary to splinting of the lung from any cause. During the evolution of proven pulmonary embolism, atelectasis always occurs. The oligemias and ill defined infiltrates being much less common.

The significant problems encountered with the chest film in pulmonary embolism are: (1) The frequent confusion of embolism and infarction. These two pathologic entities are frequently thought of interchangeably; and the nonspecific findings of embolism can occasionally mimic the findings of pulmonary infarction. (2) The nonspecific chest findings can be caused by many other disease entities.

Differential Dx. Plain film findings such as occur in pulmonary embolism can be seen in a variety of other conditions:

DIFFERENTIAL DIAGNOSIS

Pneumonia
Pleurodynia
Costochondritis
Carcinoma—primary or metastatic
Emphysema
Asthma
Acute M.I.
Pericarditis
Dressler's Syndrome
Peritonitis
Subdiaphragmatic Disease
Septicemia
Dissecting Aneurysm

Summary

The plain chest radiographic findings in pulmonary embolism, the result of a variety of events which occur when the circulation to a portion of lung is occluded, are nonspecific. The most commonly occurring changes are: elevated diaphragm due to splinting; some infiltrate or atelectasis, the former being localized areas of edema and the latter occurring secondary to splinting or an intrapulmonary shift in ventilation; and small pleural effusion. When infarction occurs, a typical hump-shaped consolidation is seen.

REFERENCES

Fleischner, F.: Roentgenology of the pulmonary infarct. *Semin Roentgenol*, 2(1):61-76, 1967.

Kerr, I. H., Simon, G. and Sutton, G. C.: The value of the plain radiograph in acute massive pulmonary embolism. *Br J Radiol*, 44:751-757, 1971.

McDonald, I. G., Hirsh, J., Hale, G. S. and O'Sullivan, E. F.: Major pulmonary embolism angiography and pathological physiology. *Br Heart J*, 34(4):356-364, 1972.

Stein, G. N., Chen, J. T., Goldstein, F., Israel, H. L. and Finkelstein, A.: The importance of chest roentgenography in the diagnosis of pulmonary embolism. *Am J Roentgenol, 81*(2):255-263.

Szucs, M. M., Brooks, H. L., Grossman, W., Banas, J. S., Meister, S. G. and Dalen, J. E.: Diagnostic sensitivity of laboratory findings in acute pulmonary embolism. *Ann Int Med, 74*(2):161-166, 1971.

Woesner, M. E., Sanders, I. and White, G. W.: The melting sign in resolving transient pulmonary infarction. *Am J Roetgenol, 111*(4):782-790, 1971.

DISCUSSION

Dr. Rosenbaum: I was interested in whether you believe the plump hilum is due to the embolus or what?

Dr. Simon: My feeling is that the plump hilum is mainly dilatation of the pulmonary artery secondary to the presence of embolus. It is possible that the embolus itself contributes to the bulge of the hilum; however, the embolus causes the bulge by dilating the pulmonary artery.

Dr. Rosenbaum: I believe so too, but if any of you have taken the recent examination of the American College of Radiology for continuing education, you would have missed a few questions by giving that answer, which I did.

Dr. Hanway (New York): The physiologists and pathologists tell us that classically we don't see the infarct in the patient with previously normal heart and lungs. How do you explain?

Dr. Simon: I felt the same way, that you should not have pulmonary infarction unless you have some compromised circulation. The patient must be in heart failure, but in the last case illustrated, as you see, those films were taken in 1971 and for about a year there were infiltrates. I performed that pulmonary angiogram myself and the patient was a colleague; I know that he was not in any trouble at all and to me that looks like pulmonary infarction. So, I have been looking at some of the patients in the Urokinase trial and over the past year I have probably looked at about 200 patients. I don't know their clinical history, but I do know that many of them, on the day after the embolus, have hump-shaped infiltrates, very dense infiltrates. Dr. Sasahara says that 41 percent have infarction, consolidation and not all those patients are in compromised circulatory status.

Dr. Dalen: I think that data actually comes from postmortem series and the problem is that most patients with pulmonary infarction don't die; therefore, the pathologists report that very few people with pulmonary embolism have pulmonary infarction and the ones that do are the ones that have underlying heart disease. That's because they are the ones that die. In our own series very similar to Dr. Sasahara's, at least 40 percent of our patients have what we consider to be pulmonary infarction and most of them don't have underlying heart or lung disease. Pulmonary infarction is very common in healthy people.

Dr. Rosenbaum: Don't you think it is fair to say though, that if you have a series of films over three or four weeks, despite your long differential diagnosis here, we can do really pretty well, suggesting a typical pulmonary infarct on chest films. I really think we are a little better than you might gather from what was said this morning. I always have to talk up radiology.

Dr. Lay (Mississippi): What actually happens to this area of infarction? Does it end up being replaced with scar tissue and concomitant loss of functioning lung tissue?

Dr. Simon: This is a pathological question I guess, but while we are talking about the difference between infiltrates and infarctions and resolution of an infiltrate, I would only give you second hand information just from what I remember reading about this partial infarction. Dr. Fleischner had a concept which I sort of adhere to, that there is very good collateral circulation in the lung and that the hemorrhagic infarction which occurs is very dense consolidation; depending on the state of the circulation, the circulation will eventually probably return, the lung will become normal, or will leave some atelectatic areas and some scars. If you do nothing to a pulmonary embolus, it will be gone in four weeks and there will be restitution of normal circulation for that lung. If the patient can live, there is enough circulating fibrinolytic activity to resolve the pulmonary embolus and as long as that lung can maintain marginal circulation to keep the cells alive and some ventilation, I suspect that you get very little residual complete damage.

Question: So you are really saying not infarction, are you not? You say just severe damage or either that are you talking about a reconstitution or a regrowth of lung tissue, it's either infarcted or not infarcted.

Dr. Simon: Lung tissue doesn't regrow. I don't know whether or not there are nonfunctioning alveoli, all I know is that the chest X-ray can look normal in patients who have had proven infarction. Most often you will see a little scar which looks like a scar of anything else.

Dr. Hirsh: Do you accept that you can get a patient with recurrent pleurisy with completely normal chest X-rays and lung scans, and if so how frequently do you find this occurring? The clinical problem with recurrent pleurisy, you think this is due to an embolus, you investigate the patient with the techniques described and are normal.

Dr. Simon: I can't talk about lung scans, because Dr. Wagner, I'm sure, still believes that nobody with an embolus has a normal lung scan. I think that is almost always true. There may be an occasional exception, so I would say if you had a normal chest X-ray and a normal lung scan and pleurisy you would have to think about other causes. The most common etiology of that syndrome which I saw a few years ago was patients on oral contraceptives who had recurrent episodes of pleuritic pain, small pleural effusions and normal scans. We angiogrammed a large series of these patients looking for emboli. They had classical symptoms that mimicked an embolus, but no embolus was seen.

Chapter 16

RADIOACTIVE TRACERS IN THE DIFFERENTIAL DIAGNOSIS OF PULMONARY EMBOLISM

HENRY N. WAGNER, JR. AND H. WILLIAM STRAUSS

OUR UNDERSTANDING of the clinical manifestations and pathogenesis of pulmonary embolism began over a century ago with the studies of Virchow,[1] Cohn,[2] and Flint.[3] Until recently most of our knowledge of pulmonary embolism came from pathological examination which created the impression that the disease is frequently fatal. During the last decade, the application of lung scanning and pulmonary arteriography as diagnostic aids made possible more accurate diagnosis of the patient with nonfatal disease, and consequently better characterized the spectrum of disease. Although at one time it was believed that pulmonary embolism was nearly always fatal, we now know that this is not the case. In the recent cooperative Urokinase Pulmonary Embolism Trial, the mortality was less than 10 percent despite the fact that the average size of the perfusion defects was equivalent of one half of one lung.[4]

Until the report of Hampton and Castleman[5] pulmonary embolism was thought to occur primarily in postoperative patients. These investigators found that the disease was more common among medical than surgical patients. After the electrocardiographic studies of McGinn and White in 1935[6] and those of Hampton and Castleman in 1940, the electrocardiogram and chest X-ray became the main diagnostic tools. Neither, however, was sufficiently sensitive or specific. Lung scanning and arteriography were sensitive and specific respectively and made possible identification of those patients who had pulmonary embolism from among those whose symptoms and signs were due to other causes, chiefly myocardial infarction or parenchymal lung disease. For example, in our patients we found that analysis of clinical manifestations, either singly or in groups, permitted correct prediction of the probability of subsequent arteriographic evidence of pulmonary embolism with a certainty of no greater than one to three. These results were obtained from the study of a patient population whose clinical manifestations of pulmonary embolism were sufficiently suggestive that an arteriogram was performed. Only one in three such patients had arteriographic evidence of pulmonary embolism.

Why is the diagnosis of pulmonary embolism difficult?

When we look at the pathophysiologic consequences of pulmonary embolism (Table 16-I), we can see that most of them result from generalized

TABLE 16-I

MANIFESTATIONS OF PULMONARY EMBOLISM

Pulmonary Hypertension
  Mechanical
  Reflex
Systemic Hypotension
  Reflex
  Decreased cardiac output
Right Ventricular Failure
  Increased work
  Decreased myocardial oxygenation
Tachypnea
  Reflex
Bronchoconstriction
  Reflex
  Low alveolar CO_2
  Humoral
Pulmonary Edema
  Reflex
Hypoxia
  Right to left shunting
  Diffusion abnormalities
  Abnormal ventilation perfusion ratio

failure of the circulation, whether the cause is failure of the myocardial pump as in myocardial infarction or obstruction of the pulmonary vascular bed as in pulmonary embolism. In Figure 16-1 A, B, the incidence of certain features of pulmonary embolism are compared in three groups of patients[7]: (1) those with specific angiographic findings of pulmonary embolism, that is, filling defects in the contrast media; (2) those with nonspecific angiographic abnormalities; and (3) those with a normal pulmonary angiogram. The patients in all three categories were so strongly suspected of having pulmonary embolism that a pulmonary arteriogram was performed as part of the diagnostic process.

Hemoptysis was present in only 15 percent of the patients with pulmonary embolism and not significantly different among the three groups of patients; pleuritic pain was present in about 40 percent of the patients with

CLINICAL FEATURES

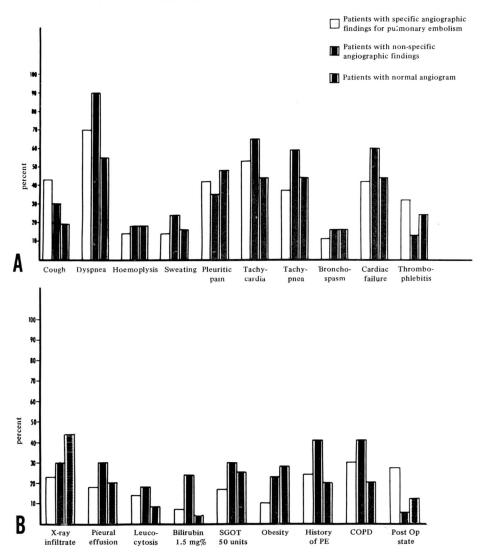

Figure 16-1. (A) Clinical findings and (B) Laboratory findings in three groups of patients undergoing pulmonary angiography for the suspected diagnosis of pulmonary embolism (after Poulose, et al. ref. no. 7).

angiographic evidence of embolism; thrombophlebitis in about 30 percent. Radiographic infiltrates were twice as common in those without angiographic evidence of pulmonary embolism as in those with pulmonary embolism. We can conclude that if the physician waits for the occurrence of the classical triad of pleuritic pain, hemoptysis and thrombophlebitis before making the diagnosis, he will frequently miss the diagnosis. Similarly, if he relies entirely on his clinical impression, he will needlessly treat about two-thirds of his patients. It seems clear that ancillary diagnostic tests are needed, although the alert clinician remains the first line in the diagnostic process. No diagnostic test is as yet so simple that it can be recommended for routine screening of even high risk populations, such as those with congestive heart failure or in a postoperative state.

What should the physician do if pulmonary embolism is suspected?

If, on the basis of clinical evidence there is a reasonably high probability of the patient's having pulmonary embolism, treatment is often begun with anticoagulant drugs and other diagnostic tests are carried out to increase or decrease the probability that the working diagnosis is correct. Figure 16-2 is a schematic illustration of the decision process as originally proposed by Sasahara.[8]

Pulmonary Thromboembolism

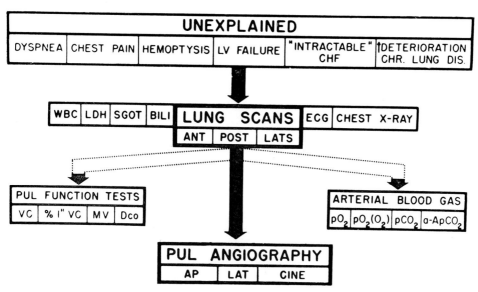

Figure 16-2. Decision process leading the physician to the diagnosis of pulmonary embolism.

In some patients, the diagnostic process will not require a pulmonary arteriogram, since the decision to treat with anticoagulants can be made without it. On the other hand, if the diagnostic certainty is not sufficiently great, an arteriogram should be performed. This will either lower the probability below the point when anticoagulation will be indicated or provide a clear-cut indication.

Does a normal lung scan rule out pulmonary embolism?

Table 16-II summarizes the results of a study that was performed soon after the introduction of lung scanning.[7] At that time, in twenty-one patients in whom a four-view lung scan was completely normal, a pulmonary arteriogram was performed on the basis of strong clinical evidence for pulmonary embolism. In none of these patients was there angiographic evidence of pulmonary embolism. On the other hand, when the scan was interpreted as indicating a high probability of pulmonary embolism, 75 percent of the patients had filling defects in the contrast media.

TABLE 16-II

SPECIFICITY AND SENSITIVITY OF LUNG SCANNING

Scan Interpretation	No.	Angiographic Diagnosis Specific P.E. %	Nonspecific P.E. %	Normal %
High probability	55	75	9	16
Low probability	32	19	53	28
Normal	21	0	5	95
Total	108	44	21	35

We can conclude that if a technically adequate four-view lung scan is completely normal, pulmonary embolism is very unlikely. Similar results were subsequently reported by Dalen and his associates.[10] Lung scanning is a very sensitive test for pulmonary embolism.

What about other examinations?

In the Urokinase Pulmonary Embolism Trial 12 percent of the patients had arterial oxygen saturation values greater than eighty mm Hg.[9] Similarly the EKG was normal in 13 percent, serum enzymes normal in 50 percent and the classical triad was present in only 4 percent. Thus, none of these were sufficiently sensitive or specific to serve as the only criteria for pulmonary embolism. Lung scanning is a more sensitive test for pulmonary embolism. On the other hand, many patients suspected of pulmonary embolism have pulmonary or circulatory disease other than pulmonary embolism that results in abnormal values for these tests.

What about the specificity of lung scanning?

Lung scanning has revealed that all pulmonary diseases, including infectious diseases, neoplasms, chronic obstructive lung disease, and diseases of unknown etiology such as sarcoidosis, are characterized by decreased pulmonary arterial blood flow.[10] This does not mean that the lesions are avascular, but that their blood supply is not arriving via the pulmonary arterial circulation. What is the mechanism of the regional reduction in pulmonary arterial blood flow? In some patients there is mechanical obstruction of the pulmonary arteries or veins; in others, there is obliteration of pulmonary parenchyma, consolidation or alveolar fluid. In other cases, the decreased blood flow is the result of functional vasoconstriction induced by regional hypoxia. As long ago as 1946, von Euler and Lilestrand, on the basis of experimental studies in cats, postulated that alveolar hypoxia resulted in decreased pulmonary arterial blood flow to the involved regions.[11] This can be shown experimentally by partial bronchial occlusion in man and animals and by having patients ventilate one lung with nitrogen rather than oxygen. For example, it was found that ventilating one lung for two minutes with 100 percent nitrogen resulted in a 16 percent decrease in pulmonary arterial blood flow to that lung. Seven minutes of ventilation with 100 percent nitrogen resulted in a 42 percent decrease in blood flow.[12] These changes have been attributed to reflex arteriolar constriction, but recent evidence raises the possibility that it may be the result of local effects of vasoactive substances such as angiotensin-II.[13]

In any case, the universality of perfusion defects in all lung diseases makes the simple finding of a perfusion defect nonspecific. In the early days of lung scanning, this resulted in a common error; if pulmonary embolism was suspected, the finding of a perfusion defect was attributed to pulmonary embolism. This resulted in many so-called "false positives." It is important to realize when we look at a lung scan that we are looking at a regional function, i.e., the relative pulmonary arterial blood flow to various regions of the lung. We must use this information intelligently to arrive at the most likely diagnosis.

How can we increase the specificity of lung scanning?

The first step toward increasing the relative specificity of lung scanning is to characterize the type, size and location of the perfusion defects. It was observed, for example, that about 70 percent of patients with proven pulmonary embolism had concave defects at the periphery of the lungs. This was not a completely specific finding, since about 30 percent of the patients with chronic obstructive lung disease had similar defects,[14] but it was a helpful sign.

When evaluating the lateral views, it becomes clear that these peripheral concave defects seen in the anterior or posterior views represent the projections of various lung segments. In interpreting lung scans, it is quite helpful to have a mental picture of the projection of the various lung segments in various views. Examples of these are shown in Figure 16-3.

In the characterization of perfusion defects, we use the following classifications: (1) segmental—corresponding to one or more segmental arteries;

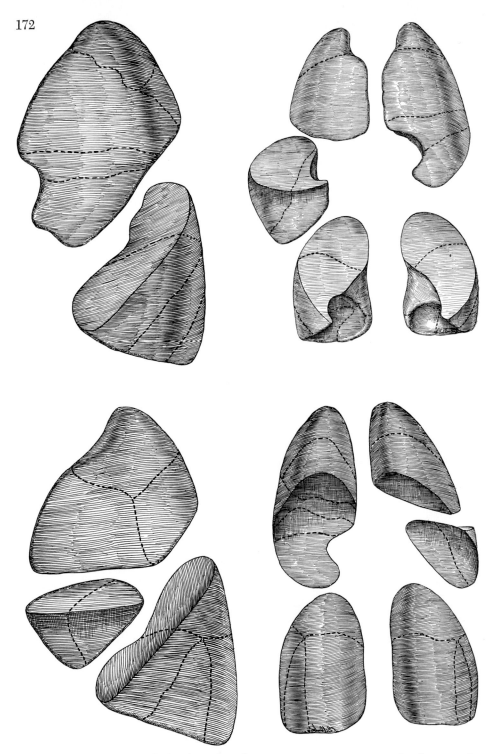

Figure 16-3. Outline of the bronchopulmonary segments as seen in the anterior, posterior and both lateral views (after DeLand and Wagner, *Atlas of Nuclear Medicine*, vol. II, W. B. Saunders Co., Publishers).

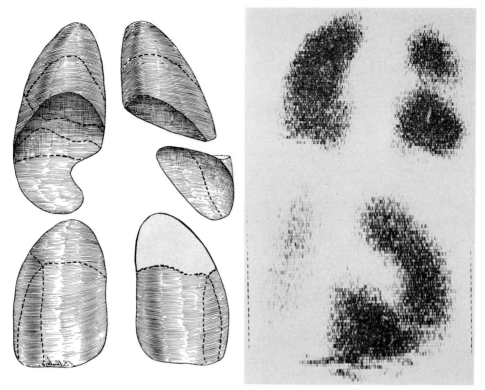

Figure 16-4. Perfusion lung scan in a patient with pulmonary embolism involving the superior segment of the right lower lobe in the posterior and right lateral projections, with accompanying diagram.

(2) nonsegmental—defects crossing the boundary between adjacent segments without corresponding to specific segments; for example, extending up the sides of the lung or symmetrically involving the apices or bases. Examples are shown in Figure 16-4.

Other patterns relatively characteristic of specific conditions are: pulmonary venous hypertension (Fig. 16-5); (b) alveolar edema and (c) pleural effusion (Fig. 16-6).[10]

What is the most reliable way to increase the specificity of lung scanning?

Soon after the introduction of perfusion lung scanning, the ventilation in patients with proven pulmonary embolism was studied with the radioactive gas xenon-133. It was found that the ventilation in those areas where the perfusion defects were observed was normal or nearly normal.[10] This finding was of great help, since it was also observed that patients with chronic obstructive lung disease or other types of parenchymal lung disease, such as pneumonia or carcinoma of the lung, had corresponding perfusion and ventilatory defects, an example of which is shown in Figure 16-7.

At present, we perform a regional ventilation study in every patient who is undergoing a perfusion lung scan because of suspected pulmonary embolism.

How are Xenon-133 ventilation studies performed?

Either a six detector system or the scintillation camera is used for these studies, depending upon the desired spatial resolution. The examination is performed by placing the patient in the supine position, with the detector(s) beneath the patient and the regional distribution of xenon-133 gas determined during: (a) an initial single breath, (b) after five minutes of equilibration of rebreathing xenon-133 from a closed system; and (c) during the clearance of xenon-133 from the lungs.

The supine position was selected for the examination, because it is the

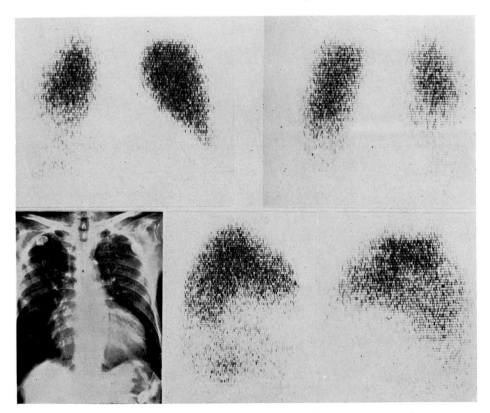

Figure 16-5. Perfusion lung scan and chest radiograph in a patient with congestive cardiac failure. There is generalized nonuniformity of tracer distribution, as seen in pulmonary edema. In addition, there is increased tracer concentration at the upper portion of the lungs compared to the bases.

same position employed for the perfusion injection, thereby facilitating correlation of regional ventilation with regional perfusion. The scintillation camera is usually used for the examination because we obtain the highest degree of spatial resolution with this instrument.

From the initial single breath distribution of the xenon, we obtain an "index of ventilation." If the patient takes his breath quickly, the alterations in ventilation caused by regional changes in airway resistance will be reflected in the distribution of the gas.[15] Unfortunately, many patients do not inhale quickly for this breath, and the distribution of the gas is not solely dependent on the distribution of ventilation. Many patients also cannot hold their breath for the fifteen to twenty seconds required to obtain an image, which makes interpretation of these results difficult in some cases.

Following the single breath, the patient breathes from the closed system

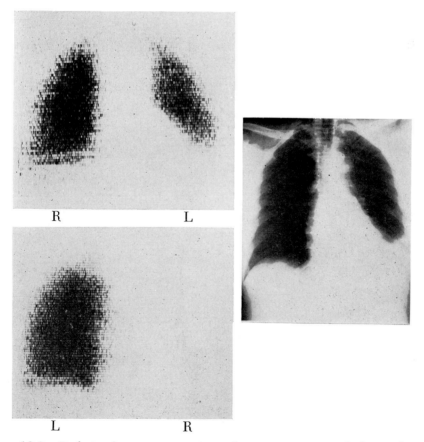

Figure 16-6. Perfusion lung scan, anterior and posterior views, and chest radiograph in a patient with pleural effusion. There is less density in the right than the left lung in the posterior view, due to absorption of the photons by the effusion.

for approximately five minutes. At the end of this time, which is sufficient for all normally ventilated regions to come to equilibrium, an image is obtained. This image represents the volume of ventilated lung.

Thereafter, the patient is disconnected from the spirometer, and the regional "wash-out" of xenon is monitored. The rate of tracer clearance is directly related to ventilation. Although means are available to convert the clearance rate to ventilation in cc/100 grams of lung or ventilation/alveolus, it is usually sufficient to simply evaluate the rate of clearance from each region of the lung as a function of the ventilatory volume to that area.

Interpretation of these images by visual inspection is difficult, because we seek to determine the alteration in the density of one zone of the lung over an interval of time, recorded on several frames of film. The eye is relatively poor at evaluating small changes in density.

One of the applications of computers in nuclear medicine was to portray regional function from scintillation camera images.[16] The computer can readily determine the precise change in counts in a region of lung, where

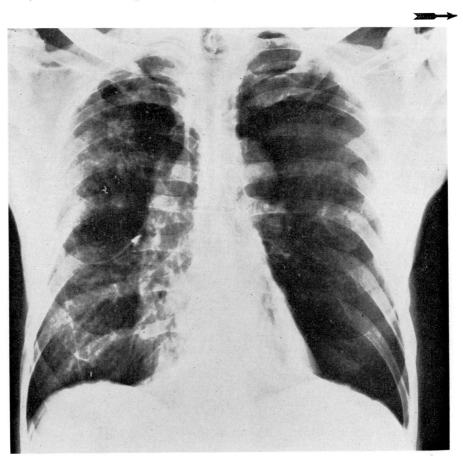

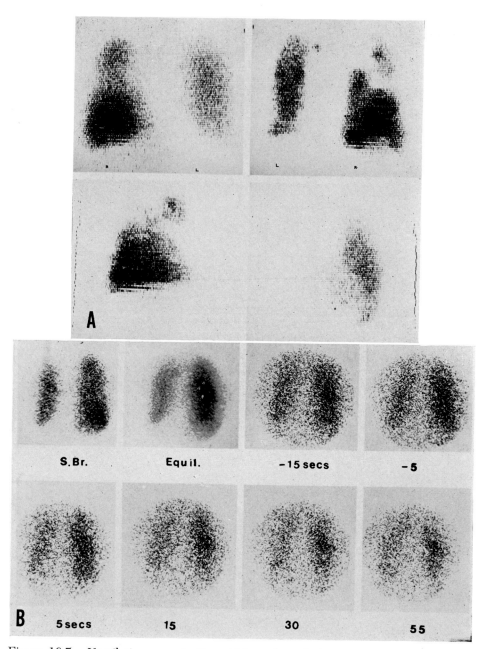

Figure 16-7. Ventilation examination (A) and perfusion examination (B) in a patient with chronic obstructive lung disease. There is a delay in the clearance of xenon from both lungs following equilibration (1), at 20 seconds of washout (2), and at 40 second of washout (3). The perfusion scan has multiple nonsegmental perfusion abnormalities on both lungs.

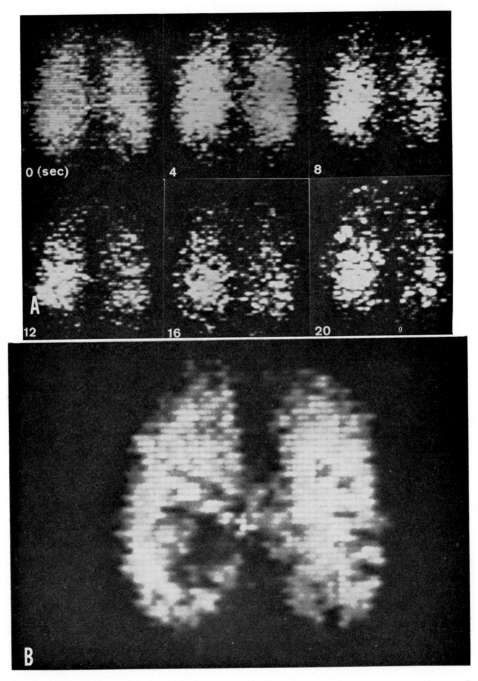

Figure 16-8. (A) Clearance portion of ventilation examination in a patient with chronic obstructive lung disease. There is a region of delayed clearance in the left lower lung field. In (B) the functional image, composed of regional rate constants obtained from the same patient. The area of delayed clearance is dark.

our eye has great difficulty in measuring these changes, and print out the regional clearance half-times. Perhaps a more useful approach that is being applied is the creation of a functional image, from the regional washout half-times. This image retains the anatomic localization obtained from the individual scintillation camera frames, while the brightness of each point within the image reflects the "ventilatory function" (Fig. 16-8). If the perfusion image is also recorded in the computer, the distribution of regional perfusion may be displayed in one color, and the "functional image" of ventilation in another. The regional distribution of perfusion and ventilation are then displayed in a single image. Imbalances in regional function are revealed as an increase in one color or the other.

The distribution of ventilation is usually measured in the posterior view only, because of the technical problems involved in performing the examination in multiple positions. The sensitivity of the technique would probably increase if anterior and lateral views were added, as proved to be the case with perfusion scans.

If there is a region of abnormal ventilation and a zone of abnormal perfusion, the likelihood of uncomplicated pulmonary embolism is greatly decreased. At times, however, pulmonary infarction can cause both abnormal ventilation and abnormal perfusion in the same region. When the perfusion is abnormal and ventilation normal, the likelihood of pulmonary embolism is greatly increased, but other diseases, such as chronic drug abuse, or periarteritis may also alter perfusion while sparing ventilation. In those instances where there is doubt about the diagnosis of pulmonary embolism, as in the patient with chronic lung disease, it is often necessary to perform an arteriogram to permit proper patient management.

What is the relationship between lung scanning and pulmonary arteriography?

The largest single experience comparing lung scans and pulmonary arteriograms was the Urokinase Pulmonary Embolism Trial.[4] In the 150 patients who had lung scans, there were no instances where the scan was completely normal in the presence of an abnormal arteriogram. It is helpful to perform the lung scan before the pulmonary angiogram, so that a selective injection can be made into the vessels supplying the lobes with the perfusion defects.

Perfusion lung scanning is not only useful for the detection of pulmonary emboli, but also in the assessment of their severity. In the UPET Trial, the correlation in the degree of perfusion abnormality as determined by pulmonary arteriography with that determined by lung scan was .68. Although there was some skew of the data toward a more severe abnormality from arteriography than from scanning, this may have been a reflection of the scoring system.

What has lung scanning taught us about the natural history of pulmonary embolism?

Lung scanning has taught us that pulmonary embolism is probably even more common, but less serious than had been thought previously. It has also increased our understanding of what happens to patients who have had pulmonary embolism. We know that a relatively small percentage die. Pulmonary embolism was the cause of sudden death in less than 1 percent of the patients in one large series.[17]

The simplicity and safety of lung scanning has permitted its application to the long-term serial evaluation of changes in pulmonary perfusion in patients sustaining pulmonary emboli. As first illustrated by Tow et al., resolution occurs to varying degrees, depending on the patient's age, general health, and the massiveness of the initial embolus.[18] In the Urokinase Trial, at thirteen days, 55 percent of the initial perfusion deficit was resolved, and by twelve months there was about 80 percent resolution. Seventeen patients had perfusion defects involving more than 10 percent of the lung twelve months after their acute embolus. One striking feature of the UPET data is the stability of perfusion defects after three months, suggesting that those regions that will reperfuse ordinarily do so within ninety days.

What about the prevention of pulmonary embolism?

This is the best approach to the pulmonary embolism. The disease usually starts in the patient's legs or pelvis and only secondarily involves the lung. The problem then becomes one of identification of the high risk patient. Although epidemiological studies are far from complete, there is considerable evidence that certain conditions increase the likelihood of venous thrombosis of the legs or pelvis and therefore pulmonary embolism. These include severe trauma, postoperative states, postpartum state, cancer and heart failure. For example, Sevitt and his co-workers dissected deep thigh and calf veins in patients without evidence of pulmonary embolism and found an incidence ranging from over 80 percent following fractures of the femur to 60 percent after severe burns and slightly less than 40 percent following head and chest injuries.[19] Using a new procedure in which the accumulation of radioiodinated fibrinogen is measured daily in the legs, Kakkar and others[20] have observed that the incidence of venous thrombosis is at least 30 percent following routine general surgical operations and has reported that over half of these complications develop on the operating table. Another approach to the problem of identifying the patient at considerable risk of pulmonary thromboembolism is that of Nossell et al.[21] who have tried to identify and quantify specific end products of fibrinogen and/or fibrin breakdown in the blood that might help identify the patient with intravascular coagulation. At the present state of development the methods are laborious and require an unusual degree of technical expertise. The approach is promising and the initial results encouraging. At present, the informed alert physician is the first line of defense in the detection of pulmonary embolism. When properly used, lung scanning can be of considerable value in confirming or refuting his working diagnosis.

REFERENCES

1. Virchow, R. L. K.: *Gessammelte Abhandlungen zur wissentschafflich.* Frankfurt-a-M, Medizin ven Meidinger Sohn u. Comp, 1856.
2. Cohn, B.: *Klinik der Embolischem Gefaasskrankheiten mit Besonderer rucksicht Auf Die Artzlich.* Berlin, Praxis, 1860.
3. Flint, A.: *A Treatise on the Principles and Practice of Medicine.* Philadelphia, Lea and Febiger, 1867.
4. Urokinase Pulmonary Embolism Trial. *Circ Suppl,* II, 37(4):AHA Monograph 39. II-1–II-108.
5. Hampton, A. O. and Castleman, B.: Correlation of chest teleroentgenograms with autopsy findings. *Am J Roentgenol Rd Ther Nucl Med,* 43:305, 1940.
6. McGinn, S. and White, P. D.: Acute cor pulmonale resulting from pulmonary embolism, *JAMA,* 104:1473, 1935.
7. Poulose, K. P., Reba, R. C., Gilday, D. L., DeLand, F. H. and Wagner, H. N., Jr.: The diagnosis of pulmonary correlative study of clinical scan and angiographic findings. *Br Med J,* 3:67, 1970.
8. Sasahara, A. A., McIntyre, K. M., Criss, A. J. and Belko, J. S.: Aggressive approach to the management of pulmonary embolism. *Cardiovasc Clin,* 1:262, 1970.
9. Dalen, J. E., Banas, J. S., Brooks, H. L., Evans, G. L., Paraskos, J. A. and Dexter, L.: Resolution rate of acute pulmonary embolism in man. *N Engl J Med,* 280:1194, 1969.
10. Wagner, H. N., Jr., Holmes, R. A., Lopez-Majano, V. and Tow, D. E.: The lung. In Wagner, H. N. (Ed.): *Principles of Nuclear Medicine.* Philadelphia, Saunders Co., 1968.
11. von Euler, V. S. and Lilestrand, G.: Observation on the effect of hypoxia on the pulmonary vascular bed. *J Physiol,* 45:135, 1946.
12. Wagner, H. N., Jr., Tow, D. E., Lopez-Majano, V., Chernick, V. and Twining, R.: Factors influencing regional pulmonary blood flow in man. *Scand J Respir Dis [Suppl],* 62:59-72, 1966.
13. Gaum, M. D. and Kot, P. D.: Response of pulmonary vascular segments to angiotensin and norepinephrine. *J Thorac Cardiovasc Surg,* 63:322, 1972.
14. Poulose, K. P., Reba, R. C. and Wagner, H. N., Jr.: Characterization of the shape and location of perfusion defects in certain pulmonary diseases. *N Engl J Med,* 279:1020, 1968.
15. Milic-Emili, J.: Radioactive xenon in the evaluation of regional lung function. *Sem Nucl Med,* 1:246, 1971.
16. Kaihara, S., Natarajan, T. K., Maynard, C. D. and Wagner, H. N., Jr.: Construction of an functional image from spatially localized rate constants obtained from serial camera and rectilinear scanner data. *Radiology,* 93:1345, 1969.

17. Cooper, M.: Unpublished data.
18. Tow, D. E. and Wagner, H. N., Jr.: Recovery of pulmonary arterial blood flow in patients with pulmonary embolism. *N Engl J Med*, 276:1063, 1967.
19. Sevitt, S., Hume, M. and Thomas, D. P.: *Venous Thrombosis and Pulmonary Embolism*. Cambridge, Harvard University Press, 1970.
20. Kakkar, V. V., et al.: Natural history of postoperative deep vein thrombosis. *Lancet*, 2:230, 1969.
21. Nossell, H. L., Canfield, R. E. and Butler, V. P.: Plasma fibrinopeptide—a concentration as an index of intravascular coagulation. Presented at the Annual Meeting of the American Society of Clinical Pathologists, 1973.

DISCUSSION

Dr. Waltman (Boston): Dr. Wagner, in normal individuals, what percentage have perfusion defects?

Dr. Wagner: There have been a couple of studies that have been done. One was done at the University of Chicago, where they found that 16 percent of normal subjects had perfusion defects that might be confused with pulmonary embolism. I'm sure if you studied patients in a Veteran's Hospital, where there is a higher than average incidence of obstructive lung disease, you will get a much higher figure than that. However, we did twenty scans in a row in people who had hip fractures with the idea that this might be a high risk population where it would be very useful to look for pulmonary embolism. We had twenty consecutive normal lung scans and gave up.

Question: Could you comment on perfusion lung scans in patients with pleuritic type complaints and question of pleuritis or pulmonary embolus who may have splinting and may have a minimal pleural effusion?

Dr. Wagner: If the patient hypoventilates one side, you will get decreased perfusion on that side, but you won't get the focal segmental type of abnormalities that are seen in pulmonary embolism. There is a very characteristic pattern in a lung scan of a patient with a pleural effusion. There is often a generalized decrease in activity on one side that is more pronounced on the posterior view than the anterior view. It is very easy to tell that from the segmental perfusion defects seen in pulmonary embolism.

Dr. Zimmerman (Rockford): Are you aware of any studies done using breathing maneuvers, such as the higher percentage of oxygen followed by a lung scan or by positioning the patient in effort to see if gravity will effect the perfusion defect, in order to sharpen the diagnostic specificity of lung scanning for pulmonary emboli?

Dr. Wagner: In 1964, we administered 100 percent oxygen in an effort to show reperfusion to an area where hypoperfusion might be on a reflex basis. The results weren't clear-cut enough that we could really use this information diagnostically. I think it is a very interesting idea. It would also be interesting to study drugs in that fashion, too.

Dr. Sasahara: There have been a lot of questions on microemboli and I realize the syndrome of microemboli is probably quite rare and I think it's more likely big clots than small clots. But if it does exist—and I suppose it does—can you conceive that a shower of emboli could be spread out evenly enough that the scan really doesn't pick it up as a segmental defect. I think that probably refers to some of the questions that we have been talking about. Is that possible?

Dr. Wagner: The smallest perfusion defects that I have seen in 10,000 or more lung scans, were in five patients who had septic emboli. Some of these emboli could be seen radiographically, but many radiographically invisible septic emboli had round areas of decreased perfusion that were one or two cm in diameter. I think that the lung scanning technique can pick up small emboli that are not visible radiographically. I was taught in medical school that patients often have showers of microemboli. I think it doesn't happen very often, that it is exceedingly rare.

Question: I'd like to ask Dr. Wagner about the apparent decrease in perfusion at the costophrenic angles that one often sees on the AP and PA lung scans, if a lateral view is not done. It is often read as compatible with a normal scan yet this is an area of lung where embolic disease is common.

Dr. Wagner: I think it is absolutely essential to do lateral views, to look for perfusion defects in the same corresponding anatomical location on multiple views. In patients who have some rounding off of the bases on the anterior or the posterior views, they almost always will have normal lateral views.

Dr. Hirsh (Hamilton): I wonder if Dr. Wagner could comment on the following: If a patient has a suspected massive pulmonary embolus and is sick enough for us to consider pulmonary embolectomy, if he got worse on medical treatment in the next few hours, then could we go straight to pulmonary angiogram without performing the scans?

Dr. Wagner: With Dr. Sautter here, I hesitate to say anything about pulmonary embolectomy. I think that in our hospital, there was a very enthusiastic approach to pulmonary embolectomy around 1964 and 1965, but I think there have been several series where patients who were equally ill who didn't have a pulmonary embolectomy survived. Pulmonary embolectomy has gone into disrepute. The answer to your question: in the days when we were doing pulmonary embolectomies at Hopkins Hospital, they occasionally would take the patient right to an arteriogram without the scan.

Chapter 17

PULMONARY ANGIOGRAPHY IN THE DIAGNOSIS OF PULMONARY EMBOLISM

ALLAN L. SIMON

PULMONARY ANGIOGRAPHY is the specific method for establishing the diagnosis of pulmonary embolism and the aim of the angiographic examination should be the definitive diagnosis or exclusion of this entity. Numerous clinical tests are available for screening patients and are discussed elsewhere in this symposium. The angiogram should be a definitive procedure for establishment of the diagnosis with minimal risk to the patient.

INDICATIONS: Improvement in the diagnostic accuracy of the lung scan has caused a revision in the angiographic approach to pulmonary embolism. At this point in time, the major indications for pulmonary angiography are: (1) The establishment of the diagnosis of pulmonary embolism in patients in whom the risk of anticoagulant therapy is great (for example, gastrointestinal bleeding, immediate postoperative period). (2) Patients requiring emergency surgery for embolism (caval interruption, caval umbrella, embolectomy). (3) Patients with preexisting parenchymal pulmonary disease in whom an abnormal lung scan on the basis of coexistent disease is assumed. (4) Any investigative procedure requiring definitive diagnosis.

(The recent cooperative study on the effectiveness of Urokinase fibrinolytic therapy upon pulmonary embolism is an example.)

TECHNIQUE OF CATHETERIZATION

(A) Premedication: Intramuscular analgesic and atropine immediately prior to the procedure.

(B) Entry site: Cut-down on the antecubital vein is preferred. Percutaneous approach via jugular or antecubital system is an alternative. Percutaneous femoral route is generally not done because of the possibility of dislodging a clot in the inferior vena cava. If the route is to be used, inferior vena cavography should precede passage of this catheter.

(C) Catheters: #7F or 8F side hole catheters (NIH or Eppendorf) or flow guided balloon tipped angiographic catheters.

(D) Catheterization: A brief hemodynamic assessment should be made at the time of catheterization of the right heart chambers and this should include measurement of the right atrial pressure including mean, right ventricular systolic and diastolic pressure, and pulmonary artery pressure, systolic, diastolic and mean. Simultaneous with the measurement of the pulmonary artery pressure, systemic pressure should be ascertained via cuff or directly.

(E) Site of Injection: The main pulmonary artery is preferred for the first injection. A contraindication to injection in the main PA is severe pulmonary hypertension. An alternative method in this case is to inject in the right atrium or to inject a smaller bolus of contrast material selectively into each pulmonary artery.

(F) Injection: fifty to sixty cc of any of the mixtures of sodium and NMG diatrizoate or iothalamate contrast agents (e.g., Renografin 76, Hypaque 75M, or Vascoray) are injected in two seconds.

(G) Filming: AP projection is used for the first survey arteriogram to allow assessment of peripheral vasculature as well as comparison of circulation times through the lungs.

Filming Sequence: At least two frames per second for four seconds followed by one frame per second for six to eight seconds so that the left heart chambers and aorta are visualized.

(H) Complications: *Arrhythmia* is the most serious complication. Multiple extrasystoles frequently occur when the catheter is passed through the right ventricle or if injection is made in the right ventricle. Treatment for this is removal of the catheter from the chamber.

Ventricular Fibrillation may occur if the tachycardia is allowed to persist. The treatment for this is electrical defibrillation.

Severe bradycardia or *arrest* may occur during the catheterization as a vaso-vagal reaction. (This risk is minimized by premedication with atropine.)

Cardiac Perforation. This most commonly occurs in the right ventricular outflow tract, and careful catheter technique generally avoids this problem. The use of a balloon-tipped (Swan-Ganz Angiographic) catheter is another method which reduces this risk. Recognition of this complication is most important and treatment should be instituted immediately if tamponade and circulatory embarrassment occur.

Dislodgement of a preexisting clot can occur if the clot is in the main pulmonary artery. A test injection is generally done as part of the angiographic procedure to eliminate the possibility of clot dislodgement as well as to insure symmetrical filling of the pulmonary arteries.

Other complications which can occur are knotting or breakage of the catheter, air embolism, and thrombosis on the catheter. All of these can be obviated by careful catheterization technique.

DIAGNOSIS OF PULMONARY EMBOLISM

There are two objective signs on which the diagnosis of pulmonary embolism can be made with certainty. Obstruction of a vessel by pulmonary embolism presents angiographically as a "cut-off." Figure 17-1 is an example of the "cut-off" sign, wherein the intermediate right pulmonary artery supplying the right middle and lower lobes is completely occluded. There is fill of the stump of the intermediate artery followed by complete occlusion.

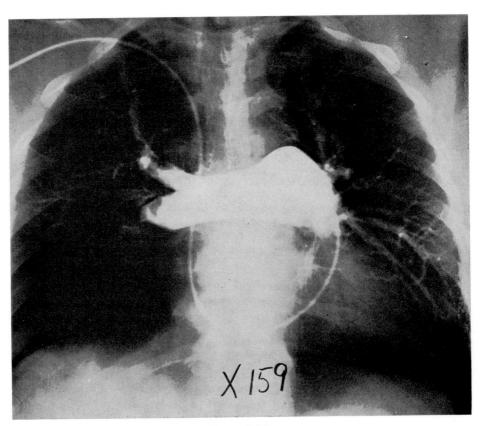

Figure 17-1.

The other sign of pulmonary embolus is the presence of one or multiple filling defects within the lumen of the pulmonary vessels as shown in Figure 17-2. Filling defects may have variable appearance. In the right lower lobe, and in the main left and left upper lobe pulmonary arteries the filling defect is freely intraluminal and a small stream of contrast material is visualized in the blood vessel on all sides of the embolus. The embolus in the right upper and left lower lobe appears to have attached itself to the intima on one side of the pulmonary vessels since no line of contrast material is visible on the lateral aspects of these emboli.

All other signs of embolus are indirect, merely circumstantial evidence for the presence of emboli. These are nonspecific and may be caused by numerous other pulmonary conditions. The indirect signs for presence of pulmonary embolus are: Delayed pulmonary arterial flow. Angiographically this appears as late fill and drainage of a pulmonary artery branch or branches, as well as late opacification of the draining veins. Although this occurs distal to a pulmonary embolus, any increase in pulmonary

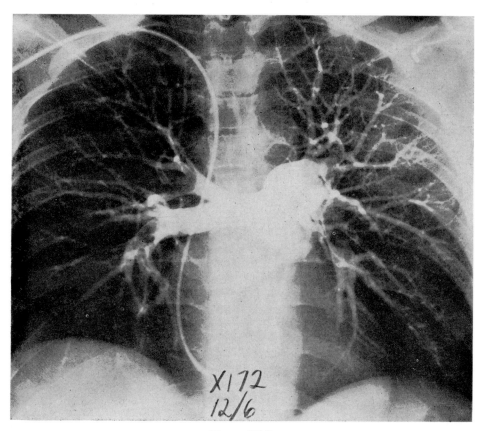

Figure 17-2.

vascular resistance can simulate this sign. Any form of pulmonary paren-chymal disease, emphysema, and even atelectasis may cause retarded flow.

Proximal arterial dilatation occurs when there is pulmonary embolism; however, pulmonary embolism is not necessary for this to occur.

Peripheral tortuosity presents as a corkscrew appearance to the distal pulmonary arteries. This is classically seen when there is loss of pulmonary volume as for example in atelectasis. However, it also occurs during re-solving pulmonary embolism.

Recognition of these indirect signs of pulmonary embolus is important, not merely to enable the angiographer to make a tentative diagnosis of pulmonary embolism but rather to direct the anigographer's attention to the region which should be studied selectively.

False-positive signs of pulmonary embolus are most often the result of vascular overlap. The summation of two vessels filled with contrast material presents a greatly increased radiodensity. The normal density of the contrast-filled vessel immediately beyond the summated image ap-pears as a filling defect. Upon closer observation, one can trace the overlapping vessels and generally exclude this entity. Frequently, however, one must resort to repeat injection with some rotation of the patient to eliminate the vascular overlap and enable the differentiation from embolus.

Nonfill of a vessel can occasionally mimic a vascular cut-off. The major differentiation between nonfill and a true embolus, however, lies in the demonstration of the stump of a vessel which has been occluded as opposed to total nonfill of the vessel.

False-negatives: Total nonfill of a vessel can result from embolism occluding a branch back to the orifice, without a resultant stump. This state of events should not result in a false-negative examination if the principles are adhered to as follows. Namely, nonfill of a vessel is recog-nized by visualization of less than the expected number of segmental branches. This is considered an indirect and nonspecific sign of embolus and leads to a selective injection in the branch pulmonary artery close to the area of the nonfilled vessel.

Large intraluminal emboli in the main and hilar pulmonary vessels have been overlooked and mentioned as a cause of false-negative examina-tion. The use of proper radiographic factors, with penetration and density adequate to visualize the major pulmonary vessels obviates this error. Simi-larly, the use of rapid serial films enables the angiographer to observe the main pulmonary artery in the diastole when there is no admixture of the contrast material with nonopacified right ventricular blood and allows the detection of these large pulmonary emboli.

SELECTIVE TECHNIQUES

Whenever there is any doubt as to the presence of pulmonary embolism, the catheter should be advanced into the main right or left pulmonary artery, or into the lobar branches for a subsequent injection. In this case, a proportional reduction in the amount of contrast material results in equally good or sometimes better visualization of the vessels. The selection of the area for injection is done after examination of the survey injection. The criteria for selective injection are as follows:

1) To attempt to demonstrate pulmonary embolism in an area of lung which manifests the indirect and nonspecific signs of embolism.

2) To rule in or out the false-positive and false-negative signs.

Selective injections are most advantageous when combined with different patient projection. The proximal right pulmonary artery is best demonstrated by slight elevation of the patient's right side (10-15 degree RAO). The proximal left pulmonary artery is best demonstrated by moderate elevation of the patient's left side (30-45 degree LAO).

Extreme obliques and the lateral projection have proved extremely valuable for the separation of segmental pulmonary vessels in the lower lobes, the right middle lobe, and the lingula.

Summary

Pulmonary angiography should be performed for the definitive diagnosis of pulmonary embolism and the technique should be aimed at this objective solely. Meticulous attention to detail results in a satisfactory procedure at minimum risk.

REFERENCES

Bookstein, Joseph J.: Pulmonary thromboembolism with emphasis on angiographic-pathologic correlation. *Semin Roentgenol, 5*(3):291-305, 1970.

Dalen, James E., et al.: Pulmonary angiography in acute pulmonary embolism: Indications, techniques, and results in 367 patients. *Am Heart J, 81*(2):175-185, 1971.

McIntyre, Kevin M.: Correlation of pulmonary photoscan and angiogram as measures of the severity of pulmonary embolic involvement. *J Nucl Med 12*(11):732-738, 1971.

Walsh, Peter N., et al.: An angiographic severity index for pulmonary embolism. *Circulation, XLVII (4)*:II-101, 1973.

DISCUSSION

Dr. Gilberts (New Jersey): Dr. Simon, on the pulmonary angiograms, 1) In a negative study, how certain can one be, assuming the study has been complete, that there aren't either smaller unresolvable emboli peripherally or that the time interval between the symptoms and the X-ray might obviate a change of making a diagnosis, 2) In the instance that you mentioned in which it is necessary to withdraw the catheter into the atrium for safety sake, how valuable is the study from that point?

Dr. Simon: I'll answer the second question first. If you do an injection in the right atrium you should be prepared to follow it up with a selective injection. The only time I would stop at the right atrial injection is if I couldn't get the catheter out where I wanted to place it. To answer your first question, there are an awful lot of vessels that you don't see with a pulmonary angiogram. You're really seeing down to segmental vessels well and may be some subsegmental vessels fairly well. It is very important that you do the angiogram at the time that the patient is suspected to have the embolic episode. If you do it two to three weeks later, you may find very nonspecific changes. I have never seen a case with proven pulmonary embolus that had a perfectly normal pulmonary angiogram. Usually they have nonspecific angiographic changes.

Chapter 18

CLINICAL MANIFESTATIONS AND DIAGNOSIS OF PULMONARY EMBOLISM

James E. Dalen

THE DIFFICULTIES encountered in making an accurate clinical diagnosis of pulmonary embolism are well known. Perhaps the best evidence that the clinical diagnosis of pulmonary embolism is difficult and often inaccurate comes from the results of pulmonary angiography. In a group of 306 consecutive patients in whom pulmonary angiography was performed because of suspected acute pulmonary embolism, we found that only 41 percent had angiographic evidence of pulmonary embolism. Fifteen percent of the studies were equivocal, but nearly half the studies, that is, 44 percent, were entirely normal.[1]

Previous studies of the clinical manifestations of acute pulmonary embolism have often been based upon postmortem studies or have been studies in which the diagnosis of pulmonary embolism was based on clinical grounds. Both of these approaches have certain limitations. The majority of patients with acute pulmonary embolism do not die. Therefore, the clinical findings in a postmortem series are not representative of all patients with acute pulmonary embolism. Since the clinical diagnosis is so frequently inaccurate, it is difficult to rely heavily on the results of studies of pulmonary embolism in which the diagnosis is made on clinical grounds.

I would like to present the findings in a series of 100 consecutive patients in whom acute pulmonary embolism was documented by selective pulmonary angiography performed at our hospital between 1964 and 1972.

The patients ranged in age from seventeen to eighty-eight, with an average age of sixty-three. Fifty-six percent were females, 44 percent were males. Whereas we often think of pulmonary embolism as being a complication of surgical procedures, only twenty of our 100 patients had acute pulmonary embolism while recovering from surgery. Twenty-three patients had acute pulmonary embolism while on the medical service, and

191

in fifty-seven cases, the episode occurred while the patient was at home or in a nursing home.

One of the most important facts about these patients is that nearly all of them had an obvious predisposition to venous thromboembolism. The factors predisposing to thromboembolism in these patients are shown in Table 18-I. The two most common predispositions were bed rest and heart disease, particularly with congestive failure. Exactly half of these 100 patients had prior heart disease and thirty-two had congestive failure prior to the episode of acute pulmonary embolism.

TABLE 18-I

PREDISPOSITION TO PULMONARY EMBOLISM IN 100 PATIENTS

Bed rest	52
Heart disease (with CHF—32)	50
Recent surgery	23
GYN or prostatic disease	19
Recent leg trauma	8
"The Pill"	4
Pregnancy	3
None of the above	16

The symptoms, physical findings, and laboratory findings in acute pulmonary embolism depend upon the sequelae of pulmonary embolism. The most common presentation of pulmonary embolism in our experience is pulmonary infarction. In other patients, pulmonary embolism presents as acute cor pulmonale. Still others, have only acute unexplained dyspnea and a smaller group presents with increasing left ventricular failure. For this reason, there is no single set of signs and symptoms that is diagnostic of acute pulmonary embolism.[2]

The symptoms in this group of 100 patients are shown in Table 18-II. The two most common symptoms were dyspnea and pleuritic pain. One or both of these symptoms occurred in ninety-four of the 100 patients.

TABLE 18-II

SYMPTOMS OF ACUTE PULMONARY EMBOLISM IN 100 PATIENTS

*Dyspnea	77
*Pleuritic pain	57
Cough	35
Hemoptysis	18
Syncope	16
Orthopnea or PND (new)	16
Palpitations	11

*Dyspnea or pleuritic pain in ninety-four patients

In our experience, the most important physical finding in acute pulmonary embolism is the respiratory rate. If the respiratory rate is counted accurately for a full minute, it will be found to be more than twenty in the vast majority of patients with acute pulmonary embolism. Ninety-four percent of our patients had a respiratory rate of greater than twenty at the time of acute pulmonary embolism.

The physical findings in the chest depend upon the patient's prior cardiovascular status and depend upon whether the patient has had pulmonary infarction secondary to pulmonary embolism. Since so many of our patients had prior heart disease, the most common physical finding in the chest was rales (Table 18-III). Seventeen patients had wheezing and twelve of these had no prior history of asthma. This is consistent with the data of Thomas et al.,[3] who have shown that experimentally, acute pulmonary embolism can cause bronchoconstriction, presumably due to the release of serotonin from platelets attached to the clot. In twenty-four of our 100 patients, examination of the chest was normal.

TABLE 18-III

PHYSICAL EXAMINATION OF THE CHEST IN 100 PATIENTS
WITH ACUTE PULMONARY EMBOLISM

Rales		56
Unilateral	17	
Bilateral	39	
*Wheezes		17
Friction rub		16
Splinting		19
Normal examination		24

*Twelve patients with wheezing had no prior history of asthma

If one considers the syndrome of dyspnea with tachypnea and a normal examination of the chest, the differential diagnosis is limited. The two most common causes of such a syndrome are the hyperventilation syndrome and acute pulmonary embolism. In this circumstance, arterial blood gas analysis should be diagnostic. The arterial pO_2 should be well within the normal range in patients with the hyperventilation syndrome, and decreased in patients with acute pulmonary embolism.

In seventy-five of our patients, blood pressure was normal at the time of acute pulmonary embolism; nine had hypotension that was transient and did not require therapy; twelve patients had hypotension requiring vasopressors. Four patients had cardiac arrest with the episode of acute pulmonary embolism. The occurrence of hypotension in the setting of acute pulmonary embolism in man is not due to reflexes; but rather it occurs only in patients with massive pulmonary embolism. Cardiac output in most patients with acute pulmonary embolism is either normal or it is high normal. If embolism has been sufficiently massive to cause acute cor pulmonale with failure of the right ventricle, then right ventricular stroke volume decreases, cardiac output decreases and finally systemic blood pressure may decrease.[4]

For these reasons, if pulmonary embolism is considered in the differential diagnosis of shock, one should measure the central venous pressure. If it is normal, it is extremely unlikely that the patient's shock is due to pulmonary embolism.

The findings by cardiovascular examination depend upon the patient's prior cardiac status, and the magnitude of the embolism. If embolism has been sufficiently massive to occlude more than 60 to 75 percent of the pulmonary circulation, one would expect to find signs of acute cor pulmonale. These findings: tachycardia, distended neck veins, S3 gallop, and parasternal heave, when they are present in a patient without prior heart disease are highly suggestive of the presence of massive pulmonary embolism.

Although there is excellent evidence to indicate that nearly all pulmonary emboli originate as thrombi in the veins of the lower extremities, the physical examination of the legs is often unrevealing. Forty-two of our 100 patients had no detectable abnormalities in their legs. Twenty-seven had a significant difference in calf size, twenty-three had leg pain, nineteen had calf tenderness and only eleven had Homan's Sign. The studies of Sevitt and Gallagher have made it very clear that if the examination of the legs is normal, it in no way excludes the presence of significant deep venous thrombosis.[5] In a group of 104 patients who died of pulmonary embolism who had been examined daily for the presence of thrombophlebitis, less than 50 percent had premortem evidence of thrombophlebitis. Yet, at postmortem examination all 104 had significant deep venous thrombosis in the lower extremities.

LABORATORY FINDINGS IN ACUTE PULMONARY EMBOLISM

Serum Enzymes and Bilirubin

Our experience had indicated that the triad of increased LDH, normal SGOT and increased serum bilirubin is quite uncommon in acute pulmonary embolism.[6] In fact, only twelve of our 100 patients with acute pulmonary embolism had this triad. It seems clear that LDH is increased in nearly all patients with acute pulmonary embolism. However, the SGOT is elevated in only one half the patients. Bilirubin is increased only if the patient had prior congestive heart failure with hepatic congestion. We know of no evidence that pulmonary embolism per se can increase bilirubin. Therefore, the only member of the triad that would appear to be relevant to acute pulmonary embolism is the LDH, which is increased in most patients with pulmonary embolism. However, it is also increased in many of the conditions that are often confused with pulmonary embolism.

Chest X-ray

The chest X-ray is very helpful in patients with acute pulmonary embolism. Seventy-five of our patients had one or more of three easily recognized abnormalities: an infiltrate, pleural effusion, and elevated diaphragm. Only twenty-five patients had a normal chest film. The infiltrate of acute pulmonary embolism is usually due to pulmonary infarction, although it could also be due to atelectasis secondary to splinting. Elevation of the diaphragm is an early sign that is associated with pleuritic pain and subsequent splinting. The pleural effusion is usually unilateral and small. It may or may not be bloody.

Arterial Blood Gases

We have found the measurements of arterial blood gases to be extremely helpful in patients with acute pulmonary embolism. As shown in Table 18-IV, 88 percent of our patients have had a pO_2 less than 80 mm Hg. It is clear that an occasional healthy patient with minor pulmonary embolism may have a normal pO_2 that is greater than ninety. However, the vast majority of people with acute pulmonary embolism have significant hypoxemia.[6,7] It is very important that the pO_2 be measured while the patient is breathing room air. It is necessary to discontinue supplemental oxygen for only five to ten minutes in order to get the baseline pO_2. The arterial pO_2 is decreased and the pH is somewhat alkalotic in acute pulmonary embolism due to hyperventilation.

TABLE 18-IV

ARTERIAL pO_2 (BREATHING ROOM AIR) IN ACUTE PULMONARY EMBOLISM

	Number	*Percent*
86-90	3	4
80-85	6	8
70-79	21	27
60-69	20	25
50-59	16	21
40-49	8	10
30-39	4	5
	78	100

Mean = 64 mm Hg

Electrocardiogram

We have found sinus rhythm or sinus tachycardia to be present in nearly all of our patients with pulmonary embolism, that is eighty-two of the 100

(Table 18-V). Sixteen of our patients had atrial fibrillation or atrial flutter, but this was a new finding in only seven patients, and five of these patients had prior heart disease. Therefore, we have found very little evidence that atrial flutter is an important tip-off of the presence of acute pulmonary embolism.[8]

TABLE 18-V

CARDIAC RHYTHM IN 100 PATIENTS WITH ACUTE PULMONARY EMBOLISM

Sinus	82
*Atrial fibrillation	14
*Atrial flutter	2
Other	2

*New AF or a flutter in seven patients
Five had prior heart disease

The EKG is very important in detecting evidence of acute right heart strain. These signs include a new S1Q3T3 pattern, right axis shift or new incomplete right bundle branch block. Twenty-seven of our 100 patients had one of these three findings (Table 18-VI). When these findings occur, it means the patient has had massive pulmonary embolism with acute cor pulmonale.

TABLE 18-VI

EKG EVIDENCE OF ACUTE COR PULMONALE IN 100 PATIENTS WITH ACUTE PULMONARY EMBOLISM

S_1, Q_3, T_3 (new)	18
Right axis shift	16
RBBB or IRBBB (new)	7
Any of the above	27

Fibrin Split Products

A new laboratory test that may well prove to be very important in the diagnosis of acute pulmonary embolism is the measurement of fibrin split products. Early data indicates that fibrin split products are significantly elevated in most patients with acute pulmonary embolism.[9] In a prospective study of forty-six patients with suspected pulmonary embolism, we found that eighteen of nineteen patients with pulmonary embolism as documented by pulmonary angiography had a fibrin split product concentration of ten micrograms/ml or greater. In twenty-two patients with a normal pulmonary angiogram, the concentration of fibrin split products was ten micrograms/ml or less in nineteen.[10] These data are shown in Figure 18-1. Further results are needed to determine the specificity of fibrin splti product elevation in acute pulmonary embolism.

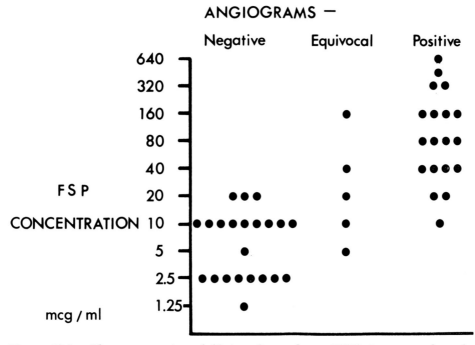

Figure 18-1. The concentration of fibrin split products (FSP) is compared to the results of pulmonary angiography in forty-six patients suspected to have acute pulmonary embolism. The average FSP concentration was 158 mcg/ml in nineteen patients with positive angiograms for pulmonary embolism as compared to eight mcg/ml in twenty-two patients with negative pulmonary angiograms (p < .001), (Rickman, F. D., et al.: Fibrin split products in acute pulmonary embolism. *Ann Intern Med*, 79:664-668, 1973.)

Lung Scans

There can be no question that the lung scan is the most useful screening test for acute pulmonary embolism. A technically adequate, entirely normal lung scan totally excludes the possibility of symptomatic acute pulmonary embolism in our opinion.[6] Over a period of ten years, we have performed pulmonary angiography in ten patients who had a normal lung scan. The pulmonary angiography was performed because the clinical suspicion of pulmonary embolism was so strong. In all ten cases, the pulmonary angiogram was normal. If the lung scan shows segmental perfusion defects that ventilate normally, pulmonary embolism is extremely likely. If the findings of the lung scan are equivocal, then one must proceed to pulmonary angiography for a definitive diagnosis.

At the present time, pulmonary angiography remains the most definitive laboratory test in the diagnosis of acute pulmonary embolism.[11]

In summary, in making the clinical diagnosis of pulmonary embolism, it is important to keep in mind that pulmonary embolism may present in at least four different ways: with pulmonary infarction, acute cor pulmonale, acute unexplained dyspnea or increasing left ventricular failure. The two most important clues from the history are the fact that patients with pulmonary embolism usually have an obvious predisposition to venous thrombosis, and that the most important symptoms are dyspnea and/or pleuritic pain. The most universal physical finding in acute pulmonary embolism is tachypnea with a respiratory rate greater than twenty. The most valuable laboratory findings are arterial blood gases which show a decreased pO_2, a decreased pCO_2 and respiratory alkalosis; the chest X-ray which shows an infiltrate, elevated diaphragm or pleural effusion in the majority of patients; and the lung scan which shows segmental perfusion defects that ventilate normally.

Most fatal episodes of pulmonary embolism are preceded by nonfatal episodes that go unrecognized. Therefore, our main hope in preventing fatal pulmonary embolism is to recognize pulmonary embolism when it first occurs.

REFERENCES

1. Dalen, J. E. (Ed.): *Pulmonary Embolism*. New York, Medcom, Inc., 1972.
2. Dalen, J. E. and Dexter, L.: Pulmonary embolism. *JAMA, 207*:1505-1507, 1969.
3. Thomas, D., Stein, M., Tanabe, G., et al.: Mechanism of bronchoconstriction produced by thromboemboli in dogs. *Am J Physiol, 206*:1207-1212, 1964.
4. Dalen, J. E., Banas, J. S., Jr. and Brooks, H. L., et al.: Resolution rate of acute pulmonary embolism in man. *N Engl J Med, 280*:1194-1199, 1969.
5. Sevitt, S. and Gallagher, N.: Venous thrombosis and pulmonary embolism: A clinicopathological study in injured and burned patients. *Br J Surg, 48*:475-489, 1961.
6. Szucs, M. S., Jr., Brooks, H. L. and Grossman, W., et al.: Diagnostic sensitivity of laboratory findings in acute pulmonary embolism. *Ann Int Med, 74*:161-166, 1971.
7. McIntyre, K. M. and Sasahara, A. A.: The hemodynamic response to pulmonary embolism in patients without prior cardiopulmonary disease. *Am J Cardiol, 28*:288-294, 1971.
8. Johnson, J. C., Flowers, N. C. and Horan, L. G.: Unexplained atrial flutter: A frequent herald of pulmonary embolism. *Chest, 60*:29-34, 1971.
9. Ruckley, C. V., Das, P. C., Leitch, A. G., et al.: Serum fibrin/fibrinogen degradation products associated with postoperative pulmonary embolus and venous thrombosis. *Br Heart J, 4*:395-398, 1970.
10. Rickman, F. D., Handin, R., and Howe, J. P., et al.: Fibrin split products in acute pulmonary embolism. *Ann Int Med, 79*:664-668, 1973.
11. Dalen, J. E., Brooks, H. L., Johnson, L. W., et al.: Pulmonary angiography in acute pulmonary embolism: indications, techniques, and results in 367 patients. *Am Heart J, 81*:175-185, 1971.

Chapter 19

THE ELECTROCARDIOGRAM IN
PULMONARY EMBOLISM

RICHARD D. ALLEN AND BORYS SURAWICZ

Introduction

ALTHOUGH THE cardiographic (ECG) changes associated with pulmonary embolism (P.E.) have been known fifty years, the reported incidence of these changes varies greatly in different studies of patients with proven, or strongly suspected P.E. Thus, in the studies of Newman[1] and Litman[2] only 10 to 20 percent of patients with P.E. had any ECG change, while in the studies of Cutforth[3] and Weber and Phillips[4] the incidence of ECG change was 76 percent. Some of this discrepancy may be explained by the transient nature of the ECG, and by the differences in the serial follow-up in different studies. This article consists of two parts: (1) a review of the subject with examples of the most characteristic ECG patterns of P.E., and (2) a retrospective study of 100 patients whose ECG diagnosis was coded as pulmonary embolism or acute cor pulmonale.

REVIEW OF LITERATURE

The earliest reports in the literature described supraventricular and ventricular arrhythmias in rabbits with experimental pulmonary emboli.[5] Subsequently, Otto[6] described T-wave inversion in dogs with total or partial occlusion of the pulmonary arteries. Buchbinder[7] found QRS and T-wave changes, but no significant shift in the electrical axis in dogs with experimental pulmonary emboli, or mechanical occlusion of the pulmonary arteries. Lundy[8] produced axis deviation, and T-wave inversion in the dog by dilatation of the right ventricle with air-filled balloons. The latter ECG changes were attributed to an acute increase in right ventricular pressure with subsequent dilatation of the right heart chambers.

In 1935, McGinn and White[9] published the first clinical paper correlating ECG changes with pulmonary embolism in man. The major points empha-

sized in this paper were: the consistency of the ECG pattern, the value of
obtaining the ECG early in the clinical course, and the contribution of the
ECG in differentiating between P.E. and acute myocardial infarction. The
ECG at that time consisted of the three standard limb leads, and in some
patients an additional single chest lead. The term "acute cor pulmonale"
characterized an ECG pattern recorded in five patients within twenty-one
hours of the clinical event suggesting P.E. This ECG pattern consisted of
prominent S-wave in lead I gradual staircase ascent of the ST segment in
lead II, Q-wave in lead III, and negative T-wave in lead III. Two patients
also had right axis deviation and an inverted T-wave in the single chest
lead. In four of these patients the diagnosis of P.E. was confirmed at
autopsy and in the other three patients the ECG became normal within
forty-eight hours, four weeks, and six weeks, respectively. Rapid resolution
of the ECG changes was thought to favor P.E. rather than myocardial
infarction. This difference has been emphasized frequently in the early
literature, and even today is considered by some investigators to be the
only contribution of the ECG to the diagnosis of pulmonary embolism.

Subsequent studies in patients with P.E. showed that the pattern of acute
cor pulmonale described by McGinn and White occurred infrequently, or
even exceptionally.[10] Love reported that ST depression in leads I and II
with T inversion in lead III and in the precordial lead was the most frequent ECG change in twelve patients with P.E. The same author reported
similar ECG changes in dogs with experimental pulmonary occlusion of
greater than 50 percent of the pulmonary arterial bed. In the first large
clinical study of ECG changes in fifty patients with P.E., Sokolow[11] found
no specific patterns.

The association between transient right bundle branch block and pulmonary embolism was initially reported by Durant.[12] In his study right bundle
branch block that regressed within twelve hours was present in three
patients in whom the ECG was recorded within three hours of the clinical
diagnosis of P.E. More recently, Szucs[13] reported an 8 percent incidence of
conduction disturbances in the right bundle branch among forty-seven
cases of angiographically documented P.E. The transient nature of this
particular ECG change may explain its infrequent documentation in most
studies. Following the introduction of multiple chest leads, Wood[14] reported sharp inversion of the T-wave in seven of ten patients with suspected P.E. in chest leads recorded at the fourth intercostal space near the
right sternal border, the apex, and a point midway between these two leads.
The amplitude of the negative T-wave and the duration of this change
decreased in the chest leads from the right sternal border to the apex.
Follow-up tracings revealed that changes in the lead at the right sternal
border sometimes persisted for several weeks. Wood observed jugular
venous distention in the seven patients with T-wave inversion, and attrib-

uted the T-wave change to "right ventricular strain." Similar T-wave changes were also found in other conditions associated with acute right ventricular "strain" including pneumonia, and exacerbation of chronic obstructive airway disease.

Early animal studies showed high incidence of supraventricular and ventricular arrhythmias in experimental P.E. However, in man ventricular arrhythmias have been found infrequently while the supraventricular arrhythmias occurred more commonly. Johnson[15] reported that twenty-five of forty-five patients with unexplained atrial flutter had P.E. Weber and Phillips[4] found atrial arrhythmias in 38 percent of patients with an autopsy-proven diagnosis of P.E. Szucs[13] found atrial flutter or atrial fibrillation in nine of forty-eight patients with angiographically confirmed P.E., but eight of those nine patients had preexisting heart disease. Of various mechanisms postulated to explain the genesis of atrial arrhythmias in P.E., none has been conclusively proven.

Recent studies of McIntyre[16] further emphasize the rare occurrence of ECG changes in patients with P.E. This study showed that of twenty-five patients free of cardiopulmonary disease prior to documented P.E., only four had ECG changes suggestive of P.E., and only one patient had an ECG pattern completely diagnostic of P.E. In these four patients, the hemodynamic findings were compatible with acute cor pulmonale: increased mean right atrial pressure, mean pulmonary artery pressure greater than thirty mm Hg, angiographically calculated obstruction of the pulmonary arteries exceeding 47 percent, increased pulmonary vascular resistance, and a cardiac index below 2.5 L/min/m². The finding of ECG changes occurring in the presence of angiographically calculated obstruction greater than 47 percent is in keeping with the earlier report by Love[10] that 50 percent obstruction was required to produce ECG changes in dogs with experimental P.E.

ECG DIFFERENTIATION OF MYOCARDIAL INFARCTION FROM PULMONARY EMBOLISM

Clinical differentiation between P.E. and acute myocardial infarction is sometimes difficult, and the ECG changes in P.E. may simulate acute inferior wall infarction, and to a lesser degree infarction of the anterior septal area. In patients with P.E. a significant Q-wave may appear in lead III and AVF, and the ST segment may be isoelectric or slightly elevated in the same leads. The degree of elevation in P.E. is usually less than would be expected with acute inferior infarction. In P.E. the T-wave is frequently negative in lead III and less frequently negative in lead AVF. Rapid regression of these changes, particularly the disappearance of the Q-waves in serial tracings, favors the diagnosis of P.E. vs. myocardial infarction.

When the ECG changes in the inferior leads are accompanied by T-wave inversion in the right precordial leads, the ECG pattern may suggest erroneously an infarction of the inferior wall and nontransmural infarction of the low anterior septal wall. Sometimes the T-wave inversion in the right precordial leads is the only ECG manifestation of P.E., or acute cor pulmonale. The rapidity of regression of these changes may be less helpful in differentiating myocardial infarction from P.E. than the regression pattern in the inferior leads. Wood[14] reported that T-wave inversion in the right precordial leads may persist for several weeks in acute cor pulmonale regardless of the etiology.

CHARACTERISTIC ECG PATTERNS IN PULMONARY EMBOLISM

The following ECG from patients with a diagnosis of acute P.E. illustrates most of the changes discussed above. The diagnosis of P.E. in these patients was made either by strong clinical evidence, lung scan, pulmonary angiography, or autopsy. Table 19-I lists the ECG changes that may occur in patients with pulmonary embolism or acute cor pulmonale. These changes may occur in any combination and appear temporally in any sequence.

TABLE 19-I

ECG CHANGES SUGGESTIVE OF PULMONARY EMBOLISM

S_1	Sinus tachycardia	P Pulmonale
Q_3	Recent axis shift	Conduction defects
Negative T_3	Negative T in 2 or more Rt. precordial leads	Atrial arrhythmias
	Clockwise rotation	

Figure 19-1 illustrates a classical ECG pattern of acute cor pulmonale in a 35-year-old man with thrombosis of the left femoral vein and clinical symptoms of P.E. The tracing on 7-26-66 shows the S1, Q3, T3 pattern, clockwise rotation, sinus tachycardia, P pulmonale, and negative T-wave in V_1-V_4. Five days later (8-1-66) the heart rate has decreased, the axis has shifted toward the left, and the S1, Q3, T3 pattern has regressed. Six weeks later (9-9-66), the T-wave is upright in V_1-V_4, the S-wave amplitude in leads V_4-V_5 is lower, and the ECG is considered to be within normal limits.

Figure 19-2 illustrates an ECG shortly after the onset of P.E. in a sixty-five-year-old man treated with X-ray irradiation for bladder carcinoma. The patient became dyspneic, cyanotic, and hypotensive, and died shortly after the ECG had been recorded. Autopsy demonstrated a large saddle embolus in the pulmonary artery. Compared to his normal ECG taken four weeks earlier (top), the pulmonary embolus produced sinus tachycardia, right

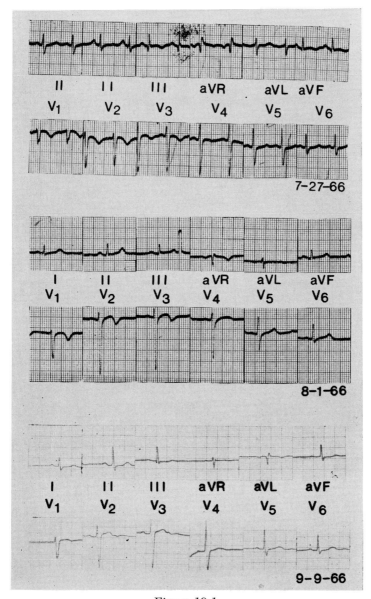

Figure 19-1.

axis deviation, clockwise rotation, QRS widening, wide S1, negative T3, and negative T-waves in all precordial leads.

Figure 19-3 illustrates less impressive ECG changes in a twenty-eight-year-old man who had multiple pulmonary emboli and total occlusion of left upper lobe pulmonary artery documented by angiography. The ECG made on the same day as the pulmonary angiogram followed the onset of

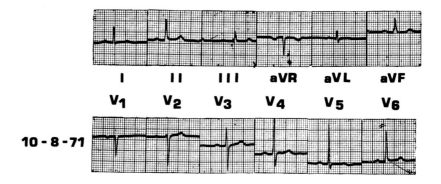

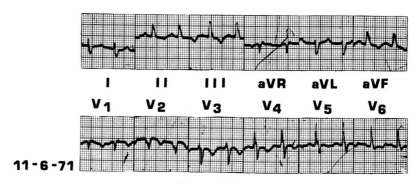

Figure 19-2.

clinical symptoms by about thirty-six hours. This ECG shows sinus tachycardia, small S1, Q3, and T-wave inversion in all precordial leads. In the absence of a strong clinical history, this ECG could not have been diagnostic of P.E. It is conceivable that more impressive changes would have been recorded if the ECG had been made earlier in the clinical course.

The ECG in Figure 19-4 were recorded from a sixty-two-year-old woman with dyspnea, tachycardia and deep venous thrombosis of the left calf. The admission ECG (12-28-65) shows atrial flutter with 2:1 A-V conduction and a ventricular rate of 170/min. There is also a prominent S1, clockwise rotation, and an incomplete right bundle branch block. In the lower tracing made two weeks later, atrial flutter is no longer present, the amplitude of S1 is lower, and the S-wave is absent in V_5-V_6. In this patient atrial flutter was thought to be secondary to P.E.

Figure 19-5 shows the value of the ECG in differentiating between acute

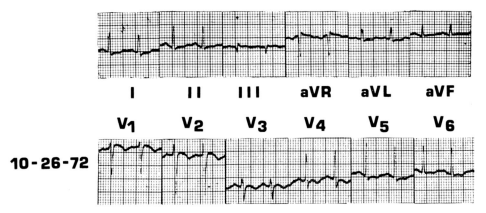

I   II   III   aVR   aVL   aVF

V₁   V₂   V₃   V₄   V₅   V₆

10-26-72

Figure 19-3.

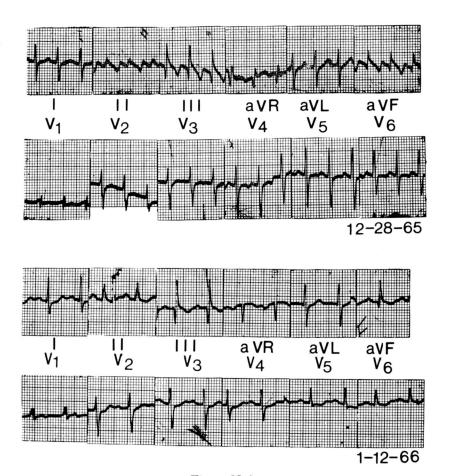

Figure 19-4.

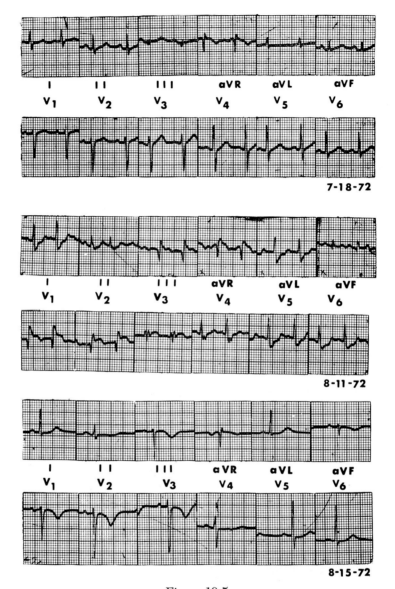

Figure 19-5.

myocardial infarction and P.E. The initial ECG (7-18-72) was recorded at the time of admission from a fifty-two-year-old-man with 30 percent second and third degree burns. This ECG reveals sinus tachycardia and is within normal limits. Twenty-four days later during physical therapy in a whirlpool the patient experienced chest pain and became dyspneic and hypotensive. The ECG obtained within fifteen minutes of the onset of symptoms (8-11-72), shows that sinus tachycardia is more pronounced, QRS duration has increased, and the S-wave in leads I and V$_5$-V$_6$ is much wider. A deep Q-wave is present in lead III, and a smaller Q-wave in lead AVF. The ST segment is elevated in leads III, AVF, V$_1$-V$_3$ and depressed in leads I, AVL, and V$_5$-V$_6$. The ECG differential diagnosis was acute P.E. versus acute myocardial infarction of the inferior and low anterior septal walls. Lung scan was consistent with multiple P.E., and the patient was clinically much improved within twenty-four hours. Four days later (8-15-72) the QRS duration became normal, and the Q-waves were no longer present in leads III and AVF. The ST segment has also returned to normal in leads III, AVF, V$_1$-V$_3$, and I, AVL, V$_5$-V$_6$. The T-wave is now inverted in leads III, AVF, V$_1$-V$_3$, and is low in leads II and V$_4$. Serial blood enzyme determination revealed no evidence of acute myocardial infarction. These evolutionary ECG changes strongly supported the diagnosis of P.E. suggested by the lung scan.

STUDY OF 100 PATIENTS

The objectives of this study were: (1) to evaluate the incidence of ECG changes in patients whose clinical history suggests P.E., and (2) to evaluate the usefulness of the ECG in the detection of clinically nonsuspected P.E. We have reviewed the hospital records and ECG's of 100 consecutive patients whose electrocardiograms suggested P.E. and acute cor pulmonale. The patients were identified by code number assigned by the electrocardiographers at the time of interpretation. The latter did not know the patients. However, all ECG requests contained an answer to the question whether P.E. was suspected or not. On the basis of this answer, two groups were established: in Group I the diagnosis of P.E. was suggested by the referring physician on the initial ECG request, and was supported by ECG changes, and in Group II, the initial diagnosis of acute cor pulmonale or P.E. was not suspected clinically but was first suggested by the electrocardiographer. Table 19-II shows the results of this study. Of thirty-six patients in Group I, in sixteen or 44 percent the diagnosis of P.E. was confirmed by lung scan, pulmonary angiography, autopsy, or a combination of these procedures. In nine patients or 25 percent the diagnosis of P.E. was made on the basis of strong clinical evidence and all of these patients were treated with anticoagulants. No other pulmonary disease was found in these patients at the time of discharge. In three patients the cause of ECG changes could not be determined, and in the remaining eight patients, or 22 percent, the clinical conditions other than P.E. could be responsible for acute cor pulmonale. The results show that in 69 percent of patients with suspected P.E. the ECG provided an evidence in support of the clinical diagnosis.

TABLE 19-II

Pulmonary embolism	Group I	Group II
Confirmed (angio, scan, autopsy)	16	3
Clinical diagnosis	9	2
Uncertain	3	13
Disproved	8	46
	36	64

Group II included sixty-four patients. In three patients in this group the diagnosis of P.E. was confirmed by autopsy, lung scan, or angiography. In two patients the ECG diagnosis was confirmed clinically, and these patients were treated for P.E. In thirteen patients or 20 percent of this group, no diagnosis was found to explain the ECG changes, and in forty-six patients or 72 percent other clinical conditions thought to explain the ECG's were present. Thus, the ECG contributed to the detection of P.E. in only five patients or 8 percent of the entire group.

Several investigators have emphasized that any conditions associated with acute right ventricular strain could produce ECG changes similar to those found in P.E. Fifty-four patients from Groups I and II had other conditions which could produce ECG changes of acute cor pulmonale. These diagnoses are listed in Table 19-III. Chronic obstructive airway disease with acute clinical deterioration was the most frequent condition, present in twenty patients. Fourteen patients had pneumonia but no evidence of underlying chronic lung disease. Pneumothorax or atelectasis was found in five patients. Less frequent causes included: pleural effusion, bronchial asthma, partial upper airway obstruction, and recent pneumonectomy. The long list of various diagnoses in Table 19-III underscores the nonspecificity of ECG changes produced by acute cor pulmonale of different etiologies.

TABLE 19-III

CLINICAL DIAGNOSIS IN PATIENTS WITH ECG
PATTERN SIMULATING PULMONARY EMBOLISM

Diagnosis	Group I	Group II	Total
Pneumonia	2	12	14
COAD	5	15	20
Bronchial Asthma	1	—	1
Post pneumonectomy	—	2	2
Pneumothorax and atelectasis	—	5	5
Pleural effusion	—	3	3
Upper airway obstr.	—	2	2
Others	—	7	7
Total	8	46	54

In Table 19-IV, thirty patients with proven or strongly suspected P.E. from both Groups I and II are compared with fifty-four patients with diagnoses other than P.E., described in Table 19-II. Since acute right ventricular strain is considered to be responsible for the ECG changes in both groups, a similar frequency of the individual ECG features would be expected in both groups. Sinus tachycardia, S1, and negative T-wave in two or more right precordial leads was present in more than 50 percent patients in both groups. A negative T-wave in two or more right precordial leads alone was also most frequently recorded in both groups. This change and clockwise rotation occurred with greater frequency in patients with P.E. than in other types of cor pulmonale but this difference is not statistically significant. The incidence of other changes which were less frequently recorded is also very similar in both groups.

TABLE 19-IV

ECG FEATURES SUGGESTIVE OF PULMONARY EMBOLUS AND ACUTE COR PULMONALE

	Proven or strongly suspected pulm. embolus (30)		Acute cor pulmonale secondary other diagnosis (54)	
	No.	%	No.	%
Sinus tachycardia	22	73	41	75
P pulmonale	10	33	17	31
Axis shift	7	23	11	20
SI	18	60	30	55
QIII	16	53	22	40
Negative TIII	6	20	13	24
Negative T 2 or more R. Precordial leads	27	90	41	75
RBBB	6	20	11	20
Supra. arrhythmia	4	13	10	18
"Clockwise rotation"	17	56	18	33

Table 19-IV shows that sinus tachycardia occurred in more than 70 percent of patients in both groups. Sinus tachycardia alone is not sufficiently specific to suspect the ECG diagnosis of P.E. or acute cor pulmonale. However, sinus tachycardia may be helpful in association with negative T-waves in the right precordial leads in differentiating between acute inferior infarction and P.E. since these two changes would not be expected to occur frequently in acute myocardial infarction.

Summary and Conclusions

The literature review presented in this paper and the results of our study, point out that no specific ECG pattern should be expected in patients with P.E. Studies in both animals and man have indicated that nearly 50 percent of the pulmonary arterial bed must be occluded to produce an ECG change. Any condition capable of producing acute right ventricular strain may simulate P.E. in the ECG. When patients with proven P.E. were compared with patients who had other causes of acute cor pulmonale, no significant difference could be found in the frequency of any ECG features.

The value of the ECG in the diagnosis of P.E. is certainly not as great as that of pulmonary angiography or the lung scan. Nevertheless the ECG supported the diagnosis in twenty-five of thirty-six or 69 percent of our patients in whom the diagnosis of P.E. was suspected clinically. This indicates that when the diagnosis of P.E. is clinically suspected, the ECG is helpful in strengthening the clinical impression in a significant number of patients. This in turn suggests that any patient suspected of pulmonary embolism should have an ECG as early as possible in their clinical evaluation. When the electrocardiographer was the first to raise the suspicion of pulmonary embolism, the diagnosis was subsequently established only in five of the sixty-four patients. Among these sixty-four patients, forty-six or 72 percent had other causes of acute cor pulmonale.

The electrocardiogram may be very helpful in differentiating between myocardial infarction from pulmonary embolism, particularly by recording serial tracings. Early loss of the Q-wave in lead III, or AVF is the most helpful diagnostic sign. Any ECG pattern resembling acute myocardial infarction of the inferior and anterior septal areas should arouse the suspicion of possible pulmonary embolism. Pulmonary embolism or other diseases with acute cor pulmonale, may cause negative T-waves in the right precordial leads, and these changes may persist for several weeks.

REFERENCES

1. Newman, D. A.: Electrocardiographic changes in pulmonary embolism. *J Fla Med Assoc*, 38:701-712, 1952.
2. Littman, D.: Observations on the electrocardiographic changes in pulmonary embolism. In *Pulmonary Embolic Disease*. New York, Grune and Stratton, 1965.
3. Cutforth, R. H. and Oran, S.: The electrocardiogram in pulmonary embolism. *Br Heart J*, 20:41-60, 1958.
4. Weber, D. M. and Phillips, J. H., Jr.: A re-evaluation of electrocardiographic changes accompanying acute pulmonary embolism. *Am J Med Sci*, 251:391-398, 1966.
5. Frommel, E.: Les troubles du rhythme cardiaque au cours de embolie pulmonaire mortelle: Etude electrocardiographique experimentale. *J Physiol Pathol Gen*, 26:247-249, 1928.
6. Otto, H. L.: The effect of a sudden increase in the intracardiac pressure on the form of the T-Wave of the electrocardiogram. *J Lab Clin Med*, 14:643-645, 1929.
7. Buchbinder, W. C. and Katz, L. N.: The electrocardiogram in acute experimental distension of the right heart. *Am J Med Sci*, 817:785-792, 1934.

8. Lundy, C. J. and Woodruff, L. W.: Experimental left and right axis deviation. *Arch Intern Med, 44*:893-907, 1929.

9. McGinn, S. and White, P. D.: Acute cor pulmonale resulting from pulmonary embolism: Its clinical recognition. *JAMA, 104*:1473-1480, 1935.

10. Love, W. S., Jr., Brugler, G. W. and Winslow, N.: Electrocardiographic studies in clinical and experimental pulmonary embolization. *Ann Intern Med, 11*:2109-2123, 1938.

11. Sokolow, M., Katz, L. N. and Muscovitz, A. N.: Electrocardiogram in pulmonary embolism. *Am Heart J, 19*:166-184, 1940.

12. Durant, T. M., Ginsburg, I. W. and Roesler, H.: Transient bundle branch block and other electrocardiographic changes in pulmonary embolism. *Am Heart J, 17*:423-430, 1939.

13. Szucs, M. M., Jr., Brooks, H. L., Grossman, W., Banas, J. S., Jr., Meister, S. G., Dexter, L. and Dalen, J. E.: Diagnostic sensitivity of laboratory findings in acute pulmonary embolism. *Ann Intern Med, 74*:161-166, 1971.

14. Wood, P.: Pulmonary embolism: Diagnosis by chest lead electrocardiography. *Br Heart J, 3*:21-29, 1941.

15. Johnson, J. C., Flowers, N. C. and Horan, L. G.: Unexplained atrial flutter: A frequent herald of pulmonary embolism. *Chest, 60*:29-34, 1971.

Chapter 20

THE NATURAL HISTORY OF PULMONARY EMBOLIC DISEASE

James E. Dalen

ONCE THE diagnosis of acute pulmonary embolism has been made, the clinician has available many different forms of therapy. He may choose from among therapeutic plans that concentrate on preventing further pulmonary embolism or forms of therapy in which the goal is to remove the emboli that have already lodged within the pulmonary circulation. The latter category includes two seemingly dissimilar forms of therapy, namely fibrinolytic therapy and pulmonary embolectomy.

In order to make an appropriate therapeutic decision, it is necessary to look carefully at the natural history of pulmonary embolic disease. What happens to the patient with acute pulmonary embolism? Which patients die acutely? Which patients are late deaths? How many and which patients go on to chronic cor pulmonale? Which forms of therapy are most likely to modify the natural course of a given patient with acute pulmonary embolism?

Reviews of cases of fatal pulmonary embolism have indicated that most of the deaths due to acute pulmonary embolism occur very rapidly. In the series from the Massachusetts General Hospital reported by Donaldson, et al.,[1] of 271 patients who died of autopsy-proven pulmonary embolism, 67 percent died within one half hour of onset of symptoms; and by one hour, a total of 75 percent were dead. Patients who die within an hour of the episode of acute pulmonary embolism almost invariably have massive pulmonary embolism occluding the main pulmonary artery or both the right and left pulmonary arteries. In many of these cases, the diagnosis is not made and therefore, therapeutic decisions are not even raised.

Even though most of the patients who die of acute pulmonary embolism die within an hour of the onset of symptoms, the vast majority of patients who have acute pulmonary embolism do not die. What happens to the patient who has acute pulmonary embolism but survives for at least an hour?

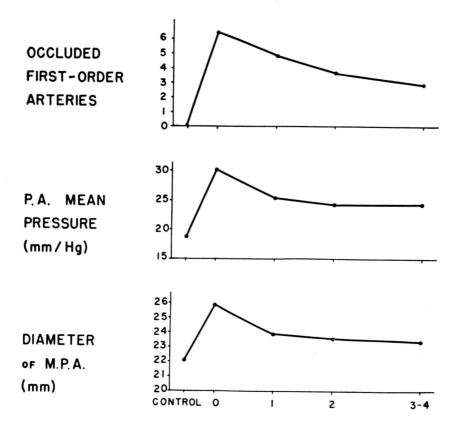

OCCLUDED FIRST-ORDER ARTERIES

P.A. MEAN PRESSURE (mm/Hg)

DIAMETER OF M.P.A. (mm)

TIME AFTER EMBOLIZATION (HOURS)

Figure 20-1. Changes after pulmonary embolization. In these three panels, the number of occluded first order arteries (top panel), average mean pulmonary arterial pressure (middle panel), and average diameter of the main pulmonary artery (bottom panel) are plotted for the control, immediate postembolization, and the one-hour, two-hour, and three-to-four-hour postembolization studies. The maximum number of occluded arteries, and the maximum pulmonary arterial pressure and size were noted in the immediate postembolization studies (plotted at 0 hours). By one hour after embolization, each of these three variables had shown significant returns toward their control values. Additional minimal improvement occurred between one and four hours after embolization.

Reprinted from: Dalen, J. E., et al., Pulmonary angiography in experimental pulmonary embolism. *Am Heart J,* 72:509-520, 1966.

We first studied the natural history of pulmonary embolism in the animal laboratory. We embolized normal dogs with autologous blood clot, and then did serial pulmonary angiograms to assess the rate of resolution of embolism without therapy.[2] The blood clots were rendered radio-opaque by the addition of dionosil. This allowed us to correlate the location and size of the emboli as visualized by plain chest X-ray, with the results of pulmonary angiography.

When we repeated pulmonary angiograms at hourly intervals up to four hours after the embolic episode, we found that even in the absence of therapy, rapid resolution occurred. That is, the number of occluded arteries progressively decreased during the hours immediately after pulmonary embolism. In many cases, slight movement of the clot would change an artery from being completely occluded to being only partially occluded. That is, we found that resolution could occur without much change in the clot size. If a completely occluded vessel becomes only partially occluded due to slight movement of the clot, it allows blood to flow by it. This causes a marked change in the hemodynamic response to pulmonary embolism. As the number of occluded pulmonary arteries decreases, pulmonary artery mean pressure decreases. This is demonstrated in Figure 20-1, which shows the number of occluded first order arteries for four hours after dogs were embolized with autologous blood clot. Figure 20-1 shows that as the number of occluded arteries decreases, the pulmonary artery pressure decreases toward normal.

When we repeated these studies two to seven days after embolization, we found that further evidence of resolution had occurred.[3] Immediately after embolization, an average of 5.2 first order arteries were occluded. Two to seven days after embolization, only 1.8 of these arteries were occluded. Oligemia due to pulmonary embolic obstruction, estimated on a scale from 1+ to 4+, decreased from an average of 2.7 immediately after embolization to 1.0 at two to seven days. Mean pulmonary artery pressure which was 20.4 mm Hg before embolization was 31.4 immediately after embolization but was back to normal (20.0) two to seven days after embolization.

These studies make it clear that in the normal dog embolism with autologous blood clot rapidly resolves without the use of fibrinolytic therapy or any other form of therapy.

Do these same rapid changes occur in patients with acute pulmonary embolism? In order to study the resolution rate of acute pulmonary embolism in man, we studied a group of fifteen patients who had definite angiographic evidence of pulmonary embolism involving both lungs.[4] None of these patients had underlying heart disease. They were treated with anticoagulation and/or venous ligation. None of the patients had pulmonary embolectomy or were treated with fibrinolytic therapy. Pulmonary angiography and right heart catheterization were repeated at varying intervals from one to thirty days after documentation of embolism by angiography.

Seven patients were restudied at one to seven days; ten were studied ten to twenty-one days and two patients were studied at thirty days after the diagnosis of embolism was documented. The repeat angiograms were classified into four categories: (1) no change—the angiogram at follow-up was unchanged from the original angiogram; (2) minimal resolution—the repeat angiogram showed detectable improvement, but major, obvious angiographic abnormalities of pulmonary embolism persisted; (3) moderate resolution—major improvement had occurred such that only minimal evidence of pulmonary embolism persisted by angiography; (4) complete resolution—the repeat pulmonary angiogram was entirely normal.

The results of the repeat pulmonary angiograms are shown in Table 20-I. Of seven patients who had repeat pulmonary angiograms one to seven days after the original study, one showed no change. Six showed minimal resolution, that is, there was evidence of some resolution but major abnormalities persisted. None of the patients had moderate or complete resolution within seven days of the original study.

TABLE 20-I

ANGIOGRAPHIC FINDINGS AT FOLLOW-UP

Angiographic change	Interval from initial study		
	1-7 days	10-21 days	> 30 days
No change	1	1	0
Minimal resolution (Marked abnormalities persist)	6	2	1
Moderate resolution (Minimal abnormalities persist)	0	5	0
Complete resolution (Angiogram normal)	0	2	1

Of the ten patients who were studied at ten to twenty-one days, one showed no change and two showed minimal change. However, five patients showed moderate resolution such that only minimal abnormalities persisted, and two patients had complete resolution, that is, the pulmonary angiogram at follow-up was entirely normal. One of the patients with complete resolution was studied fourteen days after the original study, and the other at fifteen days.

Of the two patients who were studied at thirty days, one showed only minimal resolution and the other had complete resolution.

The hemodynamic findings obtained at the follow-up studies are shown in Figure 20-2. Note that there is a good correlation between the angiographic resolution and the hemodynamic findings. That is, in the studies performed one to seven days after pulmonary embolism, there was minimal change in the pulmonary artery or right atrial pressure. In the studies performed ten to twenty-one days after embolism, right heart pressures approached normal values in the majority of patients. This correlation indicates that as pulmonary emboli resolve, the response of the right heart follows closely. This is remarkably similar to our findings in dogs embolized with autologous blood clot.[2, 3]

We concluded from these studies that pulmonary emboli resolve without fibrinolytic therapy in the majority of patients. Complete resolution may

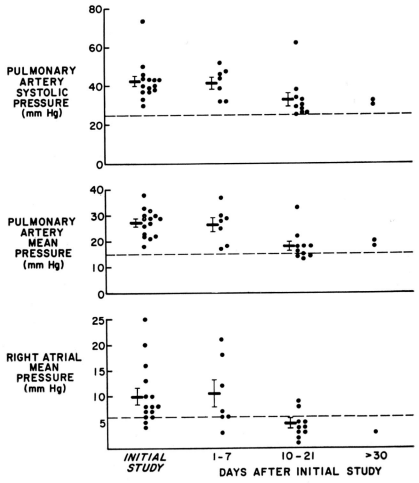

Figure 20-2. Right heart pressures are shown for the initial study, and at one to seven, ten to twenty-one, and at thirty days after the initial study. The dotted line in each panel shows the upper limits of normal for this laboratory. Note that by ten to twenty-one days, right heart pressures had decreased to near normal values. This is the same time that the pulmonary angiograms began to approach normal.

Reprinted from Dalen, J. E., et al.: Resolution rate of acute pulmonary embolism in man. *N Engl J Med, 280*:1194-1199, 1969.

occur as early as two weeks. In other patients it may take up to a month to
have complete resolution. However, there are a few patients such as the
patient who was studied at thirty days in whom resolution was still incomplete thirty days after the embolic episode. Tow and Wagner[5] utilizing
follow-up lung scans found data very comparable to our own.

The hospital mortality in patients with acute pulmonary embolism in
whom the diagnosis is made and are treated is shown in Table 20-II. Note
that in 100 consecutive patients with acute pulmonary embolism documented by angiography, eighteen died during the hospitalization. Mortality
was not related to the magnitude of pulmonary embolism. In twenty-one
patients in whom more than 50 percent of the pulmonary circulation was
occluded, the hospital mortality was 24 percent, comparable to the overall
mortality in the total group.

TABLE 20-II

ACUTE PULMONARY EMBOLISM IN 100 PATIENTS

HOSPITAL MORTALITY

	No.	Deaths	% Mortality
No heart disease	50	4	8%
Heart disease, without CHF	18	2	11%
Prior CHF	32	12	38%
Total	100	18	18%

The key factor that determines mortality in acute pulmonary embolism is
the status of the patient's cardiovascular system. Of fifty patients who had
no prior heart disease, there were only four hospital deaths for a hospital
mortality of 8 percent. Of eighteen patients with heart disease without congestive failure, there were two deaths for a mortality approximately the
same as those without heart disease, namely 11 percent. However, of thirty-
two patients who had congestive heart failure prior to the episode of acute
pulmonary embolism, twelve died for a mortality of 38 percent.

From our experience, of patients in whom the diagnosis of acute pulmonary embolism is documented and treatment is instituted, 80 percent survive and are discharged. Patients who fail to survive are primarily those
with underlying heart disease with congestive heart failure.

What happens to the 80 percent of the patients who survive pulmonary
embolism and are discharged? In order to answer this question, we studied
a group of seventy-five consecutive patients in whom a diagnosis of acute
pulmonary embolism was documented by angiogram during the time period
from 1964-1970.[6] Fifteen patients (20%) died and sixty were discharged.
The status of each of these sixty patients was determined in 1971, one to
seven years after discharge. The average duration of follow-up was twenty-
nine months.

This follow-up study was performed to determine the long-term survival rate of patients with acute pulmonary embolism, to determine the incidence of recurrent pulmonary embolism, and to find out how many patients developed chronic cor pulmonale due to unresolved pulmonary embolism.

The patients ranged in age from eighteen to seventy-two. The average age was fifty-nine. Twenty-nine of the patients had heart disease prior to the episode of pulmonary embolism and sixteen had prior left heart failure.

The treatment for the acute episode was anticoagulation, that is, Heparin followed by Coumadin, in thirteen patients; nine patients had venous interruption without anticoagulation, and thirty-six patients had anticoagulation followed by venous interruption. Two patients did not receive specific therapy for their episode of acute pulmonary embolism.

At the time of follow-up in the survivors, an interim history was taken, physical examination was performed and the patient had an ECG, chest X-ray, arterial blood gas determination and a repeat lung scan. For the nonsurvivors, the interim history was reviewed, including review of subsequent hospitalizations and physicians' records and the postmortem examination was reviewed.

Nineteen patients (33%) died during the period of follow-up. Their average survival was sixteen months. Thirty-nine (67%) of the patients were alive with an average survival of thirty-five months. Only two patients were lost to follow-up.

The causes of death during follow-up are shown in Table 20-III. Note that the most common cause of death was underlying heart disease; that is, congestive heart failure or acute myocardial infarction. None of the patients died of recurrent pulmonary embolism. One patient died of chronic cor pulmonale. This was the only patient whose death was related to pulmonary embolism.

TABLE 20-III

CAUSES OF DEATH DURING FOLLOW-UP

	No.	*Postmortem*
Congestive heart failure	4	1
Acute myocardial infarction	3	3
Postoperative complications	3	2
Pneumonia	3	2
Metastatic carcinoma	2	1
Trauma	1	0
Acute ethanol intoxication	1	0
Chronic cor pulmonale	1	1
Uncertain (died in sleep)	1	0
Total	19	10

Total mortality = 33%, Avg. survival = 16 months
Survivors = 67%, Avg. survival = 35 months

The patients who died during follow-up were compared to those who survived in regards to several factors. The patients who died were somewhat older, average age sixty-four, as opposed to those who survived whose average age was fifty-seven. The magnitude of pulmonary embolism was actually greater in those who survived than those who died during follow-up. That is, 42 percent of the patients who were alive at follow-up had obstruction of more than 50 percent of the circulation at the time of acute pulmonary embolism as compared to only 21 percent of those who failed to survive. Similarly, 28 percent of the survivors had shock with the episode of pulmonary embolism compared to only 11 percent of those who died.

The most important factor related to long-term survival after acute pulmonary embolism was the presence of prior heart disease. Eighty-nine percent of the patients who died during follow-up had had heart disease prior to the episode of acute pulmonary embolism. Only 31 percent of the survivors had prior heart disease. The impact of the presence of left ventricular failure prior to pulmonary embolism was even more striking. Sixty-eight percent of the patients who died during follow-up had had left ventricular failure prior to the episode of pulmonary embolism. Only 8 percent of those who survived had prior left heart failure.

The influence of prior left ventricular failure on long-term survival in patients who have acute pulmonary embolism is shown in Table 20-IV. Note, that of the sixteen patients who had left ventricular failure prior to the episode of acute pulmonary embolism, but survived the acute episode and were discharged, only three were alive at follow-up and only one (6%) was alive and ambulatory. This is in marked contrast to the patients who had no left ventricular failure prior to the episode of acute pulmonary embolism. Of forty-two patients who survived the acute episode and were discharged, thirty-six were alive at follow-up and thirty-three (79%) were alive and well.

TABLE 20-IV

EFFECT OF PRIOR LV FAILURE ON PROGNOSIS

STATUS 1-7 YEARS AFTER DISCHARGE

	LVF prior to PE	No LVF
No. discharged	16	42
Alive	3	36
Alive, Ambulatory	1 (6%)	33 (79%)

It seems very clear that the natural history of pulmonary embolic disease is tremendously influenced by the presence of heart disease. The acute mortality in the hospital is much higher in patients wtih prior heart disease with congestive failure and similarly, long-term survival is markedly affected by the presence of prior left ventricular failure. This data indicates that the prognosis of the patient who survives acute pulmonary embolism is essentially dependent on the prognosis of associated heart disease.

During the period of follow-up, recurrent pulmonary embolism was suspected in four patients. However, when lung scans were repeated, the diagnosis of recurrent pulmonary embolism was confirmed in only one patient. This was a patient who died of bacterial endocarditis three years after the episode of pulmonary embolism. At postmortem he had evidence of new pulmonary embolism, but it did not cause his death. None of the sixty patients died of recurrent pulmonary embolism during the period of follow-up.

The follow-up lung scans and arterial blood gas determinations were assessed to determine the late resolution of pulmonary embolism. The results of repeat blood gases in twenty-nine patients who had blood gases drawn on room air at the time of the acute episode and at the time of follow-up are shown in Figure 20-3. Note that arterial pO_2 was increased

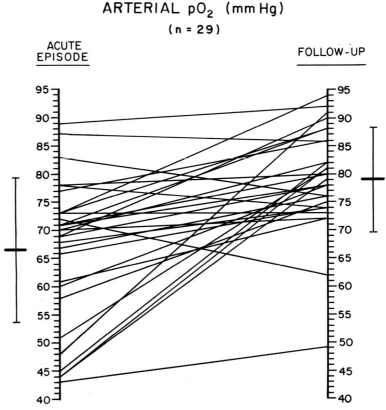

Figure 20-3. The arterial pO_2 (mm Hg) while breathing room air is shown at the time of the acute episode, and at follow-up one to seven years later in twenty-nine patients. Note the increase in pO_2 in nearly every case. The average pO_2 for the group increased from sixty-seven to seventy-nine mm Hg at follow-up.

at follow-up in almost every patient. The average increased from sixty-seven at the time of the acute episode to seventy-nine mm Hg at the time of follow-up. This is consistent with the occurrence of resolution in the majority of patients. The occurrence of late resolution was further confirmed by the repeat lung scans.

Of thirty-three patients who had follow-up lung scans, twenty-one were entirely normal and therefore, complete resolution had occurred. Eight patients had partial resolution; that is, abnormalities persisted but they were much less than had been present at the time of acute pulmonary embolism. Only four of the thirty-three patients having repeat lung scans showed persistent, unresolved embolism; that is, their lung scans were unchanged. None of these four patients had evidence of cor pulmonale by physical examination or by electrocardiogram.

Of nineteen patients who died during the follow-up, ten had postmortem examination. Seven showed no evidence of pulmonary embolism at postmortem. In two, there was minor evidence of partially resolved pulmonary embolism. Only one patient had persistent, unresolved pulmonary embolism. This patient died of chronic cor pulmonale and as noted, is the only patient who died of pulmonary embolism during the period of follow-up.

The data related to late resolution as obtained by follow-up lung scan in the survivors and postmortem examination in those who died during follow-up is shown in Table 20-V. Of forty-three patients in whom follow-up data permitted accurate assessment of the degree of resolution, 65 percent had complete resolution. Twenty-three percent had partial resolution and only 12 percent had persistent, unresolved pulmonary embolism.

TABLE 20-V

EVIDENCE OF RESOLUTION 1-7 YEARS AFTER DISCHARGE

	Follow-up lung scan	Postmortem	Total
	(33)	(10)	43
Complete resolution	21	7	28 (65%)
Partial resolution	8	2	10 (23%)
Persistent, unresolved embolism	4	1	5 (12%)

Recurrent pulmonary embolism in patients who are treated with long-term coagulation or venous interruption is quite uncommon. We documented only one case (2%) during the seven years of follow-up. Persistent, unresolved pulmonary embolism was uncommon and occurred in 12 percent. However, chronic cor pulmonale secondary to unresolved pulmonary embolism was exceedingly rare. Of our sixty patients, only one had chronic cor pulmonale secondary to persistent pulmonary embolism. This latter data indicates that definitive therapy for embolism; that is, embolectomy or fibrinolytic therapy, is not needed to prevent cor pulmonale since it is so exceedingly rare.

We conclude from these studies that long-term survival after acute pulmonary embolism is largely dependent upon the patient's cardiac status. If the patient had left ventricular failure prior to the episode of acute pulmonary embolism, his acute and long-term prognosis are poor. If he had no heart disease, his outlook is good.

REFERENCES

1. Donaldson, G. A., Williams, C., Scannell, J. G. and Shaw, R. S.: A reappraisal of the application of the Trendelenburg operation to massive fatal embolism. *N Engl J Med, 268:*171-174, 1963.
2. Dalen, J. E., Mathur, V. S., Evans, H., Haynes, F. W., Pur-Shahriari, A. A., Stein, P. D. and Dexter, L.: Pulmonary angiography in experimental pulmonary embolism, *Am Heart J, 72:*509-520, 1966.
3. Mathur, V. S., Dalen, J. E., Evans, H., Haynes, F. W., Pur-Shahriari, A. A., Stein, P. D. and Dexter, L.: Pulmonary angiography one to seven days after experimental pulmonary embolism. *Invest Radiol, 2:*304-312, 1967.
4. Dalen, J. E., Banas, J. S., Brooks, H. L., Evans, G. L., Paraskos, J. A. and Dexter, L.: Resolution rate of acute pulmonary embolism in man. *N Engl J Med, 280:*1194-1199, 1969.
5. Tow, D. E. and Wagner, H. N., Jr.: Recovery of pulmonary arterial blood flow in patients with pulmonary embolism. *N Engl J Med, 276:*1053-1059, 1967.
6. Paraskos, J. A., Adelstein, S. J., Smith, R. E., Rickman, F. D., Grossman, W., Dexter, L. and Dalen, J. E.: Late prognosis of acute pulmonary embolism. *N Engl J Med, 289:*55-58, 1973.

DISCUSSION

Dr. Dame (South Carolina): Dr. Dalen, I'm really surprised at the incidence of phlebitis that you had subsequent to clip as contrasted wtih ligation of the cava, could you comment on that please?

Dr. Dalen: First of all, it's a very small series of patients. Most of our vascular surgeons have changed over to IVC clip. There have been very few IVC ligations since 1966. It is a fact that many patients who have IVC clip come back several weeks after discharge with symptomatic thrombophlebitis and when that happens, we treat them with heparin.

Question: I'd like to ask whether you think that this experience from your hospital where this operation is done frequently would be similar to a follow-up done on a series where very little surgery was done and only medical therapy which had the same overall result in follow-up.

Dr. Dalen: I can't answer that. I would want to see what other data looks like.

Question: How do you distinguish pulmonary embolism from the early stages of a shock lung syndrome?

Dr. Dalen: Clinically, that is, of course, very difficult and pulmonary angiography would be the technique I would use.

Question: Were your patients with the clip kept on permanent anticoagulation?

Dr. Dalen: No, one of our principal indications for using venous interruption is in patients who are chronically predisposed to pulmonary embolism who do not have a reversible predisposition to embolism. We think the choice is between Coumadin forever or venous interruption. Therefore, we often choose venous interruption, and we do not treat these patients with Coumadin unless they have symptomatic thrombophlebitis in the future.

Question: Would you attempt to do bilateral venograms before proceeding on to pulmonary angiography because of the problems inherent in the procedure?

Dr. Dalen: We do pulmonary angiography first. I personally think that the time will come when we will do more venograms than pulmonary angiograms. I would expect that most people with acute pulmonary embolism would have evidence of venous thrombosis by venogram. If we could, in fact, do venograms very quickly with very little pain, yes, we would do that before pulmonary angiogram. Right now, it takes a very long time and tends to be somewhat uncomfortable.

Dr. Sasahara: I think this study with follow-up of Dr. Dalen's clearly shows that there is very little severe late impairment after pulmonary embolism. I would, however, take issue with the frequency of performing surgical venous interruption. In our own hospital, as a matter of fact, we have come around full circle from a primarily surgical interruptive approach to our current heparin anticoagulation therapy. I would not like our audience to believe that to duplicate the fine results of Dr. Dalen's, one needs to ligate the inferior vena cava, followed by initiation of warfarin therapy. In addition, it has been shown that interrupting the cava does not prevent subsequent embolization.

Dr. Dalen: I want to make it quite clear, that we're reporting the follow-up of our own patients; the majority of whom did have venous interruption. Our data does not prove that venous interruption is better, as good as, or not as good as long-term anticoagulation with Coumadin. This happens to be the result in our patients with venous interruption. I would certainly welcome someone who believes strongly in long-term Coumadin to do a similar study and see if they do as well.

Question: Certainly the evidence brought out is that most all pulmonary emboli come from the legs. Are you aware of any evidence as to how often pulmonary emboli come from other sources, such as the right heart or pelvis?

Dr. Dalen: Well, that is a very controversial question and there is no way to settle it definitively. First of all, in postmortem studies done in the United States, the leg veins are very rarely dissected and therefore very few studies in the United States have any facts on the number of people with documented pulmonary embolism who have clots in the lower extremities. The Studies from England, Sevitt and Gallagher for example, have made it clear that if you look at the leg veins at postmortem in people with documented pulmonary embolism, nearly all of them have clots. Now what do you do if a patient has clots in the lower extremities and also has a small clot in the right heart? How do you decide where the pulmonary emboli came from? I think that these are the reasons that the reported frequency of the right heart as the source of emboli is so variable. Dr. Wheeler might have an answer to this.

Dr. Wheeler: I had the privilege of studying some of Dr. Sasahara's patients who were studied for the Urokinase study. Of twenty-three who had angiographically proven pulmonary emboli, twenty-one of them had abnormal impedance in one or both legs indicating clot in the legs. Of the two who didn't, one came to post and didn't have a pulmonary embolism, but had a carcinoma of the lung. The other we studied was impedance I think, two days after Urokinase treatment. Since then, we have studied about twenty patients. I don't have the exact number with proven pulmonary embolism and all of them have had abnormal impedance findings in the legs. I think practically all of these thrombi do come from the legs and a lot of evidence supports this.

SECTION IV

PULMONARY THROMBOEMBOLISM— PREVENTION

Chapter 21

THE USE OF PLATELET SUPPRESSIVE DRUGS IN ARTERIAL AND VENOUS THROMBOEMBOLISM

Geoffrey Evans

I T IS KNOWN that platelets are important in the initiation and growth of thrombi. For this reason platelet suppressive drugs have been used in both arterial and venous thromboembolism. Sullivan, in 1970, showed that by combining dipyridamole with an anticoagulant there was a reduced incidence of thromboembolism from prosthetic heart valves compared with that of using the anticoagulant alone.[1] Harker and Slichter showed that aspirin and dipyridamole when used together normalized platelet survival.[2] However, when aspirin was used on its own it did not appear to have any effect on platelet survival. Genton, in 1970, showed that platelet survival was abnormal in those patients with prosthetic mitral valves who embolized. He showed that platelet survival could be normalized with sulfinpyrazone 200 mg four times daily and that by normalizing platelet survival there appeared to be a reduction in the incidence of thromboembolic episodes.[3] The present communication describes a further therapeutic trial with arterial thromboembolism using sulfinpyrazone 200 mg four times daily for the treatment of amaurosis fugax.

Atherosclerosis of the internal carotid artery leads to alteration of the vessel lumen which predisposes to the development of mural and occluding thrombi. The thrombi may then embolize distally and produce transient cerebral ischemia or transient blindness (amaurosis fugax). Theoretically platelet suppressive drugs might be expected to reduce the tendency to thrombosis and embolization and therefore be beneficial in the treatment of amaurosis fugax. In three detailed case reports[4, 5] aspirin has been found to be effective in the treatment of amaurosis fugax but to date there have been no comprehensive studies of the use of platelet suppressive drugs in this disorder. This controlled clinical study is a double-blind crossover study. Each of twenty patients received either sulfinpyrazone 200 mg four times daily or an identical placebo according to a prescribed randomized arrangement and after six weeks were then crossed over to the alternative therapy for a further six weeks. The arrangement was such that ten patients received sulfinpyrazone first and the other ten received placebo. There was no "washout" period between treatment periods and this could introduce a small bias against showing a benefit of sulfinpyrazone.

All patients had eye symptoms and, in addition, six had symptoms of weakness or paresthesiae of the arms or legs. Four vessel cerebral angiographic studies were performed on all patients and any with evidence of a carotid stenosis greater than 70 percent were excluded and treated surgically. Analysis of the data relating to recurrent attacks showed that the order of administration of the two treatments did not influence significantly the relative efficiency. It is appropriate therefore to assess the group of twenty patients as a whole. These twenty patients comprised five female and fifteen males with an average age of fifty-one years. Eleven had myocardial disease, seven had hypertension, eight had peripheral vascular disease, and five were diabetic. Six had bilateral disease, five had vertebral disease, and the mean carotid stenosis in the total group was 55 percent.

Table 21-I shows the observed incidence of eye symptoms in the six weeks before the trial and during the respective treatment periods there was a marked reduction in attacks during the sulfinpyrazone treatment compared with pretrial, from 3.4 to 0.5 attacks per patient (p<0.001). On the other hand, there was only a small reduction in attacks during the placebo period which was neither clinically nor statistically significant. In looking at the results for individual patients we defined a clinically significant improvement as at least a 50 percent reduction in the number of attacks compared with the six-week period immediately before the trial starter.

TABLE 21-I

INCIDENCE OF AMAUROSIS FUGAX IN A SIX-WEEK PERIOD

Treatment period	Mean number of eye symptoms per patient
Pretrial	3.4
Sulfinpyrazone	0.5
Placebo	2.7

The results are summarized in Table 21-II. It can be seen that while five patients showed improvement on both treatments and two improved on neither, the remaining thirteen patients all showed a significant improvement while on sulfinpyrazone but no improvement on placebo. This observed difference in effect is statistically highly significant (p < 0.001). In all, only five of the twenty patients had any attacks while on sulfinpyra-

TABLE 21-II

		SULFINPYRAZONE		
		Improvement	No Improvement	
Placebo	Improvement	5	0	5
	No Improvement	13	2	15
		18	2	20

zone compared with eighteen patients during the placebo treatment. Six patients had at least one transient ischemic attack exclusive of eye symptoms, in the pretrial period. The data for these patients are summarized in Table 21-III. One patient had no attacks on either treatment but for each of the other five patients the number of attacks was always less during the sulfinpyrazone treatment compared with placebo ($p < 0.05$). It is also clinically interesting to note that the three patients who each had a single attack when on sulfinpyrazone all had them when on the first week of therapy.

TABLE 21-III

NUMBER OF T.I.A.'S IN SIX-WEEK PERIOD (SIX PATIENTS)

Treatment period	*Total number of T.I.A. symptoms*
Pretrial	10
Sulfinpyrazone	3
Placebo	10

The results from this study demonstrate that sulfinpyrazone is effective in short-term reduction of symptoms of amaurosis fugax. Results in other transient cerebral ischemic attacks are promising, but the number of patients studied was small. Although the study of Acheson et al.[6] using dipyridamole was negative, the present study using sulfinpyrazone and the encouraging case reports by Harrison and Mundall suggest that a long-term randomized trial is justified.

The use of platelet suppressive drugs in the treatment or prophylaxis of venous thrombosis has been somewhat conflicting. Some of the positive results may have been associated with the method of diagnosis and it is apparent that more adequate trials have to be performed before the use of these drugs as a prophylaxis against venous thrombosis can be assessed.

The present study is related to patients with recurrent venous thrombosis. The best approach to the management of patients with this condition is somewhat nonuniform. The present study was a controlled clinical trial to evaluate sulfinpyrazone in the prevention of attacks of recurrent venous thrombosis. For the purpose of this study they were defined as more than one attack of venous thrombosis occurring per annum not precipitated by any known cause such as pregnancy or surgery. The end point in the study was a clinical recurrence of venous thrombosis manifested by pain or swelling of the affected limb.

The study was a double-blind between patient trial in which the patients were given either sulfinpyrazone 200 mg four times daily, or an identical placebo according to a prescribed randomized arrangement. Fifty patients were entered into the study, thirty into the sulfinpyrazone and twenty in the placebo group. The two groups were similarly in composition with respect to sex, age, and previous history of thrombosis. The patients were followed-up at three monthly intervals and the average duration of follow-up was twenty-four months in the sulfinpyrazone and ninteen months in the placebo group.

Eleven patients, six on sulfinpyrazone and five on placebo, dropped out of the study at times ranging from nine to twenty-four months and six to twenty-six months respectively. The results of these patients are included in the analysis summarized in Table 21-IV. This shows that three patients (10%) on sulfinpyrazone had recurrent venous thrombosis compared with eight patients (40%) in the placebo group. This difference is highly statistically significant ($p < 0.01$).

The results of this study show that administration of sulfinpyrazone 200 mg four times daily significantly reduced the incidence of recurrent attacks of clinically detected venous thrombosis. Steele, Weily, and Genton[7] have

TABLE 21-IV

	Sulfinpyrazone	Placebo	
Recurrence	3	8	11
No Recurrence	27	12	39
	30	20	50

reported on the use of sulfinpyrazone in seven patients who had recurrent venous thrombosis with reduced platelet survival while on anticoagulant therapy. They showed that these patients were clinically improved, and their platelet survival normalized. Unlike these patients, the patients on our study were not on oral anticoagulant therapy, although some had failed to respond to anticoagulant therapy before being entered into the study. The results of this study therefore suggest that sulfinpyrazone may have a place in the treatment of recurrent attacks of venous thrombosis. It is uncertain whether all patients would benefit or only those with reduced platelet survival and this aspect of sulfinpyrazone in recurrent venous thrombosis requires further study.

REFERENCES

1. Sullivan, J. M., Harken, D. E. and Gorlin, R.: Pharmacologic control of thromboembolic complications of cardiac-valve replacement. *N Engl J Med, 284:* 1391-1394, 1971.
2. Harker, L. A. and Slichter, S. J.: Studies of platelet and fibrinogen kinetics in patients with prosthetic heart valves. *N Engl J Med, 283:*1302-1305, 1970.
3. Weily, H. S. and Genton, E.: Altered platelet function in patients with prosthetic mitral valves. Effects of sulfinpyrazone therapy. *Circulation, XLII: (42):*967-972, 1970.
4. Harrison, M. J. G., Marshall, J., Meadows, J. C. and Russel, R. W. R.: Effect of aspirin in amaurosis fugax. *Lancet,* 2:743-744, 1971.
5. Mundall, J., Quintero, P., Von Kaulla, K., Austin, J. and Harman, R.: Transient monocular blindness and increased platelet aggregability treated with aspirin— a case report. *Neurology,* 21:402, 1971.
6. Acheson, J., Danta, G. and Hutchinson, E. C.: Controlled trial of dipyridamole in cerebral vascular disease. *Br Med J,* L:614-615, 1969.
7. Steele, P. P., Weily, H. S. and Genton, E.: Platelet survival and adhesiveness in recurrent venous thrombosis. *N Engl J Med,* 286:1148-1152, 1973.

DISCUSSION

Question: The Dextrans interfere with platelet adhesiveness, do they not? Have you used the Dextrans in any of the investigative studies that you have undertaken?

Dr. Evans: No, we haven't used Dextran. I think you probably know Kakkar's work on Dextran showing that there probably wasn't any difference in the incidence of postoperative venous thrombosis using iodinated fibrinogen. We have not used them at all in our arterial studies.

Dr. O'Brien: I would like to congratulate Dr. Evans on his splendid presentation. Just for the record, may I emphasize the effect of aspirin on deep vein thrombosis? Our negative results applied only to I^{125} detectable thrombi in the calf. There was quite inadequate evidence to decide whether it applied also to the clinical situation, because we did not study the patients long enough to get data on this, nor did we study enough patients. This is a much more difficult problem and aspirin is not totally excluded as a possibly beneficial drug. Indeed aspirin had no demonstratable effect whatsoever but it remains to be proved that it has no clinical effect.

Dr. Sasahara: In patients to whom we give anticoagulants, I'm sure most of us are very careful about warning patients against taking those drugs which interact with the Coumadin derivative, but I am not sure we've done this religiously about the aspirin-like compounds. Do you do this routinely on the basis of these studies?

Dr. Evans: We do this. For your information, there is a complete list of these available and it is published on pages 307-309, *Cerebral Vascular Diseases, 8th Conference,* (Ed.) McDowell and Brennan.

Question: What is the combined effect of heparin and the platelet suppressant agents in treatment of patients with thrombosis?

Dr. Evans: We don't know, but Dr. Hirsh sort of related to this yesterday. We have the impression, although we've never been able to show it experimentally, that if one combines the platelet suppressive drugs with heparin, then one does get prolongation. The interesting thing was, if it was done at critical doses using aspirin and heparin for instance, one could get increased thrombosis. This may be due to their binding capacity, as they both bind to albumin.

Question: Any data to suggest how aspirin should be used in combination with Coumadin? What dosage and what is the increased risk with that combination?

Dr. Evans: I think if you are going to use them in combination, you should use these drugs in people who have abnormal platelet survival. This is the main thing that we do and at the present time we should look at platelet survival and use these drugs in these patients only.

Dr. Hirsh: Could I comment on the question of aspirin and heparin? There is evidence that the ingestion of aspirin by patients with coagulation abnormalities, e.g., Factor IX or VIII deficiencies, results in a marked prolongation of the bleeding time. This also happens in patients who are being treated with heparin, that is the bleeding time is normal on heparin but is markedly prolonged if aspirin is added. On the other hand, there have been very few bleeding problems reported in patients who are on a combination of aspirin and oral anticoagulants provided that the prothrombin time is maintained within the therapeutic range.

Dr. O'Brien: Could I just take up a point of platelet survival which I think is important? If laboratories are not prepared to do platelet survival there is another method which may give help. If there is a rapid turnover of platelets then there will be a disproportionate number of young platelets in any given population. These young platelets are larger than the older ones and I have got a moderate amount of evidence suggesting that if you take the mean platelet size that this may well run parallel to platelet survival. An increase in size suggesting young platelets and conversely small platelets may indicate old platelets; obviously other factors may confuse this general principle.

Chapter 22

LOW DOSE HEPARIN PROPHYLAXIS

A. S. GALLUS AND J. HIRSH

THEORETICALLY, morbidity and mortality from venous thromboembolism could be reduced by treating the established episode or by preventing development of the venous thrombus.

As pointed out elsewhere in this symposium, there are limitations to the first approach. Thus, many patients with major pulmonary embolism have no premonitory clinical signs or symptoms of venous thrombosis or minor pulmonary embolism.[1] As death often occurs quickly in patients with massive embolism, there may be little time for diagnosis and effective treatment.[2] Anticoagulant treatment has been shown to prevent death from further embolism in patients with pulmonary embolism who survive the first episode[3] but is unlikely to be as effective in patients with massive embolism. In addition, anticoagulant treatment does not prevent postphlebitic symptoms in patients with iliofemoral venous thrombosis. Total lysis of venous thrombi with fibrinolytic agents may prevent postphlebitic symptoms but success depends on the age of the thrombus when treatment is begun.[4]

Prophylaxis in high risk patients is a more logical approach to the problem of venous thromboembolism. The prophylactic methods used to date, their relative effectiveness, and side effects are listed in Table 22-I. Many methods have been proposed to prevent operative and postoperative venous stasis. These include elevation of the limbs after surgery, early movement, the use of elastic stockings or bandages,[5,6] and the use of electrical or mechanical devices[7-9] to stimulate or replace the calf muscle pump. The simple measures of early mobilization, physiotherapy and leg bandaging have been shown to have only limited value.[5] Mechanical methods of improving flow have reduced postoperative venous thrombosis but have the limitation of being somewhat cumbersome. Platelet function suppressing agents, including aspirin, dipyridamole and hydroxychloroquine have been used with mixed results.[10-14] Thus, aspirin does not reduce the inci-

TABLE 22-I

EFFECTIVENESS OF AVAILABLE METHODS FOR PREVENTING POSTOPERATIVE VEIN THROMBOSIS

Prophylaxis	Reference	Evaluation°	Randomized Controlled Study	DVT Control	DVT Treated	Effective+	Side Effects
Improved blood flow:							
Elastic stockings, physiotherapy, foot of bed raised	5	F	−	35%	25%	−	Nil
	6	F/V	+	14%	4%	−	Nil
Peroperative calf muscle stimulation	7	F	+	21%	8%	+	Nil
Peroperative passive leg movement	8	F	+	28%	6%	+	Nil
Per and postoperative pneumatic compression	9	F	+	30%	10%	+*	Nil
Platelet function suppression:							
Aspirin	12	C	−	39%	14%	+	Nil
	11	F	++	22%	28%	−	Nil
Dipyridamole	12	C	−	39%	26%	−	Moderate (12%)
	13	C	++	3%	4%	−	Moderate (25%)
Hydroxychloroquine	14	C/V	++	9%	0%	+	Nil
Dextran	18	V	+	52%	4%	+	Pulmonary edema (11%)
Oral anticoagulants	19	V	++	56%	6%	++	Hemodilution (26%)
	20	F	++	11%	1%	++	Nil
	21	C/P	+	83%	14%	+	Bleeding (29%)
Low dose heparin	27	F	++	41%	15%	+++	Nil
	25	F	++	42%	8%	+++	Nil
	24	F	++	42%	8%	++	Nil
	26	F	+	24%	1%	++	Nil

°Evaluation: C = clinical examination, V = venogram, F = fibrinogen scan, P = postmortem.
*Ineffective in patients after cancer surgery.
+Effective = p<0.05

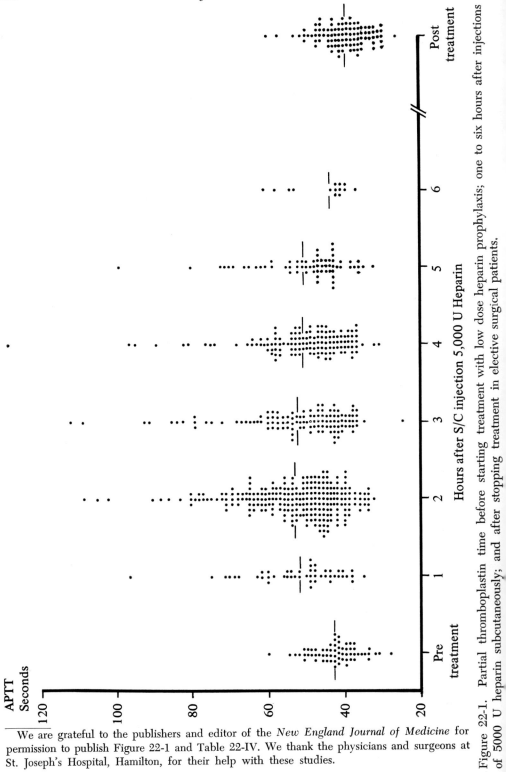

Figure 22-1. Partial thromboplastin time before starting treatment with low dose heparin prophylaxis; one to six hours after injections of 5000 U heparin subcutaneously; and after stopping treatment in elective surgical patients.

We are grateful to the publishers and editor of the *New England Journal of Medicine* for permission to publish Figure 22-1 and Table 22-IV. We thank the physicians and surgeons at St. Joseph's Hospital, Hamilton, for their help with these studies.

dence of ^{125}I-fibrinogen scan detectable venous thrombosis,[10, 11] even though it seems to suppress the clinical manifestations of leg vein thrombosis,[12] while dipyridamole has no effect on the incidence of clinically detectable thrombosis.[12, 13] On the other hand, hydroxychloroquine may be effective.[14] Dextran has a number of effects on the blood, including inhibition of platelet function, improvement of blood flow, and alteration of fibrin structure.[15-17] This agent appears to be effective if large amounts are given,[18-20] but carries a risk of fluid overload in the elderly patient.[18] Pharmacological enhancement of endogenous fibrinolytic activity has the practical limitation that it must be commenced at least three weeks before surgery and the unpublished results of a study carried out in England indicate that it is not effective in preventing postoperative venous thrombosis. Full dose oral anticoagulant treatment is effective but carries a significant risk of bleeding,[21] at least in postoperative patients, and therefore has not been widely used in North America. The purpose of this presentation is to discuss an alternative method of prophylaxis, namely low dose heparin.

Low dose heparin prophylaxis was introduced by Sharnoff and his coworkers who claimed that 10,000 units of heparin given subcutaneously twelve hours before surgery and 2,500 to 5,000 units given at six-hour intervals after surgery until the patient was mobile did not cause excess bleeding and prevented postoperative thrombosis.[22] These were uncontrolled studies using clinical and some autopsy data to diagnose thrombosis, but subsequent nonrandomized and randomized studies using ^{125}I-fibrinogen scanning to detect venous thrombosis have shown reduction of postoperative venous thrombosis without excess bleeding.[23-27] Thus, Kakkar et al.,[23-24] Gordon-Smith et al.,[25] and Nicolaides et al.[26] showed reduced venous thrombosis after elective abdominothoracic surgery in patients treated with 5,000 units of heparin two hours before surgery and 5,000 units at twelve-hour intervals after surgery starting twenty-four hours after operation, while Williams[27] showed reduced postoperative venous thrombosis in patients treated with the schedule used by Sharnoff. Failure of low dose heparin prophylaxis has been reported in patients treated after hip fracture[24] and patients admitted to hospital with myocardial infarction.[28]

We also have studied low dose heparin prophylaxis.[29] Four groups of patients were studied: (1) patients admitted for elective abdominothoracic surgery, (2) patients admitted for elective hip replacement, (3) patients admitted for surgery after fracture of the femoral neck, (4) patients admitted with suspected myocardial infarction. Four hundred ninety-seven patients have been studied. Patients in each group were separately randomized into treated or untreated categorized by cards drawn from sealed envelopes after their admission to the study. The treatment schedule consisted of 5,000 units of heparin given subcutaneously two hours before elective surgery and three times daily after surgery until the patient was mobile, starting six to eight hours after surgery. Treatment of patients with hip fracture and patients with suspected myocardial infarction was started as soon as possible after admission to the hospital.

All patients were studied with ^{125}I-fibrinogen scanning to detect thrombosis; and results with this technique agreed with those of venography in over 90 percent of cases.[29] Low dose heparin treatment produced a statistically significant reduction of venous thrombosis in all groups of patients studied except in the elective hip surgery group in which the reduction produced by heparin is not yet statistically significant. Thus venous thrombosis occurred in two (1.2%) of 167 heparin-treated patients after elective abdominothoracic surgery compared with twenty-five (14.5%) of 171 untreated patients ($p = < .001$), in one (9%) of eleven heparin-treated patients after elective hip surgery compared with five (42%) of twelve untreated patients ($p = 0.1$), in six (23%) of twenty-six heparin-treated patients after hip fracture compared with eighteen (56%) of thirty-two untreated patients ($p = .025$), and in one (3%) of thirty-eight heparin-treated patients with suspected myocardial infarction compared with nine (23%) of forty untreated patients ($p = < 0.05$) (Table 22-II).

TABLE 22-II

PROPORTION AND PERCENTAGE OF HEPARIN-TREATED AND UNTREATED PATIENTS WITH VENOUS THROMBOSIS DETECTED BY ^{125}I-FIBRINOGEN SCANNING AFTER ELECTIVE ABDOMINOTHORACIC SURGERY, ELECTIVE HIP SURGERY, SURGERY AFTER HIP FRACTURE, OR SUSPECTED MYOCARDIAL INFARCTION. P VALUES WERE CALCULATED USING FISHER'S EXACT TEST.

	Thrombosis		
Patients	*Heparin*	*No heparin*	*P*
Elective abdominothoracic surgery	2/167 (1.2%)	25/171 (14.5%)	<.001
Elective hip surgery	1/11 (9%)	5/12 (42%)	0.10
Surgery after hip fracture	6/26 (23%)	18/32 (56%)	0.025
Suspected myocardial infarction	1/38 (3%)	9/40 (23%)	<.05

These results confirm previously published conclusions about the effectiveness of low dose heparin prophylaxis in patients after elective abdominothoracic surgery,[23-27] but contrasts with the previously reported lack of effect of this prophylaxis in patients after hip fracture[24] and in patients with suspected myocardial infarction.[28]

Most venous thrombi observed in this and other studies were calf vein thrombi. The majority of asymptomatic calf vein thrombi detected with ^{125}I-fibrinogen scanning are limited to the calf and the risk of clinical pulmonary embolism in such patients is extremely small.[30] On the other hand, asymptomatic femoral and popliteal vein thrombi detected after surgery with ^{125}I-fibrinogen scanning carry a high risk of clinical pulmonary embolism if untreated.[30] Thus, it is important to demonstrate reduction of femoral and popliteal vein thrombi and, if possible, of pulmonary embolism in patients treated with low dose heparin prophylaxis before this prophylactic regime can be widely recommended for use in high risk patients. When the results in patients studied after elective abdominothoracic and elective hip surgery were analyzed together the incidence of femoral or popliteal vein thrombosis was one of 178 heparin-treated patients, compared with seven of 183 untreated patients, a statistically significant reduction (p = .04) (Table 22-III). This agrees with a similar reduction in the incidence of femoral and popliteal vein thrombosis in patients treated with low dose heparin before and after elective abdominothoracic surgery reported by Nicolaides et al.[26] Although the incidence of calf vein thrombosis was reduced in patients treated with low dose heparin after hip fracture, the incidence of femoral and popliteal vein thrombosis was not reduced in these patients. Much larger studies are needed to demonstrate an effect on the incidence of pulmonary embolism, and a cooperative study designed to answer this question is currently underway in England.

TABLE 22-III

PROPORTION OF HEPARIN-TREATED AND UNTREATED PATIENTS WITH MAJOR VENOUS THROMBOSIS DETECTED WITH ^{125}I-FIBRINOGEN SCANNING, AND PULMONARY EMBOLISM, AFTER ELECTIVE ABDOMINOTHORACIC AND ELECTIVE HIP SURGERY. P VALUES WERE CALCULATED USING FISHER'S EXACT TEST.

	Heparin	*No heparin*	*P*
Femoropopliteal vein thrombosis	1/178	7/183	.04
Pulmonary embolism	0/178	3/183	N.S.

How does this prophylactic method work? Sharnoff et al., found accelerated blood coagulation during and after surgery,[31] a change which has also been observed by others.[32] They observed that pre- and postoperative shortening of the whole blood clotting time was prevented by their low dose heparin regimen.[22] While it had been claimed that other *in vitro* coagulation tests were not prolonged by 5,000 units of heparin given subcutaneously, we found a moderate and statistically significant prolongation of the activated partial thromboplastin times for five hours after subcutaneous heparin[29] (Fig. 22-1). This observation is in keeping with more recent reports that small amounts of circulating heparin can be detected with sensitive thrombin clotting time or activated Factor X inhibitor assays for six to nine hours after subcutaneous injection of 5,000 units of heparin,[33-34] and suggests that low dose heparin prophylaxis works at least partly through the known anticoagulant effects of heparin.

Our own approach to low dose heparin prophylaxis differs a little from that of previous authors, as we give heparin two rather than ten hours before surgery, recommence treatment eight to ten hours after surgery rather than after twenty-four hours, and then give it three times rather than twice a day. This schedule was devised in an attempt to produce a sustained heparin effect during and after surgery. Kakkar et al. have recently also concluded that two subcutaneous doses of 5,000 units of heparin a day will not produce sustained elevation of the plasma heparin level after surgery.[24] The use of three doses of heparin daily, and the earlier start of prophylaxis, may account for the lower incidence of calf vein thrombosis in our patients treated after hip fracture and myocardial infarction than that reported in other studies.[24-28]

With this approach we found a moderate but statistically significant increase of blood transfusion requirement after elective abdominothoracic and elective and emergency hip operations in heparin-treated patients[29] (Table 22-IV). However, there was no increase of the proportion of patients receiving blood transfusion and excessive bleeding was not a clinically significant problem except in occasional patients in whom the partial thromboplastin time was consistently prolonged beyond sixty seconds by our regime. It is now our practice to reduce the heparin dose in such patients until the partial thromboplastin time, two to three hours after subcutaneous injection, is no greater than sixty seconds (the normal value is 40

TABLE 22-IV

BLOOD TRANSFUSION REQUIREMENT AND POSTOPERATIVE HEMATOCRIT FALL
(MEAN AND RANGE) IN TREATED AND UNTREATED SURGICAL PATIENTS.

Surgery	Heparin-treated	Untreated
Elective abdominothoracic		
patients analyzed	68	80
patients transfused	17	17
amount transfused (ml.)*	1635 (500-3500)	1117 (500-2075)
postoperative hematocrit fall (%)*	6.5 (0-19.7)	5.1 (0-14.4)
Elective hip		
patients analyzed	10	12
patients transfused	5	9
amount transfused (ml.)	1520 (600-2500)	1533 (500-3000)
postoperative hematocrit fall (%)*	11.7 (5.4-19.8)	7.7 (2.0-13.7)
Emergency hip		
patients analyzed	20	18
patients transfused	13	9
amount transfused (ml.)	1462 (500-2500)	1320 (500-4000)
postoperative hematocrit fall (%)	8.8 (2.5-18.4)	6.2 (0-13.2)

*Denotes a statistically significant difference ($p < 0.05$) between heparin-treated and untreated patients.

seconds). There was no bleeding in medical patients treated with this regimen.

The evidence therefore suggests that low dosage heparin is an effective method of prophylaxis in patients after elective surgery and in acutely ill medical patients in whom prophylaxis is started as soon as possible after admission to hospital. It does not appear to be effective in reducing popliteal and femoral vein thrombosis in patients treated after hip fracture. The complications of heparin prophylaxis include mild bruising at the injection site and occasional excessive postoperative bleeding in patients who have a marked prolongation of the partial thromboplastin time. We would recommend the use of this prophylaxis in high risk patients after elective surgery and high risk medical patients. On the other hand, more effective forms of prophylaxis need to be developed for patients after hip fracture.

REFERENCES

1. Miller, G. A. H. and Sutton, G. C.: Acute massive pulmonary embolism. Clinical and hemodynamic findings in 23 patients studied by cardiac catheterization and pulmonary arteriography. *Br Heart J*, 32:518-523, 1970.
2. Donaldson, G. A., Williams, C., Scannell, J. G. and Shaw, R. S.: A reappraisal of the application of the Trendelenburg operation to massive fatal embolism. *N Engl J Med*, 268:171-174, 1963.
3. Barritt, D. W. and Jordan, S. C.: Anticoagulant drugs in the treatment of pulmonary embolism. A controlled trial. *Lancet*, 1:1309-1312, 1960.
4. Biggs, J. C.: Thrombolytic therapy in arterial and venous thrombosis. *Aust Ann Med*, 19:Suppl 1; 19-24, 1970.
5. Flanc, C., Kakkar, V. V. and Clarke, M. B.: Postoperative deep-vein thrombosis. Effect of intensive prophylaxis. *Lancet*, 1:477-479, 1969.
6. Tsapogas, M. J., Goussous, H., Peabody, R. A., Karmody, A. M. and Eckert, C.: Postoperative venous thrombosis and the effectiveness of prophylactic measures. *Arch Surg*, 103:561-567, 1971.
7. Browse, N. L. and Negus, D.: Prevention of postoperative leg vein thrombosis by electrical muscle stimulation. An evaluation with ^{125}I-labelled fibrinogen. *Br Med J*, 3:615-618, 1970.
8. Sabri, S., Roberts, V. C. and Cotton, L. T.: Prevention of early postoperative deep vein thrombosis by passive exercise of leg during surgery. *Br Med J*, 3:82-83, 1971.
9. Hills, N. H., Pflug, J. J., Jeyasingh, K., Boardman, L. and Calnan, J. S.: Prevention of deep vein thrombosis by intermittent pneumatic compression of calf. *Br Med J*, 1:131-135, 1972.
10. O'Brien, J. R., Tulevski, V. and Etherington, M.: Two *in vivo* studies comparing high and low aspirin dosage. *Lancet*, 1:399-400, 1971.
11. Report of the Steering Committee of a Trial sponsored by the Medical Research Council: Effect of aspirin on postoperative venous thrombosis. *Lancet*, 2:441-445, 1972.
12. Salzman, E. W., Harris, W. H. and DeSanctis, R. W.: Reduction in venous thromboembolism by agents affecting platelet function. *N Engl J Med*, 284:1287-1292, 1971.

13. Browse, N. L. and Hall, J. H.: Effect of dipyridamole on the incidence of clinically detectable deep-vein thrombosis. *Lancet*, 2:718-721, 1969.

14. Carter, A. E., Eban, R. and Perrett, R. D.: Prevention of postoperative deep venous thrombosis and pulmonary embolism. *Br Med J*, 1:312-314, 1971.

15. Bygdeman, S. and Eliasson, R.: Effect of dextrans on platelet adhesiveness and aggregation. *Scand J Clin Lab Invest*, 20:17-23, 1967.

16. Gelin, L. E.: Rheologic disturbances and the use of low viscosity dextran in surgery. *Rev Surg*, 19:385-400, 1962.

17. Muzaffar, T. Z., Stalker, A. L., Bryce, W. A. J. and Dhall, D. P.: Structural alterations in fibrin clots with dextran. *Thromb Diath Haemorrh*, 28:257-267, 1972.

18. Johnsson, S. R., Bygdeman, S. and Eliasson, R.: Effect of dextran on postoperative thrombosis. *Acta Chir Scand*, 387:80-82, 1968.

19. Evarts, C. M. and Feil, E. J.: Prevention of thromboembolic disease after elective surgery of the hip. *J Bone Joint Surg*, 53A:1271-1280, 1971.

20. Bonnar, J. and Walsh, J.: Prevention of thrombosis after pelvic surgery by British dextran 70. *Lancet*, 1:614-616, 1972.

21. Sevitt, S. and Gallagher, N. J.: Prevention of venous thrombosis and pulmonary embolism in injured patients. *Lancet*, 2:981-989, 1959.

22. Sharnoff, J. G. and DeBlasio, G.: Prevention of fatal postoperative thromboembolism by heparin prophylaxis. *Lancet*, 2:1006-1007, 1970.

23. Kakkar, V. V., Field, E. S., Nicolaides, A. N., Flute, P. T., Wessler, S. and Yin, E. T.: Low doses of heparin in prevention of deep-vein thrombosis. *Lancet*, 2:669-671, 1971.

24. Kakkar, V. V., Corrigan, T., Spindler, J., Fossard, D. P., Flute, P. T., Crellin, R. Q., Wessler, S. and Yin, E. T.: Efficacy of low doses of heparin in prevention of deep-vein thrombosis after major surgery. *Lancet*, 2:101-106, 1972.

25. Gordon-Smith, I. C., Grundy, D. J., LeQuesne, L. P., Newcombe, J. F. and Bramble, F. J.: Controlled trial of two regimes of subcutaneous heparin in prevention of postoperative deep-vein thrombosis. *Lancet*, 1:1133-1135, 1972.

26. Nicolaides, A. N., Dupont, P. A., Desai, S., Lewis, J. D., Douglas, J. N., Dodsworth, H., Fourides, G., Luck, R. J. and Jamieson C. W.: Small doses of subcutaneous sodium heparin in preventing deep venous thrombosis after major surgery. *Lancet*, 2:890-893, 1972.

27. Williams, H. T.: Prevention of postoperative deep-vein thrombosis with perioperative subcutaneous heparin. *Lancet*, 2:950-952, 1971.

28. Handley, A. J.: Low-dose heparin after myocardial infarction. *Lancet*, 2:623-624, 1972.

29. Gallus, A. S., Hirsh, J., Tuttle, R. J., Trebilcock, R., O'Brien, S. E., Carroll, J. J., Minden, J. H. and Hudecki, S. M.: Small subcutaneous doses of heparin in prevention of venous thrombosis. *N Engl J Med*, 288:545-551, 1973.

30. Kakkar, V. V., Howe, C. T., Flanc, C. and Clarke, M. B.: Natural history of postoperative deep-vein thrombosis. *Lancet*, 2:230-233, 1969.

31. Sharnoff, J. G., Bagg, J. F., Breen, S. R., Rogliano, A. G., Walsh, A. R. and Scardino, V.: The possible indication of postoperative thromboembolism by platelet counts and blood coagulation studies in the patient undergoing extensive surgery. *Surg Gynecol Obstet*, 111:469-474, 1960.

32. Bergquist, G.: Changes in blood in connection with thromboembolism. An investigation regarding operation and delivery. *Acta Chir Scand* 92:Suppl. 101; 1-133, 1945.

33. Eika, C., Godal, H. C. and Kierulf, P.: Detection of small amounts of heparin by the thrombin clotting time. *Lancet*, 2:376, 1972.

34. Bonnar, J., Denson, K. W. E. and Biggs, R.: Subcutaneous heparin and prevention of thrombosis. *Lancet*, 2:539-540, 1972.

DISCUSSION

Dr. Dame (South Carolina): Dr. Hirsh, if a patient develops a bleeding problem during heparin therapy, what method do you use to determine the dose of protamine required to reverse the heparin effect?

Dr. Hirsh: This can be done most accurately by performing a protamine titration and working out the dose of protamine required from the result of this test. However, if this test cannot be performed, there are a number of guidelines that can be used to determine the correct dose. The half-life of heparin is approximately one hour and the neutralizing dose of protamine is one milligram of protamine to one milligram of heparin. Therefore, if the dose of heparin given to the patient and the time of its administration is known, the protamine dose can be readily calculated.

Question: What is your Dextran protocol?

Dr. Hirsh: Our initial protocol was to give 1,000 ml of Dextran 40 as soon as the patient was admitted to hospital with fractured hip and then to give 500 ml starting one hour before operation and then 500 ml of Dextran daily for the next three days at which time we commenced low dose heparin. However, we found that a number of patients developed heart failure when given 1,000 ml of Dextran over four to six hours and we have now modified our protocol to give 500 ml over the period of operation and then 500 ml daily for the first three days and then start low dose heparin.

Question: You mentioned in the discussion on the prevention of venous thrombosis that anabolic steroids can be used to enhance fibrinolysis. Could you expand on this please?

Dr. Hirsh: It has now been demonstrated that phenformin (an antidiabetic drug) and ethyl estranol (an anabolic steroid) when used in combination increase fibrinolytic activity in approximately 90 percent of patients. More recently, Davidson from Edinburgh has shown that the anabolic steroid Stanozolol, when used alone, can also produce a sustained increase in fibrinolytic activity. These drugs, which are given orally, take approximately three weeks to increase fibrinolytic activity.

Dr. O'Brien: I would like to speak in favor of the low dose heparin approach to prophylaxis. I think perhaps it is a little naive to think that the same dose of heparin would be effective in everybody. I am particularly impressed, looking at the literature, with the amount of heparin neutralizing activity present in patients that are thrombosis prone. Therefore, I support you strongly in feeling that the most effective approach is to monitor the effects of low dose heparin in patients receiving this prophylactic regimen. The other reason that I support this line of treatment is the fact that we showed that there was a decrease in the response of ADP in the immediate postoperative period during operation. We have no idea what this decreased response means, but it is interesting that low dose heparin reversed this effect on platelet aggregation.

Dr. Hirsh: I think that the most logical approach to low dose heparin prophylaxis is to monitor the dose according to the patient's requirements, for example, by using a partial thromboplastin time. However, we are not doing this because it is important to find out whether the much simpler standard dose approach is effective.

Question: In your series of patients on low dose heparin what operative procedures were performed?

Dr. Hirsh: These have been published in an article in the *New England Journal* (Gallus, A. S., Hirsh, J., et al.: Small subcutaneous doses of heparin in prevention of venous thrombosis, *N Engl J Med*, 288:545, 1973). The most common operation is cholecystectomy followed by gastrectomy, intestinal surgery and thoracic surgery.

Dr. Gilberts (New Jersey): As I understand it, you abandoned the low dose heparin program in patients with fractured hips because you felt that they may have formed thrombi by the time they reached the hospital. Would it not be equally important to prevent propogation of this thrombus?

Dr. Hirsh: Yes, but this low dose heparin regimen is not effective in patients with established thrombosis. To prevent propogation of established thrombosis one requires higher doses of heparin which almost certainly would be associated with operative and early postoperative bleeding in patients undergoing hip surgery.

Question: In patients treated with Dextran were there any problems in cross-matching blood?

Dr. Hirsh: No, this has not been a significant problem.

Question: Do you use low dose heparin for central venous pressure catheters to prevent clotting in the catheters, and if so, what dose?

Dr. Hirsh: We haven't been using this, but I think it would be easier to put heparin into the central venous pressure line and to deliver it by continuous infusion.

Chapter 23

VENA CAVAL FILTERS IN HIP FRACTURES

W. D. Fullen

THE SERIOUS RISK of a traumatic fracture of the hip was widely recognized prior to the report of Fitts et al. in 1959.[1] However, the magnitude of this risk was demonstrated by Fitts to be even greater than generally thought. By a follow-up study of a patient population treated for fractures of the proximal femur he found a mortality rate of 24 percent within six months of the injury. In spite of many advances in anesthesia, fluid management, respiratory care and many other aspects of patient care since that time the mortality rate of hip fractures has been only modestly reduced. Mulholland et al.[2] reported a 23 percent mortality within four months of operation during the period from 1959 to 1971.

Even more disastrous results occur in elderly patients already suffering from other diseases, particularly those which lead to the need for institutional care. Niemann et al.[3] in 1968 reported their experience with 190 previously hospitalized patients in whom hip fractures occurred. In this group the one year survival was only 33 percent. In comparable patients without hip fractures the one year survival was 71 percent and in the normal population of similar ages 90 percent. Similar findings were reported by Gordon[4] studying 202 patients treated from 1966 through 1968. If dependency is defined as confinement to bed or chair most of the time and partial dependency being confined indoors but able to move about, marked differences in survival were seen (Table 23-I).

The causes of death in these patients are complex but many investiga-

TABLE 23-I

202 PATIENTS—COMBINED DEGREES OF DEPENDENCY

Survival at One Year:	Independent	Partially Dependent	Dependent
After fracture	82%	44%	33%
Life table	93%	85%	86%

245

tors have shown that a high incidence of thromboembolic phenomena is seen in this patient group. Sevitt and Gallagher[5] found an incidence of venous thrombosis of 83 percent in patients who died after hip fracture. Pulmonary emboli were present in 46 percent of these patients. Fitts et al.[6] in 1964 in a large series of autopsy studies showed pulmonary emboli to be the most common cause of death in fractured hip patients. Subsequently, a number of reports[7, 8] have shown clinically evident thromboembolism in patients with fractured hips in incidences ranging from 15 to 48 percent.

Because of the high frequency of venous thrombosis in this patient group, the unequivocal role of pulmonary emboli as the cause of death in some and the suspicion of a major contributing role of small emboli in the development of "pneumonia" in many others a variety of prophylactic medicinal approaches have been tried and reported with conflicting reports of success or failure.

The treatment of proven pulmonary emboli with anticoagulant drugs was clearly shown to be efficacious by Barritt and Jordan[9] in 1960 through a randomized trial using heparin and nicoumalone in the test group versus untreated controls. The treated group survived in a highly statistically significant proportion compared to the controls (Table 23-II).

TABLE 23-II

73 PATIENTS WITH PULMONARY EMBOLI

    a. 35 patients randomized for anticoagulants
       Versus no anticoagulant
       1. Mortality: 5 of 19 untreated
       2. Mortality: 1 of 16 treated

    b. 38 additional treated
       1. Total treated mortality: 2 of 54

Because of the age group at greatest risk to hip fracture and the associated diseases common in this group, treatment of established pulmonary emboli is not as effective as in younger patient groups. Thus there is a strong stimulus for prophylaxis of pulmonary embolism focused on efforts to prevent the initial formation of thrombi in the leg or pelvic veins.

Salzman, Harris, and DeSanctis in 1966[10] reported an early randomized evaluation of the use of anticoagulants (warfarin) in patients with fractured hips who were randomly assigned to a treated group or an untreated (with reference to anticoagulants) group. Using standard clinical criteria for the diagnosis of thrombosis and embolism a markedly lower incidence of both was noted, thrombophlebitis 7 percent versus 22 percent and pulmonary embolism 1.2 percent versus 7 percent. If the thesis that pulmonary emboli were the major cause of death in these patients was true then such dramatic differences in phlebitis and clinical pulmonary emboli should have produced a marked reduction in mortality. However, the treated group mortality was 24 percent, which when compared to the control group mortality of 27 percent was not a statistically significant improvement. Others[11] had found similar results in fractured hips.

Subsequently, Harris, Salzman, and DeSanctis[12] made a similar evaluation of warfarin in elective hip surgery. In this much better risk group of patients, only one of 116 patients died. Thromboembolic complications occurred in 36 percent of the controls but in only 9 percent of the treated group. A deliberate bias in favor of the treated group was established in the protocol, however, in that all patients with anticoagulant contraindications were excluded from the test group. Later the same authors reported a comparison of the use of aspirin, dextran (40,000 molecular weight) and dipyridamole with warfarin, again in elective hip surgery.[13] Statistically significant differences were not shown in relation to warfarin. A retrospective comparison with the untreated control of the 1967 paper showed statistical superiority of all but dipyridamole. In contrast, Pinto[14] in England using I^{125}-labeled human fibrinogen as the diagnostic tool showed no difference between warfarin treated patients undergoing elective hip surgery compared with untreated controls. Others (Evarts et al.)[15] have reported marked reduction of thromboembolic complication in elective hip surgery with dextran using venography as the major diagnostic tool.

While the status of anticoagulants or platelet aggregation inhibitors in elective surgery appears promising, albeit somewhat confusing, no convincing reduction of mortality has been accomplished by these agents in the high risk population of hip fracture patients. Since pulmonary emboli have been clearly implicated as a cause of death, any reduction which may be accomplished by anticoagulants has apparently not been sufficient to change this high mortality rate. It is likely that thrombosis has occurred prior to anticoagulant therapy in many of these patients and that the anticoagulants do not prevent many smaller emboli which ordinarily would be tolerated well but not by this fragile group. The report of Kistner et al.[16] showing a 52 percent embolic rate in patients with proven thrombophlebitis treated aggressively with intravenous heparin lends evidence to this thesis. Especially convincing was the obscurity of most of these emboli (72% asymptomatic in these younger patients).

Faced with results comparable to other general hospitals with a large percentage of fracture patients from institutional situations, we had experienced no improvement with anticoagulation, dextran or aspirin although we had not critically tested these agents. The results of our treatment program in 1970 during which these agents were used in many cases showed a 26 percent mortality rate (Table 23-III).

TABLE 23-III

CINCINNATI GENERAL HOSPITAL

1970 Hip Fractures

	Number of Patients	%
a. Mortality	29	26%
b. Pulmonary emboli	33	30%
c. Mortality in patients with pulmonary emboli	17	51%
Total	110	

A modest but highly successful experience with a transvenous inferior vena caval filter in problem patients with pulmonary emboli encouraged us to employ this device as a prophylactic measure in patients with hip fractures.[17]

To evaluate the effectiveness of such prophylaxis a randomized study was begun in March 1971 and concluded in August 1972. During that period 129 patients with fractures of the proximal femur were admitted to the Cincinnati General Hospital. All patients were assigned to either a control group or a test group by a predetermined selection based on odd and even hospital numbers. Fifty-nine patients had even hospital numbers and were assigned to the control group. Seventy patients with odd hospital numbers were assigned to the test group. Those assigned to the test group were informed of the nature of the inferior caval filter and our experience with its use. They were also informed of the risk of thromboembolism in hip fractures. In addition, the uncertainty of the role of vena cava filters as a prophylactic measure was emphasized. Of the seventy patients assigned to the test group twenty-two refused the insertion. In seven patients technical difficulties prevented insertion so that filters were not placed. These were excluded from the study. A total of forty-one patients had vena caval filters inserted in a prophylactic fashion. No medicinal prophylaxis was employed in the controls although several received aspirin in varying doses. Any evidence of thrombophlebitis or pulmonary embolism was treated in a standard fashion with anticoagulants as the initial therapy.

The vena caval filters were inserted during the first twenty-four hours of hospitalization in most cases although occasionally a longer interval supervened. Fracture care was not altered in any way by the study. Internal fixation was employed as the primary fracture management in most cases.

The vena caval filters were inserted via a right transverse supraclavicular incision under local anesthesia with continuous cardiac monitoring and fluoroscopic control of the filter insertion. A preliminary intravenous pyelogram was performed in all patients in the test group. If aberrant anatomic arrangements were suspected, the renal veins were identified by venographic techniques. The filter was inserted just distal to the level of the renal veins as more distal insertion increases the risk of thrombosis cephalad to the filter. Postoperatively the patients were monitored by serial hematocrits to detect any significant retroperitoneal bleeding. No anticoagulants were used postoperatively unless pulmonary emboli were diagnosed.

The diagnosis of pulmonary embolism in elderly patients with hip fractures is hindered by the logistical and technical difficulties in performing the standard diagnostic tests in such patients who do not tolerate extensive manipulation and in whom the risk of pulmonary angiography is considerably increased when compared with younger patients. Since detailed information was not available in each patient, the reliability of the diagnosis of pulmonary embolism was classified as definite, probable and possible. Those patients in whom clinical symptoms or signs and laboratory data suggesting pulmonary embolism were supported by positive lung scan with negative chest X-rays were categorized as definite. In addition, those patients in whom pulmonary angiograms or autopsy diagnosis of pulmonary embolism were present were also considered definite. When a lung scan was negative the diagnosis of pulmonary embolus was considered to be ruled out. In the event that lung scan or pulmonary angiography was not performed but a chest film was interpreted by the staff radiologist as consistent with pulmonary embolism and clinical symptoms and signs also suggested the diagnosis, such circumstances were classified as probable pulmonary emboli. If neither lung scan nor pulmonary angiogram was done and the chest film was normal in the presence of clinical or laboratory evidence for pulmonary emboli, the event was classified as a possible embolus.

Of the total of 129 patients seen during the study period with fractures of the proximal femur, seventy were offered inferior vena caval filters while fifty-nine were placed in the control group. Of the seventy offered vena caval filters, twenty-two refused the surgical procedure and in addition seven patients had failure of insertion of the inferior vena caval filter due either to a narrow jugulosubclavian vein confluence or difficulty in traversing the right atrium. The difficulty in traversing the right atrium was generally noted in small, very elderly females with severe dorsal kyphosis. Attempts to manipulate the inserter in such patients were limited in view of the study nature of the technique in this circumstance and the risk of initiating a cardiac arrhythmia should the inserter cross the tricuspid valve. As a result, a total of 100 patients were studied, fifty-nine

TABLE 23-IV

PATIENT DISTRIBUTION

Total patients with hip fractures		129
a. Vena caval filter group		41
b. Control group		59
c. Excluded from study		29
A. Refused filter	22	
B. Unable to insert	7	

controls and forty-one patients in whom the filter was inserted (Table 23-IV).

The two groups were roughly comparable when examined from the point of view of their ages and associated diseases. However, the control group was favored slightly in that the average age of the filter group was sixty-nine years and the control group sixty-seven years. Similar discrepancies in favor of the control group existed in the number and severity of associated disease present. These differences were accounted for by the fact that of the seventy patients offered the inferior vena caval filter, twenty-two elected not to partake in the study. The patients who refused this technique were younger patients with better general state of health and apparently therefore less concerned with the risk of pulmonary emboli.

The vast majority of patients were transferred to Cincinnati General Hospital from nursing homes and only nineteen of the 100 patients had no serious associated disease. Arteriosclerotic heart disease was encountered in 60 percent of the filter group compared with only 26 percent in the control group. Decompensated congestive heart failure was present in 20 percent of the filter group and only 7 percent of the controls. Neurologic diseases consisting of senile dementia as well as other neurologic problems were present in 24 percent of both groups. Chronic obstructive bronchiopulmonary disease was also common, being present in 17 percent of the filter group and 12 percent of the controls.

The type of fracture suffered by the patients in the control and filter group were essentially similar in distribution among femoral neck, intertrochanteric or subtrochanteric sites. The frequency and type of operative fixation of these fractures was not significantly different between the two groups. The median time delay from admission until the day of internal fixation was four days in both the filter and control groups and was no different in those patients who lived or died in either group. The length of hospital stay was thirty-four days in the filter group and thirty-three days in the controls who survived. There was essentially no difference also in the length of time between admission and death of the nonsurvivors in either group.

Since these patients represented the group of people in whom the more accurate diagnostic tests for the complication of thromboembolic diseases are difficult to perform and in fact were not performed to any great extent, the most definitive measure of the effectiveness of the vena caval filter was also the most tragic; that is, failure to survive the traumatic insult of the fractured hip. In the group of forty-one patients in the test group who received the vena caval filter there were four deaths, constituting a mortality of slightly less than 10 percent. Only one death of the four was related to a pulmonary embolus and this occurred in a patient who developed the signs and symptoms of an acute pulmonary embolus within a matter of a few hours after admission to the hospital and approximately two hours prior to the insertion of the vena caval filter. She subsequently died of a series of complications largely relating to the pulmonary embolus and of course could not be considered as a failure of the filter device. The three other nonsurviving patients in this group died of septic complications—two of which had their origin in urinary tract infections and one from an infection in the operative wound for the internal fixation of hip fracture (Table 23-V).

TABLE 23-V

RESULTS

	Filter	Control
Mortality	4-10%	14-24%
Pulmonary emboli		
Definite	0- 0%	7-12%
Probable	1 prior to filter insertion	5- 8%
Possible	3- 7%	7-12%
Total	4-10%	19-32%

In contrast the fifty-nine patients who constituted the control group had a mortality of 24 percent. Fourteen of the fifty-nine patients died. Of this group of fourteen patients, eight appeared to have died as the result of pulmonary emboli or subsequent complications related to the occurrence of a pulmonary embolus. Of these eight patients, five of the pulmonary emboli were definitely diagnosed. Four of them were proven at autopsy. The diagnosis of pulmonary embolism in three patients was classified as probable and one possible embolus. The last four unfortunately were not examined postmortem. The remaining six deaths in the control group were due to a variety of problems. Four patients had pneumonia as the initial event in a series of complications eventuating in death. One was due to sepsis arising in the urinary tract and one patient died due to an assocated head injury.

The mortality rate in the control group of 24 percent is essentially the same as the mortality rate for fractured hips in our hospital in the years prior to the study. It should be emphasized that each of these patients was treated aggressively with the standard therapeutic approach for any complications which were recognized, specifically those patients who developed signs of pulmonary embolism or thrombophlebitis were treated with aggressive anticoagulant therapy.

Evaluation of the series in relation to the development of pulmonary emboli alone is less reliable, but nevertheless shows dramatic differences in the two groups using the same criteria of diagnosis. In the filter group there was one probable pulmonary embolus which occurred in an eighty-one-year-old woman two hours prior to the insertion of her inferior vena caval filter. She subsequently developed pneumonia and died as a result of this pulmonary infection. Otherwise no definite or probable pulmonary emboli were detected in the inferior vena caval filter group after the filter insertion. Possible pulmonary emboli were seen in three of the forty-one patients in this group. Of the fifty-nine patients in the control group, there were seven definite pulmonary emboli encountered and five probable emboli for a total incidence of 20 percent. An additional seven patients had criteria satisfying the possible presence of pulmonary embolus such that there was an overall total incidence of 32 percent of embolic phenomena in the control group versus 10 percent in the filter group.

The complications suffered by the two groups were similar with the exception of the difference in pulmonary embolic complications. The incidence of phlebitis occurring either unilaterally in the opposite leg or bilaterally was noted in five of the forty-one patients in the filter group and six of fifty-nine patients in the control. There were no serious complications noted in the patients in whom the inferior vena caval filter was inserted, specifically there was no filter migration, no malposition of the filter, no detectable retroperitoneal hematoma and no perforation of the gastrointestinal or urinary tract structures.[18] The only complications related to the filter were those of insertion difficulties which again were encountered primarily in very elderly women of small stature. These difficulties appeared to be related to the small size of their venous structures or their severe kyphosis.

As a result of this randomized study, we feel that inferior vena caval filter placement is superior in the prevention of pulmonary emboli to the standard forms of leg elevation wrapping, exercise, etc. Its effectiveness in comparison to the variety of anticoagulant or antiplatelet prophylactic programs now being reported and tested is unclear. We hope to randomly evaluate the filter in relation to a series of such medicinal prophylactic plans. However, at this point we feel assured that in the high risk elderly hip fracture patients in whom anticoagulant therapy is contraindicated due to some bleeding problem, the evidence from this study supports the effectiveness of the inferior vena caval filter as a prophylactic measure in such a circumstance. This is particularly applicable if deep venous thrombosis is shown to be present.

REFERENCES

1. Fitts, W. T., Jr., Lehr, H. B., Schor, S. and Roberts, B.: Life expectancy after fracture of the hip. *Surg Gynecol Obstet, 108*:7-12, 1959.
2. Mulholland, R. C. and Gunn, D. R.: Sliding screw plate fixation of intertrochanteric femoral fractures. *J Trauma, 12*:581-591, 1972.
3. Niemann, K. M. W. and Mankin, H. J.: Fractures about the hip in an institutionalized patient population. *J Bone Joint Surg, 50-A*:1327-1340, 1968.
4. Gordon, P. C.: The probability of death following a fracture of the hip. *Can Med Assoc J, 105*:47-51, 1971.
5. Sevitt, S. and Gallagher, N.: Venous thrombosis in pulmonary embolism: A clinico-pathological study in injured and burned patients. *Br J Surg, 48*:475-489, 1960.
6. Fitts, W. T., Jr., Lehr, H. B., Bitner, R. L. and Spelman, J. W.: Analysis of 950 fatal injuries. *Surgery, 56*:663, 1964.
7. Evarts, C. M. and Feil, E. I.: Thromboembolism after elective surgery of the hip. *Orthop Clin North Am, II*:167-174, 1971.
8. Freeark, R. J. and Fardin, R.: Venographic study of the lower extremity in patients with fracture of the hip. *Surg Forum, XVII*:444-446, 1966.
9. Barritt, D. W. and Jordan, S. C.: Anticoagulant drugs in the treatment of pulmonary embolism: A controlled trial. *Lancet, 1*:1309-1312, 1960.
10. Salzman, E. W., Harris, W. H. and DeSanctis, R. W.: Anticoagulation for prevention of thromboembolism following fractures of the hip. *N Engl J Med, 275*:122-130, 1966.
11. Sevitt, S. and Gallagher, N. G.: Prevention of venous thrombosis in pulmonary embolism in injured patients. *Lancet, 2*:981, 1959.
12. Harris, W. H., Salzman, E. W. and DeSanctis, R. W.: The prevention of thromboembolic disease by prophylactic anticoagulation. *J Bone Joint Surg, 49-A*:81-89, 1967.
13. Salzman, E. W., Harris, W. H. and DeSanctis, R. W.: Reduction in venous thromboembolism by agents affecting platelet function. *N Engl J Med, 284*:1287-1291, 1971.
14. Pinto, D. J.: Controlled trial of an anticoagulant in the prevention of venous thrombosis following hip surgery. *Br J Surg, 57*:349-352, 1970.
15. Evarts, C. W. and Feil, E. J.: Prevention of thromboembolic disease after elective surgery of the hip. *J Bone Joint Surg, 53*:1271-1280, 1971.
16. Kistner, R. L., Ball, J. J., Nordyke, R. A. and Freeman, G. C.: Incidence of pulmonary embolism in the course of thrombophlebitis of the lower extremities. *Am J Surg, 124*:169-176, 1972.
17. Fullen, W. D., Miller, E. H., Steele, W. F. and McDonough, J. J.: Prophylactic vena caval interruption in hip fractures. *J Trauma, 13*:403, 1973.
18. Fullen, W. D., McDonough, J. J. and Altemeier, W. A.: Clinical experience with vena caval filters. *Arch Surg, 106*:582-587, 1973.

DISCUSSION

Dr. Hirsh: It was a very impressive paper. What about the question of clotting of the filter? Do you treat these people with anticoagulants and if not, I presume you haven't, what about this program?

Dr. Fullen: Well, we did not use anticoagulants in any patients in either group unless they subsequently developed thrombophlebitis or a pulmonary embolism, then they were treated in the standard fashion. We use intravenous heparin, not continuous but intermittant. We didn't try to keep the filters open, and I am quite certain that they do not stay open under that routine in any significant percentage. We have had the opportunity to examine some of these filters at autopsy, both in this group and in patients who are treated with pulmonary emboli. There is consistently, with occasional exception, a thrombus on the superior aspect of the filter. That thrombus generally is small, just the size of the depression in the superior aspect of the filter, but clearly in one patient we had a large thrombus above. That worries me, and I would wish Dr. Mobin-Uddin success in fashioning one that will prevent it. As far as flow through the vena cava, I think unless you give them anticoagulants it is not going to be present, and I am not totally convinced that even with anticoagulants that it will be present.

Dr. Mobin-Uddin: Let me ask. What was the incidence of leg edema in these patients who had the filter?

Dr. Fullen: Well, if we take these patients it's almost impossible to answer that because most of these patients never walked before they came and they never walked subsequent to coming, so nearly all had leg edema on the leg that was fractured. Phlebitis occurred in six in the control group and five in the test group. We just reported a series published in *Archives of Surgery* of our experience with eighty patients in whom we have placed the filter. There was an incidence of 14 percent of subsequent phlebitis, either opposite leg or both legs, or demonstrably worse in the leg with initial trouble.

Question: In the mortality rates that you described in the comparison of the treated and controlled group, what was the incidence of hospital deaths?

Dr. Fullen: These are all hospital deaths. This is not a long-term follow-up. We hope to follow these patients and tabulate their long-term follow-up. The hospital stay for the two groups in the survivors was essentially the same, thirty-four days in the filter group and thirty-three days in the controlled group. The time till death in the nonsurvivors was essentially the same in the two groups.

Question: Is there going to be a subsequent follow-up study on the survival of these patients after six months and a year?

Dr. Fullen: I hope so.

Dr. Hanway (New York): Dr. Mobin-Uddin has told us that he used anticoagulants for three months as I recall to prevent this proximal clot and therefore your studies should provide us with some evidence that this is or isn't needed. If, for instance, your one year mortality catches up to the untreated, this would suggest that the proximal clot is a major factor whereas, if your one year mortality is unchanged obviously or unchanged from the life table that would suggest that Dr. Mobin-Uddin's program is not necessary and that maybe the heparin bonding is not necessary.

Dr. Fullen: I'm not sure that is true, because the filters we have examined at postmortem some months after they were inserted were well endothelialized and well fixed. I think that the risk is one that is there in the first weeks after it is inserted and that's when I think that thrombus can break.

Dr. Brown: In your cases that died of pulmonary emboli, did they die suddenly in the control group?

Dr. Fullen: A few of them died suddenly, but the bulk of them had a major embolus recognizable clinically, were scanned and a relatively certain diagnosis of pulmonary embolus made. Then they just developed what our residents call the dwindles. In this kind of patient the reserve to withstand that insult is not adequate as Dr. Dalen demonstrated.

Question: Did you then stick to your protocol and not change as far as treatment of pulmonary emboli?

Dr. Fullen: No, the protocol never included any restriction about the treatment of pulmonary emboli. Any reasonable suspicion of pulmonary emboli was then followed by aggressive anticoagulant treatment as we would for any patient. There was no change in treatment in any way other than the use of the filter in the test group.

SECTION V

PULMONARY THROMBOEMBOLISM — THERAPY

Chapter 24

ANTICOAGULANT THERAPY IN VENOUS THROMBOEMBOLIC DISEASE

William W. Coon

DURING THE past forty years the gradually increasing utilization of heparin and oral anticoagulants for the prevention and therapy of thromboembolic disease has made these drugs one of the most widely used groups of pharmacologic agents. We have estimated that, in the United States, more than 200,000 patients receive anticoagulants for the treatment of clinically recognized venous thromboembolism yearly.

The objective of anticoagulant therapy in the treatment of established venous thromboembolism is to inhibit propagation of a preexisting thrombus and thus lessen the hazard of further pulmonary embolism and the morbidity from postphlebitic sequellae resulting from venous valvular destruction.

There is no good evidence that anticoagulants have a significant effect upon acceleration of the dissolution of thrombi; a friable, free-floating thrombus remains a source of potential embolism until the process of organization has fixed it to the vein wall. Heparin may have an additional beneficial effect in alleviating the postulated acute vasoconstrictive and bronchoconstrictive effects of pulmonary embolism. Gurwich et al.[1] have shown that pulmonary embolism from fresh autologous venous thrombi in rabbits produces a rise in central venous pressure which can be prevented by a dose of 200 units of heparin per kg body weight. This effect appears to be related to inhibition of accretion of platelets on pulmonary emboli, brought about by blocking by heparin of thrombin-platelet interaction. The bronchoconstriction observed in pulmonary embolism in animal models has been attributed to platelet release of serotonin;[2] heparin has been shown to inhibit effects of serotonin upon smooth muscle contraction. However, whether this vasoconstriction and bronchoconstriction play a significant physiologic role in the morbid effects of pulmonary embolism in man is still debatable.

Although anticoagulants have been widely used for many years, decisions concerning the proper regimen of therapy have often been empirical. Since animal models are poor simulators of the clinical condition, judgments concerning that program of treatment which will minimize morbidity and mortality from both recurrent thromboembolism and from hemorrhage must be based upon clinical data. For more than twenty-five years a group of internists and surgeons at the University of Michigan have collaborated in a program of research and consultation in the diagnosis and management of thromboembolic disease. Information has been collected from each patient concerning diagnostic criteria, epidemiologic factors, drug dosages and prothrombin activity, thromboembolic and hemorrhagic complications during and after therapy, duration of follow-up and autopsy findings. Any new symptom or sign compatible with the diagnosis of deep venous thrombosis or pulmonary embolism, appearing after the first dose of heparin or oral anticoagulant, was considered a complication. Factors which might influence results of therapy have been periodically assessed, and our approach to treatment has been gradually modified in an attempt to lower thromboembolic complication rates and lessen morbidity from hemorrhage.

For many years our usual program of anticoagulant therapy included initial heparinization only until prothrombin activity (Quick) had reached therapeutic levels; then administration of heparin was discontinued, and oral anticoagulants were given for ten days or more. When data from a twenty-year interval prior to 1965 were assessed, the mean duration of anticoagulant therapy in the hospital was 16 ± 11 days (standard deviation). During 639 courses of treatment for pulmonary embolism, possible pulmonary embolic complications during the period of hospitalization were recognized in 4.9 percent (fatal in 1.3%). By comparison, of the 1388 courses of therapy for deep venous thrombosis alone, embolic complications were diagnosed in 3.2 percent (0.14% fatal).[3] The risk of subsequent death from pulmonary embolism was almost ten times as high in patients with a preexisting pulmonary embolus at the time treatment was instituted.

During these earlier experiences one of the unanswered problems which concerned us was the importance of the intensity of oral anticoagulant therapy in influencing thromboembolic complication rates. In 1956 an eight and one-half year prospective randomized trial was begun, treating one half of the patients at a range of prothrombin activity between 30 and 49 percent and the others at a range of 10 to 29 percent by the Quick method.[3] We found that patients with an initial diagnosis of pulmonary embolism who were treated more intensively (in the lower range of prothrombin activity) had fewer complications (3.0%) than those treated less vigorously (7.4% complications); $p < 0.1$. No recognizable difference in rate

of complications was observed in those subjects with deep venous thrombosis alone. In 1965 we terminated this study because we felt that although
these observations merited the utilization of the more intensive program
of oral drug therapy, extension of the duration of heparin administration
might be more important.

In another attempt to assess epidemiologic and therapeutic elements
influencing the development of thromboembolic complications during
treatment in the hospital, eighty-two patients with thromboembolic complications during hospital treatment were matched with controls selected
according to the following criteria: same sex, age within fifteen years, same
indication for treatment, year of treatment within five years, equivalent
duration of therapy, no thromboembolic complication during treatment.[4]
A preliminary analysis showed that many more controls had received
heparin as the sole therapeutic agent; for this reason, other controls were
selected to match subjects for principal therapeutic agent (heparin or oral
anticoagulant) as well. The most important findings from multiple statistical analyses were that the controls had received more days of herapin
treatment and higher doses of heparin ($p < .05$). Their oral anticoagulant
treatment had also been maintained at lower levels of prothrombin activity
($p = .09$). These results prompted a basic modification of our program of
hospital treatment to include longer periods of therapy with heparin.

Another problem was to attempt to define the optimum total duration
of anticoagulant treatment required to minimize the frequency of recurrent
thromboembolism developing after the patient is discharged from the hospital. Some of our earlier studies had shown that duration of treatment
had a significant influence upon the rate of development of recurrent
thromboembolism within twelve weeks after hospital discharge. Complication rates were significantly different in three groups of subjects: (1)
those receiving "incomplete" treatment in the hospital (therapy prema-
turely discontinued because of need for operation, bleeding, etc.)—12.5
percent; (2) "complete" treatment in the hospital—7.2 percent; and (3)
outpatient anticoagulant treatment of variable duration added—4.6 percent
($p < .025$).[3] These data had shown the value of continuing treatment after
the patient left the hospital but did not provide sufficient information to
make a judgment concerning the optimal duration of ambulatory therapy.

We have recently completed estimates of risk of development of recurrent thromboembolism in relation to the time after hospital discharge.[5]
The curve for risk of recurrence is hyperbolic in configuration, being very
high immediately after hospital discharge and gradually decreasing to
reach a plateau after a period of three years. For example, the recurrence
rate is eighty-three episodes per 1000 patient-months of observation during
the first week after hospital discharge, decreasing to 4.0 episodes at five

months and 2.2 episodes after three years. During the period of this study most of the patients receiving continued outpatient anticoagulant therapy were treated for a period of only six to twelve weeks. When those patients receiving ambulatory treatment were compared to those who were not treated after hospital discharge, the subjects receiving continued therapy had one-half to one-fourth the number of recurrences during the various weekly intervals up to ten weeks. Since the overall frequency of recurrence drops to a rate of four episodes per 1000 patient-months after four months, a practical compromise which might lessen the rate of recurrence without inordinate prolongation of treatment would involve therapy for a minimum period of four months after hospital discharge. A possible exception to this recommendation includes those patients with a prior history of thromboembolism (one or more episodes prior to the one for which treatment is instituted) since these subjects continue to have a rate of recurrence about double that observed in individuals without such a history.

After more than 1000 separate statistical comparisons of various measures of intensity of anticoagulant therapy in the hospital between 236 patients with thromboembolic recurrences after hospital discharge and matched controls, we could find no evidence that intensity of treatment in the hospital affected the frequency of development of these "late" recurrent episodes.[5] Unlike the patients who developed another episode of thromboembolism while under treatment in the hospital, the critical element affecting those individuals who developed "late" recurrences was total duration of treatment.

These observations, in combination with data concerning the clinical pharmacology of anticoagulants, can be utilized to develop a program of therapy which may serve to lessen the number of fatal and nonfatal complications. The duration and intensity of heparin treatment should be increased. Animal studies have shown that heparin is more effective than oral anticoagulants in preventing the formation and propagation of experimental thrombi. In experiments with serum thrombosis in rabbits, Wessler and Morris[6] have shown that the antithrombotic effect of usual doses of Dicumarol is negligible unless the drug has been administered for one week or more before thrombosis is produced. This delay in development of antithrombotic effect is probably related to the fact that five to seven days must elapse from the time of initiation of oral anticoagulant treatment before maximum depression of vitamin K-dependent clotting factors other than Factor VII occurs. Our current program for anticoagulant treatment of the usual patient with venous thromboembolism is as follows:

1. Intermittent intravenous injection of 10,000 to 15,000 units of heparin every six to eight hours for ten or more days.

2. Simultaneous administration of moderate daily doses of oral anti-

coagulant (e.g., 10-15. mg. daily of warfarin) until prothrombin activity (Quick) reaches a therapeutic level of 15 to 29 percent. Then proper daily maintenance dosage is determined.

3. Several days prior to hospital discharge, the oral anticoagulant dosage is modified to maintain prothrombin activity in the 25 to 40 percent range in order to lessen the risk of bleeding in the more active ambulatory patient.

4. Ambulatory therapy is continued for a minimum of four months after hospital discharge. Initially prothrombin activity is checked once or twice weekly. When the proper dose for maintenance of a stable prothrombin activity has been ascertained, the period between determinations is gradually lengthened to no longer than once every four weeks. The patient is asked to return promptly if bleeding or intercurrent illness occurs and is warned about taking any other drug, including aspirin, without prior consultation with his physician. The many drug interactions which affect anticoagulant dosage requirements have been discussed elsewhere.[7]

Alternative methods for heparin administration should be reserved for circumstances in which oral anticoagulants are not simultaneously administered since these other techniques prevent the obtaining of reliable estimates of one-stage prothrombin time. When heparin is given by continuous infusion or by subcutaneous injection, levels of circulating heparin are often high enough to produce a heparin-induced prolongation of prothrombin time.

Continuous intravenous infusion of heparin is chosen as initial therapy in patients with unusually extensive or refractory thrombotic processes. Regulation of rates of infusion to maintain a relatively constant anticoagulant effect is difficult unless a constant infusion pump is used. After the period of greatest risk is past, oral anticoagulant administration is initiated and the patient is switched to intermittant intravenous therapy for at least an additional week to allow for maximum reduction in levels of vitamin K-dependent clotting factors before heparin treatment is discontinued. Administration of concentrated aqueous heparin by subcutaneous injection in doses of approximately 250 units per kg. lean body mass every twelve hours is restricted to situations in which heparin is the sole therapeutic agent. Such a choice might be made when long term oral anticoagulant treatment is contraindicated because of an uncooperative patient, the absence in the patient's home area of accurate laboratory estimates of prothrombin time or an unacceptable risk of hemorrhagic complications during ambulatory therapy.

Heparin is monitored with thrombin clotting times which are easier to perform and more reproducible than Lee-White clotting times. The usual objective is to obtain a two to three-fold prolongation of thrombin time about two hours prior to the next dose of intravenous heparin. In monitoring the effect of subcutaneous heparin, the dose is adjusted so that just prior to a subsequent injection the thrombin time is about 1.5 times normal.

As O'Reilly et al.[8] have pointed out, the use of more prolonged combined heparin and oral anticoagulant therapy permits the utilization of smaller loading doses of oral drug; this approach should lessen the hazard of bleeding brought about by excessive prolongation of prothrombin time resulting from too large an initial dose. Instead of administering thirty to fifty mg of warfarin as a single dose, one may give more moderate doses (10-15 mg. daily) until prothrombin activity has reached the desired level. Although several additional days may be required before the therapeutic range of prothrombin activity is reached, this longer interval appears to reflect differences in rate of depression of Factor VII, while activities of Factors II, IX and X fall almost as rapidly as with single large induction doses. Since heparin is being administered concurrently, adequate anticoagulant protection is provided during this interval.

Repeated and careful monitoring of anticoagulant effects can keep hemorrhagic complications of therapy within limits acceptable on a risk-benefit basis. During 3862 courses of anticoagulant treatment in the hospital major episodes of bleeding occurred in 2 percent of courses and minor episodes in 4.8 percent.[9] Major bleeding is defined as hemorrhage of sufficient severity to require blood transfusion or termination of treatment. During either heparin or oral anticoagulant treatment the rate for major bleeding was approximately 2.8 episodes per 1000 days at risk. In the course of this experience, four deaths attributed to anticoagulant-induced bleeding were encountered (about one per 1000 courses of treatment). The presence of certain associated conditions precludes the use of anticoagulants, especially recent operations upon the brain, spinal cord or eye and during the first several days after operations involving bladder or prostate. Other diseases in which risk versus benefit must be assessed on an individual basis include severe hypertension, recent stroke, esophageal varices and ulcerative lesions of gastrointestinal and genitourinary tracts. The use of heparin alone is preferable in the management of patients with severe hepatic disease.

Reversal of the effects of heparin on the clotting mechanism occurs within one to two minutes after administration of a proper dose of protamine sulfate. The administration of vitamin K_1, either orally or intravenously, will usually lessen the excessive anticoagulant effect produced by coumarin or indandione derivatives within four to twelve hours. Route of administration and dose of vitamin K_1 should be determined by the severity of the bleeding. If control of mild or moderate bleeding is to be followed by further anticoagulant therapy, small doses of vitain K_1 (2.5 to 15 mg) should be used. Larger amounts of vitamin K$_1$ may make the patient very refractory to subsequent oral anticoagulant therapy for a period of several weeks or longer. Severe bleeding can be controlled with larger doses of vitamin K$_1$ (two to three injections of 25 mg at four- to six-hour intervals) plus administration of plasma or whole blood as needed. The currently available concentrates of vitamin K-dependent clotting factors are reserved for very unusual circumstances since this plasma fraction may contain the virus of serum hepatitis. Each patient receiving ambulatory oral anticoagulant therapy is given several tablets of vitamin K$_1$ to ingest if severe bleeding occurs, and he is asked to return to see his physician immediately.

These observations made during the course of the past twenty-five years describe the evolution of a changing approach to the management of venous thromboembolism by anticoagulant therapy. The principal changes which have led to our current therapeutic regimen include the use of higher doses of heparin for longer periods of time, the induction of oral anticoagulant therapy by administration of smaller doses of drug and, whenever possible, the continuation of coumarin treatment for a minimum of four months after the patient leaves the hospital. Other members of this symposium will describe several newer agents and techniques valuable in the management of selected patients with deep venous thrombosis and pulmonary embolism. In the great majority of instances, whenever no serious contraindication exists, these other modalities of treatment should be accompanied or followed by anticoagulant therapy.

REFERENCES

1. Gurewich, V., Cohen, M. and Thomas, D. P.: Humoral factors in massive pulmonary embolism: An experimental study. *Am Heart J, 76*:784-794, 1968.
2. Cobb, B. and Nanson, E. M.: Further studies with serotonin and experimental pulmonary embolism. *Ann Surg., 151*:501-560, 1960.
3. Coon, W. W., Willis, P. W., III and Symons, M. J.: Assessment of anticoagulant treatment of venous thromboembolism. *Ann Surg, 170*:559-568, 1969.
4. Coon, W. W. and Willis, P. W., III: Thromboembolic complications during anticoagulant therapy. *Arch Surg, 105*:209-212, 1972.
5. _____: Recurrence of venous thromboembolism. *Surgery, 73*:823-827, 1973.
6. Wessler, S. and Morris, L. E.: Studies in intravascular coagulation. Effect of heparin and dicumarol on serum-induced venous thrombosis. *Circulation, 12*:553-556, 1955.
7. Coon, W. R. and Willis, P. W., III: Some aspects of the pharmacology of oral anticoagulants. *Clin Pharmacol Ther, 11*:312-336, 1970.
8. O'Reilly, R. A., Aggeler, P. M., Kowitz, P. E., Kropatkin, M. and Leong, L. S.: New approaches to the initiation of long-term anticoagulant therapy. *Clin Res, 13*:94, 1965.
9. Coon, W. W. and Willis, P. W., III: Hemorrhagic complications of anticoagulant therapy. *Arch Intern Med, 133*:386-392, 1974.

DISCUSSION

Question: How do you monitor patients on heparin therapy?

Dr. Coon: Although many clinicians are using the activated partial thromboplastin time, we prefer the thrombin time which is simpler and more reproducible in our hands. One may measure the prolongation of thrombin time by varying amounts of heparin and construct a curve which will reflect "units of heparin per milliliter of plasma." The Lee-White clotting time presents many problems in reproducibility and accuracy; most physicians have abandoned it for one of these other procedures.

Dr. Silver (Durham): If you were going to be anticoagulated with coumadin, what level would you want to be kept at? My impression is 30 percent is worthless. I've always thought between 10 percent and 15 percent was ideal. What is your impression?

Dr. Coon: We've looked at all sorts of therapeutic ranges of prothrombin activity. The only way one can do this is by computer analysis of large numbers of patients. Our statistical studies have not shown any significant differences in thromboembolic complication rates in the range of 15 to 30 percent prothrombin activity. When prothrombin activity is below 15 percent, the rate of hemorrhagic complications increases markedly. I would rather maintain the patient in the 15 to 30 percent range to balance the risks of recurrent thromboembolism against the risk of a hemorrhagic complication.

Chapter 25

A CONTROLLED TRIAL OF THROMBOLYSIS IN PULMONARY EMBOLISM: THE NATIONAL HEART AND LUNG INSTITUTE EXPERIENCE

ARTHUR A. SASAHARA, THOMAS M. HYERS, CHRISTINE M. COLE,
G. V. R. K. SHARMA, KEVIN M. MCINTYRE AND JOHN S. BELKO*

Introduction

ALTHOUGH significant advances have been made in the early diagnosis of pulmonary embolic disease, particularly with the routine application of radioisotope lung scanning and in many instances pulmonary angiography, relatively little new has been added to therapy. Medical therapy, however, has improved through earlier and more frequent use of heparin followed by the oral administration of anticoagulants for varying periods of time. Currently, intravenous heparin is the treatment of choice for the

*We would like to acknowledge the other principal investigators from the many institutions involved in this Trial: Dr. John R. Blackman (University of Washington); Dr. Richard D. Sautter (Marshfield Clinic Foundation); Dr. Henry N. Wagner, Jr. (Johns Hopkins Medical Institutions); Dr. Noble O. Fowler (Cincinnati General Hospital); Dr. Edward Genton (University of Colorado Medical Center); Dr. Joseph V. Messer (Boston City Hospital); Dr. Donald Silver (Duke University Medical Center); Dr. Park W. Willis III (University of Michigan Medical Center); Dr. James E. Dalen (Peter Bent Brigham Hospital); Dr. Nanette K. Wenger (Emory University School of Medicine); Dr. Frank P. Hildner (Mount Sinai Hospital of Greater Miami); Dr. Robert N. Cooley (University of Texas Medical Branch); and Dr. Robert M. Stanzler (Cook County Hospital).

We also wish to acknowledge the helpful guidance of Dr. Sol Sherry, Chairman, Policy Board; Dr. James M. Stengle, Director, National Blood Resource Branch, National Heart and Lung Institute; and Dr. Peter N. Walsh, former liaison officer, UPET Project, National Heart and Lung Institute.

We are also indebted to the following members of our local UPET team who have been available on a twenty-four-hour basis: Scan and Biochemical Team: Robert G. Simpson, Paul F. Godin and Curtis E. Wrenn; Angiographic Team: Gail Gardner, Paula Fierro, James Flaherty, John Lynch and Leo Barron; Blood Analysis Team: Virginia A. Burleson, Helen Guilford and Nazarene Mondello. We thank Mrs. Donna Kantarges for invaluable editorial assistance.

acute phase of pulmonary embolism. Its advantages are the rapidity of action, predictability of response, the ability to block platelet-thrombin interaction and the empiric fact that it is the most effective anticoagulant in use today. Although heparin has been effective in reducing the frequency of thromboembolic episodes, no direct effect on the thromboembolus itself has been identified. Nor has there been any evidence that heparin accelerates the dissolution of thrombi at the site of origin in the deep venous system. What dissolution of clot occurs is probably a reflection of natural fibrinolysis activated by the thrombotic process. In addition, heparin may induce serious hemorrhage. For these several reasons, heparin is not the "ideal" drug to treat thromboembolism. Two drugs, both plasminogen activators, have emerged from laboratory investigations to the stage where extensive clinical testing was necessary to assess their applicability in the treatment of thromboembolic disorders. Streptokinase (SK) was initially and extensively used by investigators,[1,3,8,12] but until recently, its antigenicity and pyrogenicity have limited its use in this country. In 1964, the Committee on Thrombolytic Agents of the National Heart and Lung Institute identified urokinase (UK), the naturally occurring plasminogen activator present in human urine as the most promising agent for thrombolysis. UK has been shown by several lines of investigation to be identical, or nearly so with the plasminogen activators released from human tissue.[2,30] Urokinase possesses several important properties which characterize it as an excellent thrombolytic agent: it is not antigenic, being of human origin; it is not pyrogenic, having been sufficently purified to remove trace contaminants; and its use does not appear to require strict dosage or cautious laboratory control which is generally required when SK is being administered. The principal disadvantage, however, is the prohibitive cost of production currently precluding its use on a routine basis. Streptokinase, in contrast, is antigenic, being a foreign protein of bacterial origin; it is also pyrogenic, although improved modern methods of purification have minimized the frequency and intensity of febrile reactions; and finally it requires greater individualization of dosage and rather more extensive laboratory control.[3] The clinical feasibility of administering UK in clinical pulmonary embolism was established from several early trials in this country.[5,7,9] Observations on the ease of administration, standard dosage and duration of infusion, safety and laboratory monitoring were made in a number of patients who suffered mild to severe pulmonary embolism. These experiences established that UK administered in amounts sufficient to produce an active fibrinolytic state was tolerated even in critically ill patients. In addition the evidence suggested that thrombolytic therapy was capable, at times dramatically, of dissolving thromboemboli in the pulmonary circulation and restoring normal or near normal hemodynamics. As a consequence, the National Heart and Lung Institute sponsored a carefully controlled, multi-center-study, the UK-Pulmonary Embolism Trial to compare the results of UK followed by anticoagulant therapy with the use of anticoagulant therapy alone. This study, which accessed patients with acute pulmonary embolism to the Trial in random fashion was modified double-blind in design to observe differences in the rate and degree of clot resolution in the pulmonary circulation. The three parameters used to assess these changes included control and postinfusion pulmonary angiography, hemodynamic measurements and serial perfusion lung scanning. In addition, other clinical and laboratory abnormalities due to pulmonary embolism were observed for differences in rate of change towards normal in the two treatment groups.

Because the mortality of patients with pulmonary embolism treated with anticoagulants is relatively low, it was not anticipated that a sample size necessary to demonstrate differences in clot resolution would be large enough to demonstrate differences in mortality. Nor was it expected that an accurate comparison of mortality frequency in the two treatment groups could be made in the follow-up period since protocol therapy could not be controlled for such long periods of time. The primary purpose of the Trial, therefore, was a comparison of the rate and degree of resolution of thromboemboli in the two treatment groups. However, clinical assessment and serial perfusion lung scanning were performed at three-, six-, and twelve-month intervals. This report is based on the official publication of the National Heart and Lung Institute Urokinase Pulmonary Embolism Trial which was recently published in its entirety.[11]

MATERIALS AND METHODS

One hundred and sixty patients with acute pulmonary embolism from fourteen participating centers were admitted to this Trial from October, 1968, to August, 1970. The National Heart and Lung Institute, as the coordinating and sponsoring agency, supervised the development and implementation of a standard protocol and later audited records of the participating centers for adherence to the protocol. Criteria for admission included: (1) clinical history of pulmonary embolism within five days of anticipated therapy; (2) abnormal lung scan compatible with pulmonary embolism; (3) positive identification of pulmonary embolism by selective pulmonary angiography; (4) no bleeding diathesis or current bleeding; and (5) signed informed consent by the patient. Patients excluded from the Trial were those with operations within ten days of anticipated thrombolytic therapy, cerebral vascular accidents within two months of anticipated therapy and finally any contraindication to anticoagulant or thrombolytic therapy. Procedures, methodology and techniques, standardized in the fourteen institutions, were carefully monitored by a visiting Methods Team. The three major parameters used to assess drug efficacy included pre- and postinfusion pulmonary angiograms, right heart and pulmonary artery pressures, and serial perfusion lung scans. In addition, cardiac outputs, systemic arterial pressures, arterial blood gas determinations and biochemical tests were also performed before and after therapy.

The protocol was designed not only to compare the thrombolytic capability of urokinase with heparin but also to permit study of the disease model, pulmonary embolism. Since the patients in this Trial constituted a unique sample with angiographically proven pulmonary embolism with clinical and laboratory data recorded prospectively in a standard fashion, it seemed important to assess the presenting clinical and laboratory findings and to document the course of the disease.

Patients randomized to the UK group were given a loading dose of 2,000 CTA (Committee on Thrombolytic Agents) units/pound body weight, followed by a sustaining dose of 2,000 CTA units/pound/hour for twelve hours. Patients randomized to the heparin group (H), received a loading dose of seventy-five units/pound body weight followed by ten units/pound/hour for twelve hours by constant pump infusion. Following completion of the twelve-hour constant infusion, all patients received heparin intravenously for five or more days, followed by oral anticoagulants. Long-term observations included interval history, physical examination and lung scanning at three-, six-, and twelve-month intervals.

Statistical significance was established by calculating "critical ratios" (treatment difference/standard error), 2.5 being of borderline significance and 3.0 being of full significance.

Of the 160 patients entered into the Trial, seventy-eight patients received heparin and eighty-two urokinase. (One patient was randomized to urokinase but died before therapy was begun; she has been excluded from all data tabulation.) Table 25-I describes the patient population which was reasonably well matched. There were, however, several slight imbalances: the urokinase patients were found to be slightly younger and also had slightly greater preinfusion pulmonary angiographic, lung scan and hemodynamic abnormalities. Patients who were normotensive during their acute pulmonary embolism were grouped as Class I while those patients who had varying periods of hypotension were grouped into Class II. S (submassive) and M (massive) are angiographic estimates of the degree of pulmonary vascular obstruction: S involving at least one segmental pulmonary artery and M involving two or more lobar arteries.

Fibrinolytic Activity

Figure 25-1 shows in general terms, the fibrinolytic pathway. Urokinase

UPET: PATIENT POPULATION

		HEPARIN	UROKINASE	TOTAL
TOTAL		**78**	**82**	**160**
SEX	Male	45	47	92
	Female	33	35	68
AGE	<50	35	46	81
	>50	43	36	79
CHF	(clinical)	27	29	56
ANGIO SEVERITY	Minimal	16	11	27
	Moderate	24	19	43
	Severe	17	26	43
CLASS	I-S	35	33	68
	I-M	38	40	78
	II-S	1	2	3
	II-M	4	7	11

TABLE 25-I

is shown on the left, interacting with plasminogen which is then converted to the active lytic fraction plasmin which in turn lysis fresh clots. The levels of plasminogen and euglobulin clot lysis times were used to reflect the degree of thrombolysis achieved. No significant changes in plasminogen or fibrinogen levels in the heparin group were noted (Table 25-II). Whereas in the urokinase (UK) group, plasminogen was reduced 72 percent and fibrinogen 48 percent from the control levels. Whole blood euglobulin lyses times showed active thrombolysis at two hours following institution of urokinase, which was then maintained throughout the infusion of UK. Although some variability did exist among individual patients, 85 percent of the patients on UK had a satisfactory biochemical response to the drug.

Pulmonary Angiogram

The pulmonary angiograms, performed pre- and postinfusion, were interpreted independently by an "expert panel" which had no knowledge of treatment regimen or patient and hospital identification. Methods of analyses were developed, both subjective and objective, which permitted quantitative evaluation of the pulmonary vasculature obstruction. Figure

25-2 shows the average control or baseline severity of angiographic obstruction and the subsequent change following drug therapy. Both groups were judged moderately severe in vasculature obstruction, which corresponded to approximately one lobar artery occlusion. In the H group, minimal improvement was noted at the twenty-four postinfusion assessment, whereas in the UK group the improvement was considered moderate. The difference in mean change between the two groups produced a critical ratio of 5.2, which was highly significant. Although few patients showed striking improvement, many more patients improved on UK than on H therapy. Figure 25-3 is a representative example of a "good result" following urokinase therapy.

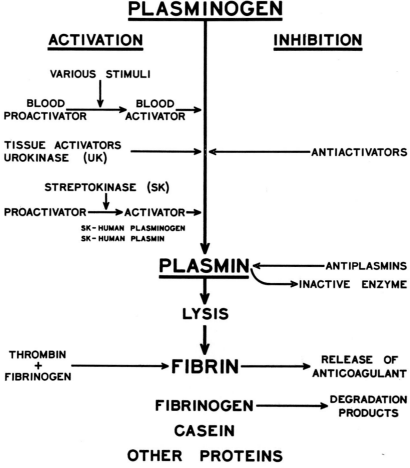

Figure 25-1. Diagrammatic representation of the fibrinolytic process, indicating the presumed site of action of urokinase and streptokinase.

Figure 25-4 shows the difference in severity change when the patients are subgrouped according to massiveness of pulmonary embolism: the improvement following UK therapy was considerably greater in those who sustained massive embolism, compared to those with submassive embolism.

Hemodynamic Assessment

Figure 25-5 summarizes the hemodynamic changes measured before and following drug infusion. The abnormalities noted most frequently were elevation of right ventricular systolic pressure (greater than 25 mm Hg) and lowering of arterial oxygen tension (less than 90 mm Hg) which occurred in 96 percent and 94 percent of the patients respectively (Fig. 25-6). The right ventricular systolic pressure averaged forty-five mm Hg, but 15 percent had systolic pressures in excess of sixty mm Hg. Significant

MEANS OF PRE AND POST INFUSION LEVELS

	HEPARIN MEAN (S.D.)	UROKINASE MEAN (S.D.)
PLASMINOGEN [CTA Units/ml.]		
PRE – :	2.17 (0.57)	2.12 (0.59)
POST – :	2.24 (0.64)	0.60 (0.42)
Δ :	+ 0.07 (0.32)	– 1.52 (0.64)
FIBRINOGEN [mg %]		
PRE – :	493 (159)	515 (200)
POST – :	529 (167)	268 (138)
Δ :	+ 36 (78)	–248 (174)
WBELT [minutes]		
PRE – :	—	200 (168)
2 hrs. :	—	32 (63)
6 hrs. :	—	19 (42)
12 hrs. :	—	16 (19)

TABLE 25-II

improvements in six of the eight measurements in the UK group were noted, while in the remaining two measurements, arterio-venous difference and cardiac index, no significant difference was noted between the two groups. The greatest change occurred in total pulmonary resistance which, because of the wide range of values, was expressed as the natural logarithm of the resistance. It was of great interest to note that in the twenty-four-hour period following drug infusion there was little change in the hemodynamic status of the patients treated with heparin.

Perfusion Lung Scanning

The pre- and postinfusion perfusion lung scans were also evaluated independently by an expert panel which had no knowledge of treatment regi-

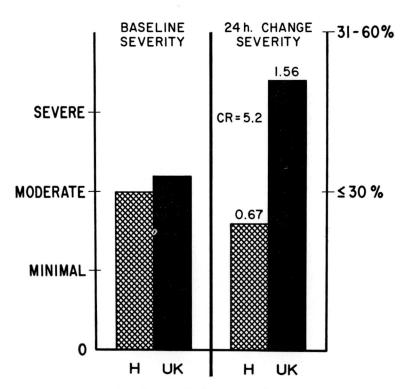

UPET: ANGIOGRAM BASELINE AND CHANGE

Figure 25-2. Angiogram baseline and change in the two treatment groups. The UK-group had slightly more vascular occlusion than the H-group. The 24-hour change shows greater resolution with UK which was highly significant (critical ratio 5.2). (Courtesy of *J Louisiana State Med Soc, 124*:1, 1972).

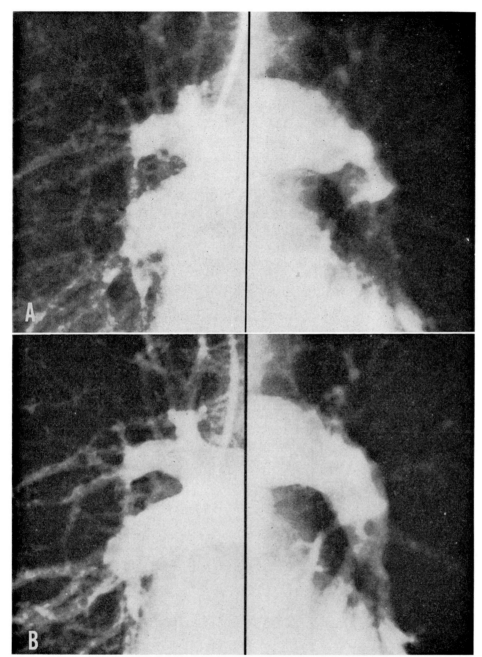

Figure 25-3.   A. Preurokinase angiogram of patient showing cut-off of upper and lower lobar arteries. The right panel shows irregular filling of the descending left lobar pulmonary artery, indicative of a filling defect. B. Posturokinase angiogram showing the marked improvements in the affected areas. Some residual defects are visible.

men and patient or hospital identification. The lung scans were assessed by visual techniques and the perfusion defects were expressed as a percentage of total normal perfusion of both lungs. The mean control perfusion defect in both groups was approximately 25 percent which corresponds to a perfusion defect of one half of one lung. The percentage of the control lesion which resolved during the first twenty-four hours following the beginning of therapy was 8.1 percent in the H group and 22.1 percent in the UK group (Fig. 25-7). This is a significant difference which parallels the improvement noted in the angiogram and hemodynamics measurements. At the fifth and fourteenth days, however, there was no significant difference in the percentage resolution of perfusion defects.

Although not all patients in Class II-M (massive with shock) had perfusion lung scans performed, four treated with UK showed percent resolutions ranging from 33 to 69 percent, while the only patient in this category receiving heparin showed a percent resolution of 6.2 percent.

Treatment Complications

Although no febrile, anaphylactic or other untoward reactions were ob-

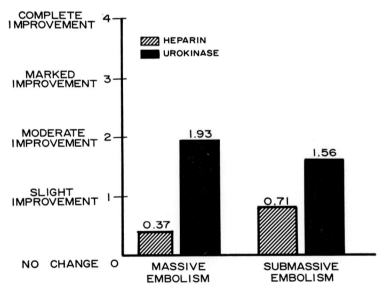

Figure 25-4. Comparison of the degree of resolution in massive and submassive pulmonary embolism. Note the greater improvement in the 24-hour period with massive embolism.

served with UK administration, overt bleeding or unexplained falls in hematocrit were frequently noted. Twenty-one (27%) in the H group and thirty-six patients (44%) in the UK group had bleeding complications which were classified as moderate (blood loss of approximately 150-1500 ml; hematocrit fall of 5-10%; blood transfusion of 2 units or less) or severe (exceeding the moderate criteria) (Table 25-III). A large majority of patients in the UK group who bled did so in the early period, i.e. within the first twenty-four hours while urokinase was being infused. Thereafter, there was no increase in bleeding compared to the H group. In the H group, a similar number bled early in the infusion period as did in the later period. It is of interest to note that during the later period, although the number bleeding in each treatment group was not significantly different, the UK group had more severe bleeding. Further analysis (Table 25-IV) showed that the increased frequency of bleeding in patients receiving UK therapy was associated with cutdown and arterial puncture sites. Spontaneous

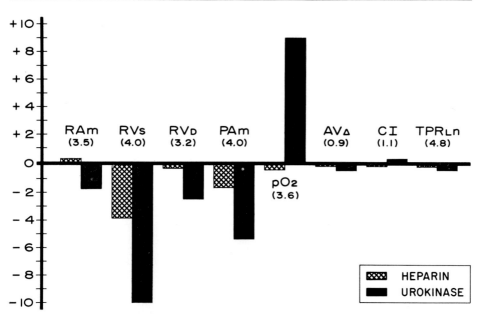

UPET: HEMODYNAMIC DATA — MEAN CHANGES IN 24 h.

Figure 25-5. Eight hemodynamic parameters with their mean changes in 24 hours are depicted here for the two groups. The scale is in the appropriate units: mm Hg for pressures and gas tensions; volumes percent for AV differences; liters/min/M² for cardiac index and natural logarithms for total pulmonary resistance. The wide range of resistances necessitated using natural logs. The most significant changes were noted in the pulmonary resistance. Only arteriovenous difference and CI were not significantly different. (Courtesy of *J Louisiana State Med Soc, 124*:1, 1972).

hemorrhage, on the other hand, occurred with equal frequency in both groups. However, when spontaneous hemorrhage occurred, it tended to be more severe in the UK group. In both treatment groups, bleeding from the venous cutdown site was more troublesome than the arterial puncture. It was difficult, in most instances, to maintain perfect hemostasis around the indwelling angiocatheter as well as to maintain the optimal amount of pressure at other invasive sites. The obese patient was particularly suscep-tible to vigorous oozing from the deep invasive sites. In patients treated with urokinase who had bleeding complications, there was no relationship to the degree of thrombolytic activity as assessed by the whole blood euglobulin lysis time (WBELT) (Table 25-V). In patients treated with heparin, however, there appeared to be a significant relationship between bleeding and heparin anticoagulant activity. When the Lee-White clotting time (LWCT) was greater than sixty minutes, 20 percent of the patients in this group bled, whereas in those patients with a LWCT less than thirty minutes, no patient had bleeding complications (Table 25-VI.)

Recurrence of pulmonary embolism within the first two weeks of therapy was noted in fifteen patients in the heparin group and eleven patients in the urokinase group. While recurrences were generally well tolerated by the patients, one was fatal for a patient who had received urokinase ten days before the event. It was of interest to note that 16 percent of those patients who were judged to be adequately anticoagulated had recurrence while 35 percent of those patients considered to be inadequately antico-

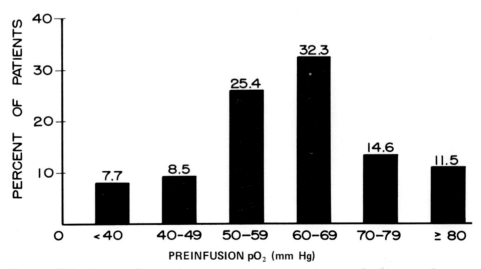

UPET: ARTERIAL $P_a O_2$ FINDINGS

Figure 25-6. Range of arterial oxygen tensions in patients with proven pulmonary embolism. Note the 12 percent of patients with arterial PaO_2 greater than 80 mm Hg.

UPET: % RESOLUTION BY LUNG SCANS

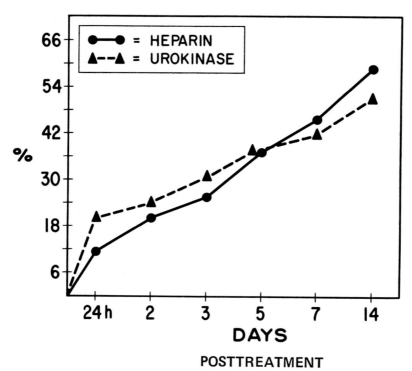

Figure 25-7. Mean percent resolution for both groups estimated by scans. Note the small but significant improvement in scan resolution in the first 24 hours, which diminishes by the fifth day. (Courtesy of *J Louisiana State Med Soc, 124:1, 1972*).

UPET: HEMORRHAGIC COMPLICATIONS

	HEPARIN	UROKINASE
TOTAL	**21** (27%)	**36** (44%)
EARLY { MODERATE	4	15
EARLY { SEVERE	5	13
LATE { MODERATE	6	0
LATE { SEVERE	6	8

TABLE 25-III

agulated had recurrence (Table 25-VII). Adequacy of anticoagulation in this study was defined as a LWCT greater than twenty minutes or a prothrombin time greater than eighteen seconds. In addition, there appeared to be no difference in the recurrence rate of those patients who received

UPET: HEMORRHAGIC COMPLICATIONS

	HEPARIN	UROKINASE
CUTDOWN	**6**	**20**
moderate	2	13
severe	4	7
SPONTANEOUS	**15**	**16**
moderate	7	2
severe	8	14
HCT FALLS (Idiopathic)	**20** (26%)	**20** (24%)
moderate	19	15
severe	1	5

TABLE 25-IV

UPET: BLEEDING & UROKINASE

WBELT	%
<10 min	34
10–30 min	36
>30 min	38

TABLE 25-V

heparin for two weeks in contrast to those patients who received heparin for the required five days and then subsequently maintained on warfarin for the two weeks. There were six deaths in the UK group and seven in the H group in the two-week observation period (Table 25-VIII). Analysis of mortality by subgroups shows that the great majority of patients grouped in Class I with a massive or submassive survived the embolic insult. In addition, only two of eleven patients in shock with massive embolism died, whereas, all three in shock with submassive embolism died. The latter three patients were seriously ill with cardiopulmonary failure prior to emboliza-

UPET:
BLEEDING & HEPARIN

MEAN INFUSION LWCT	%
> 60 min	20
30 – 60 min	5
< 30 min	O

TABLE 25-VI

UPET: RECURRENT PE AT 2 WEEKS

ANTICOAGULATION		% PATIENTS
ADEQUATE*	20/123	16
INADEQUATE	12/34	35
HEPARIN-2 WEEKS	8/44	18
HEPARIN → WARFARIN	12/79	15

*(LWCT > 20min; PT ≥ 18sec)

TABLE 25-VII

tion and deteriorated rapidly with less than massive amounts of pulmonary vasculature obstruction. The overall mortality of this Trial was 8.1 percent, which is in keeping with other previously reported series of treated pulmonary embolism.

Clot Resolution Rate

Follow-up perfusion studies performed in most patients up to one year revealed no significant difference in mean absolute improvement in perfusion in the two treatment groups as shown in Figure 25-8. While improvement in perfusion lung scan was significantly better in the UK group at twenty-four hours, it was approximately the same at day 7, day 14, three months and at the end of one year. In the one year follow-up analysis, eighty-eight patients had no significant residual defect by lung scan examination (less than 10 percent defect), while seventeen patients had residual defect equal to or greater than 10 percent. Only two factors appeared to contribute to the presence of a significant residual defect (Fig. 25-9).

UPET: OTHER COMPLICATIONS

	HEPARIN	UROKINASE
PE (recurrent)	15	11
definite	2	3
probable	13	8
ACUTE MI	1	O
IVC PROCEDURES	9	3
EMBOLECTOMY	O	O
DEATH	7	6

I-S : 4/68 (5.9%)
I-M : 4/78 (5.1%)
II-S : 3/3 (100%)
II-M : 2/11 (18.2%)

TABLE 25-VIII

Thirty-five percent of those with a residual defect equal to or greater than 10 percent had previous pulmonary embolism and 59 percent had previous cardiopulmonary disease, whereas in those patients without residual defect, only 18 percent had previous pulmonary embolism and 34 percent had previous cardiopulmonary disease. The other factors appeared to have no influence on the presence or the absence of residual defects.

DISCUSSION

This first phase of the National Heart and Lung Institute study of pulmonary embolism was terminated when data from the three parameters used in analysis showed significant differences in treatment improvement with one drug in comparison with the other. These data indicate that a twelve-hour infusion of urokinase significantly accelerated the dissolution of pulmonary emboli, improved pulmonary perfusion, and returned right heart and pulmonary artery pressures toward normal levels. Angiography, which was the most sensitive indicator in this study, showed significantly

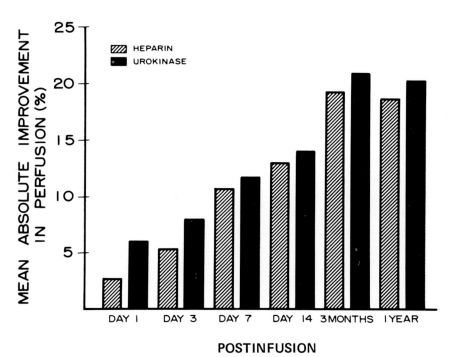

Figure 25-8.   Perfusion status at one year following therapy. From day 7, no significant difference was found in the extent of reperfusion.

ONE YEAR SCAN STATUS:
POSSIBLE CONTRIBUTING FACTORS
(COMBINED UK—HEPARIN PATIENTS: 105)

	Without Residual Defect (<10%) NO. %	With Residual Defect(≥ 10 %) NO. %
NUMBER OF PATIENTS	88	17
PREVIOUS P. E.	16 (18)	6 (35)
PREVIOUS CP DISEASE	30 (34)	10 (59)
CXR INFARCT	33 (38)	4 (24)
AGE ≥ 50 YEARS	44 (50)	11 (65)
EMBOLI AGE ≥ 48 HOURS	46 (52)	11 (65)
PERFUSION DEFECT > 35%	16 (18)	5 (29)
RECURRENT P. E. (I YEAR)	25 (28)	4 (24)

Figure 25-9. Possible contributing factors relating to residual scan defects noted at one year. Significance was established only for previous pulmonary embolism and cardiopulmonary disease leading to residual defects equal to or greater than 10 percent. The size of the initial perfusion defect did not appear to influence eventual resolution.

greater clot resolution in patients treated with urokinase. Hemodynamic measurements which included right heart and pulmonary arterial pressures also showed significantly greater return towards normal with UK as compared to H. Finally, lung scans showed significantly greater return of perfusion with urokinase than with heparin treatment. Of the patients who received UK, 31 percent had a "large" improvement at twenty-hours in their angiogram, lung scan and pulmonary artery mean pressure. No patient treated with H had comparable improvement. The absence of a significant effect on mortality was not unexpected in view of the low mortality of treated pulmonary embolism and the relatively small number of patients entered into this Trial. However, UK appeared to have a greater effect on both the angiographic and pulmonary artery mean pressure improvement when the embolism was massive. Urokinase thus may be of particular value in patients with massive pulmonary embolism in shock. Survival among such patients who have undergone pulmonary embolectomy has been very low; "medical embolectomy" with thrombolytic therapy may prove preferable. In fact, eleven patients from several institutions were not entered into this Trial because of massive pulmonary embolism. It was felt on a clinical basis that these patients could not tolerate the necessary studies required for admission into the Trial. All patients were subjected to pulmonary embolectomy with an operative mortality of 73 percent. Although this group may not be comparable to the Class II-M patients, the striking difference in mortality (73% against 18%) suggests that pulmonary embolectomy may not be the preferred treatment in most patients with shock due to massive embolism. A therapeutic trial comparing thrombolytic therapy with operative pulmonary embolectomy in such patients is probably indicated.

The perfusion lung scan and concomitant chest roentgenogram provide an ideal noninvasive screening method to diagnose pulmonary embolism. When a scan perfusion defect corresponds to a vascular segment or subsegment, the diagnosis of pulmonary embolism is highly probable. Perfusion lung scanning was accomplished quickly without morbidity; dual-head scanners and newer radiopharmaceuticals permitted multiple-view lung scans in about twenty minutes.

Pulmonary angiography, which entails somewhat more complexity and morbidity than perfusion lung scanning, remains the definitive diagnostic method, particularly when the scan abnormalities are equivocal. Right heart catheterization and pulmonary angiography did not prove detrimental to the patients, including those in shock. It was performed 310 times; there were five episodes of ventricular arrhythmias which required treatment and one case of cardiac perforation, but the procedure caused no fatalities and no residual disability.

The administration of intravenous heparin during the diagnostic procedures was encouraged and is recommended in all patients with suspected pulmonary embolism in whom anticoagulation is not contraindicated.[6] Prolongation of the Lee-White Clotting Time (LWCT) to twenty-five minutes or more at all times was recommended. The usual daily dose of heparin was equal to or greater than 30,000 units (10 units/pound body weight/hour). Oral anticoagulants (generally warfarin) were permitted only after day five.

The single proven benefit of anticoagulation of patients with pulmonary embolism is the prevention of recurrence. To determine the adequacy of anticoagulation, the incidence of recurrent pulmonary embolism during the fourteen-day observation period was examined. The majority of patients who had recurrence either had a LWCT below twenty minutes during heparin therapy or had a prothrombin time of eighteen seconds or less during oral anticoagulation (35%); in patients with longer LWCT or prothrombin time, the recurrence rate was 16 percent. Although these data indicate a minimal level of "adequate" anticoagulation, it is recommended that enough heparin be administered to maintain a LWCT of at least twenty-five minutes at its lowest level or oral anticoagulant to maintain a prothrombin time of at least twenty seconds. There was no significant difference in the recurrence rate of pulmonary embolism between patients treated with heparin alone for the fourteen days and those who received heparin for the first five days followed by oral drugs alone. Because this observation differs from the clinical experience of many investigators who believe that heparin is more effective in preventing recurrence of pulmonary embolism, further study and confirmation appears warranted before this observation can be accepted as a clinical fact.

Inferior vena cava (IVC) ligation or plication was performed nine times in this Trial when pulmonary embolism occurred in patients on anticoagulant therapy. These procedures may entail considerable risk, particularly in patients with heart failure and do not always prevent recurrent embolism. A newer, nonoperative technique of IVC interruption[4] with transvenous insertion of an IVC "umbrella" markedly reduces the risk of this procedure but was not employed in this Trial.

Pulmonary embolectomy was not performed on any patient in this Trial. Because of the high mortality rate associated with this procedure, it should probably be reserved for the rare patient with cardiac arrest due to massive pulmonary embolism or massive pulmonary embolism and shock whose cardiopulmonary status could not be stabilized by vigorous medical therapy. In this study, two-week mortality for patients with massive pulmonary embolism and shock was 18 percent (2 of 11 patients).

In summary, ideal therapy for patients with pulmonary embolism includes adequate anticoagulation and an effort to alter any characteristic that predisposes to pulmonary embolism; immobilization, congestive heart failure, trauma, use of oral contraceptives, etc. Urokinase or a similar thrombolytic agent may prove valuable in treating patients with massive pulmonary embolism in shock who were previously considered candidates for emergency pulmonary embolectomy. Although data which would support the use of thrombolytic therapy in all patients with pulmonary embolism were not available from this study, there appears to be some basis for this recommendation. In our own hospital, for the past several years of the Trial, complete pulmonary function studies including the diffusing capacity as well as its component parts, the pulmonary capillary blood volume and membrane diffusion, were performed in all patients entered into the Trial. These studies were performed in the recovery period of pulmonary embolism when the patients were ambulatory. Particular attention was paid to those patients with pulmonary embolism who had no prior heart or lung disease which might compromise the lung function studies. It was interesting to note in a small number of patients in the heparin group that although the routine lung volume and air flow studies returned to normal in the recovery period, the single-breath carbon monoxide diffusing capacity and pulmonary capillary blood volume continued to remain below normal levels. The membrane component of diffusion, however, was within normal limits. In contrast, those patients previously normal who were treated with urokinase, showed in addition to their normal lung volumes and air flow studies, a normal diffusing capacity as well as a normal pulmonary capillary blood volume measurement. These preliminary observations suggest that patients treated with heparin alone do not reestablish complete patency of the pulmonary circulation (which can only be detected by the sensitive measurement of pulmonary capillary blood volume) whereas in those patients treated with UK, virtual complete restoration of the integrity of the pulmonary circulation was achieved. If these observations are indeed correct, the basis for the application of thrombolytic therapy in all patients with pulmonary embolism will have been established.

REFERENCES

1. Browse, N. L. and James, D. C. O.: Streptokinase and pulmonary embolism. *Lancet,* 2:1039, 1964.
2. Fletcher, A. P. and others: The development of urokinase as a thrombolytic agent: Maintenance of the sustained thrombolytic state in man by intravenous infusion. *J Lab Clin Med,* 65:713, 1965.
3. Hirsh, J., O'Sullivan, E. F. and Martin, M.: Evaluation of a standard dosage schedule with streptokinase. *Blood,* 35:341, 1970.
4. Mobin-Uddin, K. and others: Transvenous caval interruption with umbrella filter. *N Engl J Med,* 286:55, 1972.
5. Sasahara, A. A. and others: Urokinase therapy in clinical pulmonary embolism. *N Engl J Med,* 277:1168, 1967.
6. Sasahara, A. A. and others: Diagnostic requirements and therapeutic decisions in pulmonary embolism. *JAMA,* 202:553, 1967.
7. Sautter, R. D. and others: Urokinase for the treatment of acute pulmonary thromboembolism. *JAMA,* 202:215, 1967.
8. Schmutzler, R. and others: Thrombolytic therapy of recent myocardial infarction. *Dtsch Med Wochenschr,* 91:581, 1966.
9. Tow, D. E. and others: Urokinase in pulmonary embolism. *N Engl J Med,* 277:1161, 1967.
10. Urokinase, editorial. *N Engl J Med,* 277:203, 1967.
11. Urokinase Pulmonary Embolism Trial: A national cooperative study. *Circulation* [*Suppl*] No. II, April, 1973.
12. Verstraete and others: Feasibility of adequate thrombolytic therapy with streptokinase and peripheral arterial occlusions: I. Clinical and arteriographic results. *Br Med J,* 1:1499, 1963.

Chapter 26

STREPTOKINASE THERAPY IN PULMONARY EMBOLISM

J. Hirsh, A. S. Gallus and J. F. Cade

Pulmonary embolism is the commonest preventable cause of death in hospital patients. Although the purpose of this presentation is to discuss streptokinase therapy, it should be emphasized that the major objective in the management of venous thromboembolism is to prevent the disorder from developing to the state where it requires treatment with streptokinase. This can be achieved by a combination of adequate prophylaxis in high risk groups,[1] early diagnosis of both asymptomatic and symptomatic venous thrombi, and early and adequate treatment of venous thrombosis and minor pulmonary embolism with heparin.[2, 3]

The aims of treating established pulmonary embolism are (1) to prevent death from the acute episode, (2) to prevent chronic venous insufficiency from the frequently associated deep vein thrombosis and (3) to prevent thromboembolic pulmonary hypertension.

Death from acute pulmonary embolism may occur as a consequence of the acute episode or as a consequence of further embolism. Treatment with streptokinase is probably of little value in preventing recurrence although there is evidence that the incidence of recurrence can be markedly reduced by adequate heparin therapy.[3] On the other hand, streptokinase treatment accelerates lysis of pulmonary emboli[4, 5] and therefore there is reason to believe that this form of therapy may reduce mortality from major pulmonary embolism.

The evidence that streptokinase accelerates lysis of major pulmonary embolism is derived from both experimental and clinical studies. In 1964, Browse and James[6] compared the lysis of experimental pulmonary emboli in streptokinase treated and untreated dogs and demonstrated that streptokinase accelerated lysis of these pulmonary emboli. In a recent study Dr. Cade, in our department,[7] compared the effects of streptokinase, heparin and no treatment on the resolution of pulmonary emboli in dogs. Radioactive sublethal emboli were injected into the pulmonary circulation of dogs and the dogs were treated with enough heparin to prolong the partial thromboplastin time to twice control levels, with streptokinase in a dose which produced a brisk thrombolytic effect, or with saline for twenty-four hours. The dogs were then heparinized, exsanguinated and the lungs homogenized and the residual radioactivity assessed. Streptokinase produced a marked increase of the amount of dissolution in twenty-four hours and was superior to heparin. In addition, more resolution occurred in the heparin treated group than in the saline treated group (Fig. 26-1). Using the same experimental model, it was shown that heparin, combined with streptokinase in doses that produced only a mild systemic effect and that were not associated with surgical bleeding, accelerated the rate of lysis of pulmonary emboli to the same extent as full dose streptokinase without heparin (Fig. 26-1).

There is now good evidence that most major pulmonary emboli seen clinically resolve within weeks or months. The results of the NHLI study comparing the effects of heparin and urokinase on the resolution of major

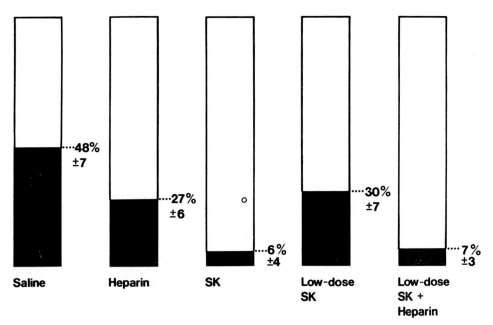

Figure 26-1. The amount of residual embolism after twenty-four hours is illustrated by the black portions of the columns. There was a significant difference between the heparin and saline-treated animals. The animals treated with high dose streptokinase alone or low dose streptokinase plus heparin showed significantly less residual embolism than the saline or heparin-treated animals.

pulmonary emboli have demonstrated early acceleration of lysis in the urokinase group.[8] This study has now been extended to a comparison of the effects of streptokinase and urokinase on resolution of major pulmonary emboli but the results are not yet available.

We have compared the degree of early resolution of major pulmonary embolism after heparin therapy with that occuring after streptokinase therapy.[4] (Table 26-I and 26-II) Patients in both groups were well matched for age, sex, previous thromboemboli and severity of pulmonary embolism. All had pulmonary hypertension and the pulmonary angiograms showed filling defects in proximal pulmonary arteries with severe obstruction to both sides. The hemodynamic and angiographic changes were assessed in ten patients before and after twenty-four hours of heparin treatment and in fourteen patients before and after twenty-four hours of streptokinase therapy. All patients in both groups had treatment started within twenty-four hours of their most recent episode of major pulmonary embolism. Seven of ten patients treated with heparin showed no angiographic change, two showed slight improvement and there was angiographic deterioration in one. In contrast, eight out of fourteen patients in the streptokinase group showed marked improvement. Seven of the patients in the heparin group who showed no angiographic change after twenty-four hours of heparin, were then treated with streptokinase. Four showed marked angiographic improvement and three showed moderate improvement. Measurement of pulmonary artery pressure and total pulmonary vascular resistance paralleled the angiographic findings in that there was no significant change of either of these two measurements in the heparin-treated group but significant improvement in the streptokinase-treated patients. It is of interest that although there was improvement in pulmonary arterial pressure and pulmonary vascular resistance after streptokinase, the degree of improvement in these measurements appeared to lag behind the marked improvement seen angiographically.

TABLE 26-I

COMPARISON OF STREPTOKINASE AND HEPARIN IN ACUTE MAJOR PULMONARY EMBOLISM—*ANGIOGRAPHIC CHANGES* Hirsh et al. 1971

	Heparin	*Streptokinase*	*Total Streptokinase*
Marked improve	0	8	12
Moderate improve	0	4	7
Slight improve	2	2	2
None	7	0	0
Deteriorated	1	0	0
Total	10	14	21

TABLE 26-II

COMPARISON OF STREPTOKINASE AND HEPARIN IN ACUTE MAJOR
PULMONARY EMBOLISM—*HEMODYNAMIC CHANGES* Hirsh et al. 1971

		Heparin	*Streptokinase*	*Total Streptokinase*
Number		10	14	21
Mean PAP	Before	27.1	30.0	28.6
	After	24.7	21.3*	20.2*
Total PVR	Before	5.8	6.6	6.1
	After	5.9	4.5*	4.3*

If it is accepted that streptokinase accelerates lysis of major pulmonary emboli, does it necessarily follow that it will save the lives of patients who have sustained a major pulmonary embolus? Theoretically, accelerated lysis of major pulmonary embolism could reduce morbidity and mortality in two ways, namely (1) by preventing acute deaths from the obstructive effects of major pulmonary embolism and (2) by preventing chronic thromboembolic pulmonary hypertension.

It has been shown that most patients who die from major pulmonary embolism do so within two hours of the embolic episode, consequently before they can be adequately investigated and treated either by surgery or thrombolytic therapy.[9,10] Most patients who survive the initial episode of major pulmonary embolism long enough to be investigated by pulmonary angiography survive if further pulmonary embolism can be prevented by adequate heparin treatment.[4,5] However, a small group of patients survive the initial episode long enough to be adequately investigated but die in the next twenty-four to forty-eight hours from the effects of severe obstruction.[11] Theoretically, these patients should benefit from thrombolytic therapy. Proof of this supposition would require the establishment of a randomized study either using a very large number of patients with major pulmonary embolism or admitting patients to the trial on clinical diagnosis and then proving their eligibility by subsequent angiography.

Short of definite proof, it is reasonable to suggest, on the basis of current evidence, that thrombolytic therapy may reduce mortality in (1) patients with massive pulmonary embolism who are critically ill with severe mechanical obstruction if treatment is started shortly after the embolic episode, (2) small groups of patients who survive for twenty-four to forty-eight hours after the embolic episode but who continue to suffer from the effects of persistent pulmonary embolic obstruction, and (3) patients with underlying cardiac or respiratory disease who have a reduced reserve and in whom spontaneous resolution is often delayed. Resolution with streptokinase treatment in this group may not only improve the immediate mortality from the recent episode of pulmonary embolism but may decrease morbidity from the consequences of persistent embolic obstruction.

The second possible indication for streptokinase therapy in venous thromboembolism is the prevention of chronic venous insufficiency in patients with iliofemoral thrombosis. Although iliofemoral thrombi may recanalize, the lumen is not fully restored and the valves are permanently damaged. This results in interference with venous outflow, with the production of venous hypertension, chronic oedema, venous claudication and recurrent leg ulceration. Theoretically, this complication could be prevented by rapid and complete lysis of the acute iliofemoral thrombosis. There have now been at least five well controlled studies comparing the effects of heparin and streptokinase on the resolution of acute venous thrombi judged by phlebography. All show that the incidence of both complete and partial lysis is greater following streptokinase than following heparin therapy. Combining the results of these five studies, twenty-two out of forty-seven patients (47%) achieved complete lysis after twenty-four to forty-eight hours streptokinase therapy while only five of forty (12.5%) achieved complete lysis after heparin therapy. Kakkar and associates did follow-up ascending, functional cinephlebography at six to twelve months and demonstrated that valve function was normal in patients in whom complete lysis had been achieved.[12] These results suggest that streptokinase therapy may reduce the incidence of chronic venous insufficiency in patients with iliofemoral venous thrombosis.

REFERENCES

1. Gallus, A. S. and Hirsh, J., et al.: *N Engl J Med*, 288:545, 1973.
2. Barritt, D. W. and Jordan, S. C.: *Lancet*, 1:729, 1961.
3. Basu, D., Gallus, A. S., Hirsh, J. and Cade, J. F.: *N Engl J Med*, 287:324, 1972.
4. Hirsh, J., McDonald, I. G., Hale, G. S., O'Sullivan, E. F. and Jelinek, V. W.: *Can Med Assoc J*, 104:488, 1971.
5. Miller, G. A. H., Sutton, G. C., Kerr, I. H., Gibson, R. V. and Honey, M.: *Br Med J*, 2:681, 1971.
6. Browse, N. L. and James, D. C. O.: *Lancet*, 2:1039, 1964.
7. Cade, J. F., Hirsh, J. and Regoeczi, E.: (in press) *J Clin Invest*, 1974.
8. Urokinase pulmonary embolism trial. *JAMA*, 214:2163, 1970.
9. Donaldson, G. A., Williams, G. and Scannell, J. G., et al.: *N Engl J Med*, 268:171, 1963.
10. Rosenberg, D. M., Pearle, C. and McNulty, J.: *J Thorac Cardiovasc Surg*, 47:1, 1964.
11. Gorham, L. W.: *Arch Intern Med*, 108:418, 1961.
12. Kakkar, V. V., Howe, C. T., Laws, J. W. and Flanc, C.: *Br Med J*, 1:810, 1969c.

Chapter 27

VENA CAVAL INTERRUPTION FOR THE PREVENTION OF PULMONARY EMBOLISM

Alton Ochsner

My interest in pulmonary embolism began early in my career during my training as an exchange surgical resident at the Städtisches Krankenhaus at the University of Frankfurt, Frankfurt Am Main, Germany. In the spring of 1924, I attended the meeting of the German Surgical Congress in München at which meeting Professor Kirschner[1] presented to the Congress the first successful pulmonary embolectomy ever performed. Trendelenburg[2] had described the operation in 1908 as an anatomical procedure and it was hoped that it might be possible to restore life in many individuals who had died of massive pulmonary embolism. Twenty reported attempts previously had been made but none had been successful until Professor Kirschner successfully performed pulmonary embolectomy on a thirty-eight-year-old woman who had been operated on three days previously for an incarcerated femoral hernia. Kirschner had had ten previous unsuccessful cases. The presentation of the patient electrified the entire Congress. It was the first time a patient had been brought back to life after having "died" from pulmonary embolism. Because of this success, there was immediately greatly renewed interest in the possibility of successful pulmonary embolectomy. In many Germanic and Scandinavian clinics, including the one at Frankfurt, in cases in which fatal pulmonary embolism was likely (those having had a nonfatal pulmonary embolism), the so-called Trendelenburg set, which consisted of all the instruments used in the operation, was placed in the patient's room and a skeletal staff waited for the fatal embolus to occur. Being a young resident in the Clinic, the lowest man on the totem pole, I sat through a number of these vigils as in a wake. If a massive embolus did occur, it was possible to immediately operate upon the generally unconscious patient, usually without anesthesia, and occasionally successfully remove the obstructing embolus. After spending a number of such nights waiting for the final catastro-

293

phe to happen, it occurred to me there must be a better way to accomplish the desired result, than waiting for the massive fatal pulmonary artery occlusion, and then attempting to extract the embolus and restore life. Although it was then not generally known that most emboli originated in the veins of the pelvis and/or lower extremities, it occurred to me that vein ligation on the cardiac side of area of involvement would prevent the thrombus—if it became detached—from being carried to the heart and lungs. Moreover, I did not know until years later that Trendelenburg[3] in 1902 was the first to employ vein ligation in puerperal sepsis by ligating the hypogastric vein, ligation and partial resection of the ovarian veins.

Pulmonary embolism in the twenties and thirties, although frequent, was not as common as it is today and although many patients recovered, many did not. Some clinicians still maintain that pulmonary embolism is rare and that fatalities are unusual in their institution, to which I reply that either they see few really sick people or that autopsies are seldom performed. Pulmonary embolism is increasing. According to Berger et al., "Ten percent of an autopsied adult population died from pulmonary embolization, while emboli of varying sizes were found at autopsy in 64 percent."[4] Soloff and Rodman[5] stated, "Acute pulmonary embolism is probably the commonest lethal pulmonary disease in the United States today—the primary cause of at least 50,000 fatalities annually and a contributing cause to the death of several times that number of additional patients." Smith et al.[6] (Peter Bent Brigham Hospital in Boston), Daicoff et al.,[7] and Thomas[8] believe that pulmonary embolism is the most commonly found pulmonary lesion at autopsy in large general hospitals. Bergan et al.[9] state, "Unfortunately the frequency of pulmonary embolus has not decreased during the past fifty years despite increased interest in the condition, improved diagnostic methods, and apparently improved methods of therapy. Ochsner, DeBakey, and DeCamp[10] found the incidence increased at the Charity Hospital in New Orleans from less than 100 per 100,000 admissions in the period from 1938 to 1939 to 250 in 1948 to 1949. Ochsner and DeBakey[11] found that the expected incidence of fatal pulmonary embolism at Charity Hospital was one in every 878 patients operated upon and one in every 502 nonsurgical patients. According to Ludbrook[12] pulmonary embolism occurs once in every 200 hospital admissions and deep vein thrombosis is not recognized in more than 5 percent of patients in a general hospital. According to Coon and Willis[13] 47,000 persons die annually in the United States from pulmonary embolism and in more than 50 percent of the fatal cases, there is no previous evidence of venous thrombosis. Dalen and Dexter[14] stated, "Few diseases are as common, as potentially lethal, and yet as frequently unrecognized as is pulmonary embolism. When pulmonary emboli have been carefully sought at postmortem examination, the incidence can be found to be in excess of 25 percent." They found that at the Peter Bent Brigham Hospital in Boston, pulmonary embolism was one of the three most common causes of death, and the antemortem diagnosis is made in only about 50 percent of the cases. According to Doran, White, and Drury,[15] "The risk of dying from a postoperative pulmonary embolus is now (1970) twice as great as it was twenty years ago. . . . Modern methods of diagnosis using phlebograms and ^{125}I-fibrinogen have established that 35 percent of all surgical patients over the age of forty develop a deep vein thrombosis." Freimann,[16] in autopsy studies at the Beth Israel Hospital in Boston, found that pulmonary embolism incidence has increased as follows: In the period 1951-1954, 22 percent; 1955-1957, 28 percent; 1958-1960, 44 percent; 1960-1962, 40 percent; and from 1963-1965, 45 percent. In a series of 500 consecutive adult autopsies performed between January 1963 and March 1965, only ten of sixty-four cases (15.6%), in which pulmonary emboli were found in the major arterial branches, were diagnosed clinically.

Sevitt and Gallagher,[17] in a series of 125 autopsies, found by venous dissection that 65 percent had venous thrombosis. These did not include the cases with pulmonary embolism. Teviotdale and Gwynne[18] in 100 unselected necropsy cases found by careful dissection of deep veins of the calf, recent thrombi in forty-seven cases and old thrombi in a stage of organization in an additional fifteen cases. The incidence of pulmonary embolism was 25 percent. Hackl[19] in 7,797 autopsies in which massive pulmonary embolism was found in 590 (7.5%), determined the origin of the embolus as follows: right femoral and iliac, 63 percent; left femoral and iliac, 58 percent; both femorals and both iliacs, 34 percent; right auricular appendage, 5 percent; right ventricle, 2 percent; and other veins, 6 percent. In Kaufmann and Keresztes'[20] 1,280 cases, the site of origin of the embolus was as follows: deep calf veins, 74.2 percent; femoral veins, 15 percent; prostatic plexus, 5 percent; pelvic veins, 5.54 percent; and right heart, 0.16 percent. Horwitz and Tatler,[21] in a series of 10,991 autopsies performed at the Los Angeles County Hospital from 1961 to 1965, found pulmonary embolism was the cause of death or major contributory cause in 316. Thus, pulmonary embolism was found in one third of all autopsies and was the cause of death in 3 percent. In only 11.5 percent of patients dying of pulmonary embolism was the diagnosis made clinically. Twenty-one and eight-tenths percent had been diagnosed as dying of myocardial infarction; 14.9 percent of cerebrovascular accidents; 14.2 percent of pneumonia; and 13.2 percent of heart disease other than myocardial infarction. Sandritter and Felix[22] found that the incidence of pulmonary embolism as determined at autopsy varied according to the various countries as follows: Europe, 2.3 percent; United States, 2.5 percent; Canada, 5.12 percent; South America,

0.34 percent; Africa, 0.18 percent; Asia, 0.22 percent; Australia, 1.92 percent. Ludbrook[23] found that venous thrombosis and pulmonary embolism are increasing in New Zealand. He stated, "In prosperous communities pulmonary embolism is fast becoming the greatest single cause of death in hospitals."

Pulmonary embolism is frequently found in patients with massive trauma. Sevitt[24] found pulmonary embolism in 20 percent of 468 patients who reached necropsy after a wide variety of injuries which correspond to a frequency of fatal pulmonary embolism of about 1 percent among inpatients, excluding those admitted to short stay wards. "Pulmonary embolism was the most frequent single cause of death in the elderly injured." He also stated that, in a recent study:

> Nineteen of 250 patients who reached necropsy after road accidents had major pulmonary embolism. . . . Seventeen of the cases of embolism were among the sixty subjects over forty-five years old who lived more than four days (28%). Thrombosis occurred in 19 percent of twenty-six patients who died within the first three days of injury, 44 percent of those who died between the fourth and seventh days, and between 79 and 88 percent among those who died between the second, third, and subsequent weeks.

Study further showed that thrombosis was diagnosed clinically in thirteen of forty-one subjects who died later, but thirty-two of forty-one (including all 13 with limb swelling) and significant thrombosis at necropsy. Sixty percent of those who died of pulmonary embolism had no antemortem symptoms. Flesch[25] found among 91,690 patients treated at the Erlanger-Nürenberg Surgical Clinic, that there were 3,794 deaths of which 378 (4.13%) were from pulmonary embolism. Out of 60,849 patients operated upon, 270 (4.45%) died of pulmonary embolism.

Pulmonary embolism is almost invariably the result of detachment of a clot in the veins of the pelvis and/or extremity originating in phlebothrombosis. Although pulmonary embolism can and does occur in thrombophlebitis, this is unusual because the clot in thrombophlebitis is firmly attached and does not become detached. In the short segment of vein between the attached thrombus (white thrombus) and the next proximal venous radical, in which blood is stagnant, a nonadherent coagulation thrombus can occur which can become detached and produce embolism. It, however, is usually relatively small and seldom if ever is large enough to produce severe symptoms. The other instance in which pulmonary embolism can occur in thrombophlebitis is suppurative thrombophlebitis when as a result of liquifaction of the clot, septic emboli can break off producing sepsis. In such cases, death, when it occurs, is usually from sepsis and not from massive pulmonary embolism as in phlebothrombosis. This is a situation that can occur in septic thrombophlebitis of the pelvic veins associated with puerperal sepsis or other septic conditions in the pelvis. The mortality rate is usually high unless there is interruption of the venous drainage of these areas, namely the vena cava and the ovarian or spermatic veins. As mentioned previously, Trendelenburg in 1902 advocated ligation of the hypogastric and ovarian veins in treatment of puerperal sepsis.

Pulmonary embolism is increasing because the incidence of phlebo-thrombosis is increasing. Phlebothrombosis is the result of two factors which favor intravenous clotting, i.e., increased blood coagulability and slowing of venous flow. As a result of tissue injury (the cause of injury—operative trauma, accidental trauma, destruction of tissue by neoplastic disease, or infection—is immaterial), alterations in blood constituents occur which favor clotting. This is a protective, desirable mechanism to keep one from bleeding to death. Phlebothrombosis, almost without exception, occurs in deep veins of the lower extremities and/or pelvis, because it is in these areas that venous circulation is frequently slowed. The combination of the increased clotting tendency plus the slowing of venous flow favors the development of a coagulation, nonadhered, clot. Slowing of blood flow in the veins of the lower extremities occurs because the principal factors which are responsible for the movement of venous blood are diminished in the sick individual. The principal factor is the contraction of the peripheral muscles and the sick individual who is usually lying supine in bed, although using his upper extremities from time to time, is very un-likely to move the lower extremities. Another factor responsible for the movement of venous blood is the negative pressure within the thorax. If for any reason, such as pain, there is decrease in the respiratory move-ments, the aspiratory effect of the negative pressure within the thorax becomes lessened. If there is abdominal distention or tight application of an abdominal bandage, pressure on the inferior vena cava is increased which tends to slow the blood flow from the lower extremities. Finally, as a result of the relative inactivity of the lower extremities, there is a de-crease in the arterial and capillary circulation in the lower extremities resulting in the decreased *vis a tergo* through the capillary bed and de-creased flow in the venous system.

In contradistinction to thrombophlebitis in which the symptoms are evident and obvious (the patient usually makes the diagnosis), the clinical manifestations in phlebothrombosis are minimal or absent. An important finding is an increasing pulse rate out of proportion to any other manifes-tation such as fever (Mahler's sign), which the Germans have described as "step ladder pulse." Also, frequently the patient has a sense of impend-ing disaster which is justified because he is a potential fatality. It is difficult to explain what is its cause but when present it is real. I have seen a num-ber of patients who have had the apprehension of impending disaster, until proximal ligation of the involved vein, when it disappeared, even though the patient was unaware of what was done.

The clot in phlebothrombosis is a nonadherent coagulation thrombus similar to the clot that occurs in a test tube when blood is withdrawn and is allowed to clot. It is only slightly attached to the wall of the vessel and can be easily detached, producing an embolus which may produce either nonfatal or fatal pulmonary embolism. Once a diagnosis of phlebothrombosis is made, either the thrombus should be removed by a thrombectomy, (which is a procedure of some magnitude and should only be done by those trained in the procedure) or the vein should be ligated on the cardiac side of the involvement. Administration of anticoagulants, although useful in preventing further coagulation, will not prevent the detachment of an already existing thrombus. Anticoagulation may be hazardous in that the physician is given a false sense of security that something is being done when in reality it will not prevent pulmonary embolism. Moreover, there is also the hazard of bleeding. Sautter et al.[26] warn against anticoagulation with sodium warfarin for venous thrombosis in pregnancy because of an 18 percent fetal mortality rate. Nothing short of mechanical interruption of the venous return from the site of the thrombus can prevent pulmonary embolism.

For a number of years we[27, 28] advocated superficial femoral vein ligation which could be done under local analgesia, and even in bed. In this way we were able to prevent many cases of pulmonary embolism, but because in some eleven cases in which superficial femoral vein ligation had been done, subsequent pulmonary embolism developed, we now prefer inferior vena caval interruption. This has been our method of treatment for over three decades. The condition of very few patients is too critical to undergo a caval ligation. In such a case, however, femoral vein ligation could be done under local analgesia in bed as we previously did.

Caval ligation is done only as a lifesaving procedure and, if done properly, carries little or no risk and is attended with few or no sequelae if proper measures are taken to prevent them. If there is no swelling before ligation, if the extremities are wrapped from the toes to the groin using elastic adhesive bandages on the thigh because of its conical shape, and if the patient is mobilized immediately after the operation, usually no sequelae develop.

In 1943, DeBakey and Ochsner[29] stated, "Although ligation of the vena cava may seem a very radical procedure and far too extensive to be justified, our results demonstrate that not only is the operation lifesaving, but also it is attended with little risk and few if any sequelae."

We have observed no untoward cardiovascular effects of caval ligation even in extremely ill individuals. Usually it can be performed through a rightsided extraperitoneal approach with simple mobilization of the cava in order to insert a curved instrument around it so that a ligature can be slipped around and quickly tied. Manipulation is minimal and the operating time extremely short in contrast to the dissection, manipulation, and time for mobilization of the cava necessary for application of a clip or the plication of the cava. As a result of inferior vena caval ligation, the venous pressure distal to the ligature is increased causing a tremendous demand for the opening of the collaterals. Also the increased venous pressure distal to the ligature tends to prevent detachment of the nonadherent thrombus in the distal veins. Although originally we felt that the principal objection to the incomplete interruption of the cava was the additional time and risk involved, we have subsequently become convinced that these procedures are even more hazardous as far as the subsequent sequelae are concerned than is caval ligation. Our experience with incomplete interruption of the cava is limited to twenty-eight cases, all of whom had caval plication or clip application. In each instance following the incomplete interruption of the cava, phlebograms showed the compartmentalization of the cava to be adequate and that the venous flow was normal. Although in all instances the cava was open immediately after the partial occlusion, in twelve the cava became occluded in less than a week; in eight more it became occluded after a week. When the occlusion occurred, it was almost invariably associated with severe massive swelling of one or both extremities which we have never seen after ligation of the cava. Two of the cases developed such severe phlegmasia cerulea dolens that thrombectomy was necessary to save the patient's life, which has never been necessary after caval ligation. The reason, we believe, that the undesirable sequelae are more severe and more frequent after incomplete caval interruption is because the grid or plication does not completely interrupt the caval flow. There is no increased pressure distally which would tend to prevent detachment of a clot which may be present and there is no demand for the opening of collaterals. If and when the clot does become detached, which is likely because of normal venous pressure, it is stopped by the compartmentalization thus preventing pulmonary embolism but because of the sudden occlusion and blocking of all collaterals not previously dilated, massive thrombosis within the veins of the lower extremity occurs. Only four of our twenty-eight patients with incomplete caval interruption had persistently patent cavae.

The advocates of incomplete interruption of the cava[30-36] almost invariably start out with the premise that caval ligation is usually followed by disabling sequelae, which is not correct. Our experience is substantiated by that of Cranley[37] who states, "I have never seen—repeat, *never seen,* the postphlebitic syndrome develop in a patient following thrombophlebitis with or without venous interruption if the swelling was controlled." He correctly emphasized that the swelling following vena caval ligation is more directly related to the extent of the venous thrombosis than to the ligation of the vein itself, with which I thoroughly agree. Bergan et al.[9] performed caval plication in eleven cases with one death, four subsequently developed new edema or worsening of their edema and in nine patients in whom cavograms were done, the cavae were found to be closed in six. They concluded, "The apparent advantages to vena caval plication over vena caval ligation were not upheld by this study. Both operations protect the patient against pulmonary embolism and neither is associated with marked morbidity. Surprisingly, caval patency was preserved in only one third of the plication patients." Moran et al.[38] in an experience with twenty-five cases of caval ligation and twenty-nine treated by the Miles' teflon clip state:

> In our experience the severe postoperative sequelae usually attributed to vena caval ligation have not been observed in either the immediate or late postoperative period. In fact, early postoperative leg swelling and fluid sequestration are seen somewhat more frequently with clips than after ligation, probably because of the embolization to the clip site. . . . In the late follow-up studies stasis changes in the legs of patients with ligation have been indistinguishable from those of partial occlusion. . . . The one patient in this review with considerable leg swelling had a caval clip and recurrent bilateral leg swelling which suggests obstruction at the clip site and this has been established by venography.

Spencer et al.,[35] early advocates of partial caval interruption, at Johns Hopkins Hospital stated, "Plication procedure was developed because ligation of the vena cava has been effective in preventing pulmonary embolism but has also caused permanent venous insufficiency in the lower extremity with varices, edema, and ulceration." Subsequently, DeMeester et al.[39] reviewed fifty-six patients at the Johns Hopkins Hospital, thirty-four of whom had been treated by caval plication, twenty had clips applied, and two had the cava stapled, with seven postoperative deaths (9%). They state that fifteen of forty-nine patients surviving the plication had extensive ileofemoral thrombosis, five of which required ileofemoral thrombectomy, resulting in massive retroperitoneal hematoma in two. A total of thirty-five of the forty-four surviving patients, with plications of the inferior vena cava, were studied for subsequent sequelae for a period of from one month to six years. Only eight were free from venous problems preoperatively and remained so postoperatively. Of thirty-five patients followed for from one month to six years, twenty-five (71%) had persistent edema; ten required elastic stockings; twelve had recurrent phlebitis; six had leg ulceration; and only eight (23%) were free from symptoms. Examinations either by phlebography or at autopsy showed that 40 percent of the veins treated by clips had occluded. There were three proved and three suspected pulmonary emboli after plication, three of which were fatal. They concluded, "On the basis of this study, considering the observed mortality and morbidity, we are unable to justify the liberalization of the indications for inferior vena caval plication for prevention of pulmonary thromboembolism." It is interesting that Spencer's original cases were included in this series.

Harjola et al.,[40] in a well-controlled experimental investigation in dogs, demonstrated that caval compartmental channels of 3.5 to 5.5 mm openings freely permitted passage of radio-opaque emboli. Smaller channels interfered with the blood flow through the cava. They conclude, "On the basis of these results, it seemed that total freedom from recurrent embolism could not be guaranteed by partial compartmentation unless the channel diameter is so small that flow and pressure effects are almost the same as after caval ligation." Annetts et al.[41] concluded from the results of their study as follows: "Our results and those of DeMeester et al. suggest that plication offers little advantage over ligation as far as the lower limbs are concerned, and the latter provides at least in theory more adequate protection against further embolization." Crane,[42] in reporting the experience of the Peter Bent Brigham Hospital, found that of 104 patients treated by caval ligation, 1 percent had further embolization and only 10 percent had marked edema postoperatively.

Since 1934, we have carefully followed 315 cases having venous interruption of which 91 percent had caval ligation, 8 percent caval clips, 1 percent caval plication, 8 percent femoral vein ligation, 7 percent ovarian vein ligation, and 2 percent thrombectomies. Of the 315 patients, ninety are known to be dead (28.3%). Five (1.59%) were in extremis when operated upon and died during the operation or immediately afterward. Obviously the operation should not have been done in these cases, but it was done as a last resort to save the patient's life and it was not felt that the ligation itself in any way contributed to the fatal outcome. Twenty-four died within two weeks (7.6%) all from the condition which had caused the phlebothrombosis; twenty-seven (8.5%) died from two weeks to a year, and thirty-four (10.8%) died after one year and had been followed from one to over twenty years. Two-thirds of the patients had been followed from two to thirty years. One hundred and eighty-eight (59.6%) living patients had been followed from one to 360 months. Sequelae in these cases were as follows: immediate edema, 50 percent; edema after one week, 12.8 percent; disappearance of edema, 21 percent; persistent mild edema, 33 percent; persistent severe edema, 3.9 percent. One percent developed varices, 9 percent recurrent phlebitis, 9.7 percent ulceration, none had recurrent pulmonary embolism, and 40 percent had no sequelae. The final long-term results were classified as follows: excellent, 73 percent; good, 27 percent (those who had some swelling but it was easily controlled by packings or compression bandages); fair, 5 percent (persistent edema which could be controlled, however, and not resulting in incapacitation). None of them had any poor result as far as the sequelae following ligation was concerned. One percent of the entire series were incapacitated but these were incapacitated because of the quadraplegia which was the original cause of their trouble. In a small group of cases having plication, or clip, 21 percent had immediate edema, another 21 percent after a week, 9 percent persistent mild, 25 percent persistent severe, and the edema disappeared in only 4 percent. One case had recurrent nonfatal pulmonary embolism, 21 percent had ulceration, and only 28 percent had no sequelae. The results were considered excellent in 54 percent, good in 21 percent, fair in 21 percent, and poor in 4 percent, incapacitation in 4 percent.

Conclusion

Phlebothrombosis and pulmonary embolism is increasing, mainly because more individuals are subjected to severe tissue injury caused by operative and accidental trauma, infections, and neoplastic disease. Once phlebothrombosis occurs, pulmonary embolism is possible unless the thrombus is removed (thrombectomy) or the venous system on the cardiac side of the thrombus is interrupted. The easiest, most expeditious and safest way to interrupt the venous drainage is by inferior caval ligation, which can be done safely on even the extremely ill patient in approximately ten minutes. If there is no swelling before ligation, the lower extremities are wrapped from the groin to the toes and mobility of the lower extremities instituted. Few or no sequelae follow caval ligation. None are disabling. Incomplete caval interruption (plication, application of clips, or intravenous introduction of umbrellas), although theoretically sound, are more hazardous, associated with much more severe sequelae and a higher incidence of subsequent pulmonary embolization.

REFERENCES

1. Kirschner, M.: Ein dursh die Trendenburgsche Operation gehalter Fall von Embolie der Art pulmonalis. *Arch Klin Chir, 133*:312-359, 1924.
2. Trendelenburg, F.: Ueber die operative Behandlung der Embolie der Lungenarterien. *Arch Klin Chir, 86*:686-700, 1908.
3. _____: *Münch med Wochenschr,* 1902. Cited by Krotoski, J.: Zur Venenunterbindung bzw—extirpation bei der puerperalen Allgemaininfektion von chirurgischern Stand Punkt der Chirurg. 425-439, 1902.
4. Berger, R. L., Ryan, T. J. and Sidd, J. J.: Diagnosis and management of massive pulmonary embolism. *Surg Clin North Am, 48*:311-325, 1968.
5. Soloff, L. A. and Rodman, T.: Acute pulmonary embolism. A review. *Am Heart J, 74*:710-724, 1967 and 74:829-847, 1967.

6. Smith, G. T., Dexter, L. and Dammin, G. J.: Postmortem studies in pulmonary thromboembolism. In Sasahara, A. A. and Stein, M. (Eds.): *Pulmonary Embolic Disease*. New York, Grune and Stratton, 1965.

7. Daicoff, G. R., Ranninger, K. and Moulder, P. V.: The diagnosis and management of massive pulmonary embolism. *Surg Clin North Am, 48*:71-88, 1968.

8. Thomas, D. P.: Treatment of pulmonary embolic disease. A critical review of some aspects of current therapy. *N Engl J Med, 273*:885-892, 1965.

9. Bergan, J. J., Kaupp, H. A. and Trippel, O. H.: Critical evaluation of vena caval plication. Prevention of pulmonary embolism. *Arch Surg, 88*:1016-1020, 1964.

10. Ochsner, A., DeBakey, M. E. and DeCamp, P. T.: Venous thrombosis. *JAMA, 144*:831-834, 1950.

11. Ochsner, A. and DeBakey, M. E.: Thrombophlebitis, phlebothrombosis, and pulmonary embolism. In *Lewis-Walters Practice of Surgery*, vol. XI. Hagerstown, W. F. Prior Co., 1965, pp. 1-54.

12. Ludbrook, J.: The prevention of pulmonary embolism. *NZ Med J, 68*:379-382, 1968.

13. Coon, W. W. and Willis, P. W.: Deep venous thrombosis and pulmonary embolism. Prediction; prevalence and treatment. *Am J Cardiol, 4*:611-621, 1959.

14. Dalen, J. E. and Dexter, L.: Pulmonary embolism. *JAMA, 207*:1505-1507, 1969.

15. Doran, F. S., White, M. and Drury, M.: A clinical trial designed to test the relative value of two simple methods of reducing the risk of venous stasis in the lower limbs during surgical operations, the danger of thrombosis and a subsequent pulmonary embolus, with a survey of the problem. *Br J Surg, 57*:20-30, 1970.

16. Freimann, D. G.: Venous thromboembolic disease in medical and malignant states. In *Thrombosis*. Washington, National Academy of Science, 1969, pp. 5-18.

17. Sevitt, S. and Gallagher, N.: Venous thrombosis and pulmonary embolism. A clinicopathological study in injured and burned patients. *Br J Surg, 48*:475-489, 1961.

18. Teviotdale, B. M. and Gwynne, J. F.: Deep calf vein thrombosis and pulmonary embolism. A necropsy study. *NZ Med J, 66*:530-534, 1967.

19. Hackl, H.: Ueber das Vorkommen von Pulmonalembolism. *Med Klin, 62*:44-46, 1967.

20. Kaufmann, F. and Keresztes, A.: Bericht über die fulminante todliche Lungenembolie des Obduktionsmaterials der Jahre. 1952 bis 1965. *Wien Klin Wochenschr, 79*:155-161, 1967.

21. Horwitz, R. E. and Tatler, D.: Lethal pulmonary embolism. In *Thrombosis*. Washington, National Academy of Science, 1969, pp. 19-28.

22. Sandritter, W. and Felix, H.: Geographical pathology of fatal lung embolism. *Pathol Microbiol (Basel), 30*:742-746, 1967.

23. Ludbrook, J.: The prevention of pulmonary embolism. *NZ Med J, 68*:379-382, 1968.

24. Sevitt, S.: Venous thrombosis in injured patients. *Thrombosis*. Washington, National Academy of Science, 1969, pp. 29-49.

25. Flesch, R.: Die Prophylaxe der tödlichen Lungenembolie durch Vena-Cava Durch Trennung. *Thoraxchirurgie, 16*:30-34, 1968.

26. Sautter, R. D., Fletcher, E. W., Lewis, R. F. and Wenzel, E. J.: Inferior vena caval and ovarian vein ligation for antepartum pulmonary thromboembolism. *JAMA, 196*:290-292, 1966.

27. Ochsner, A. and DeBakey, M. E.: Therapeutic considerations of thrombophlebitis and phlebothrombosis. *N Engl J Med, 225*:207-227, 1941.

28. Ochsner, A., DeBakey, M. E., DeCamp, P. T. and DeRocha, E.: Thromboembolism. An analysis of cases at the Charity Hospital in New Orleans over a 12-year period. *Ann Surg, 134*:405-419, 1951.

29. Ochsner, A. and DeBakey, M. E.: Intravenous clotting and its sequelae. *Surgery, 14*:679-690, 1943.

30. Adams, J. T. and DeWeese, J. A.: Comparative evaluation of ligation and partial interruption of the femoral vein in the treatment of thromboembolic disease. *Ann Surg, 172*:795-803, 1970.

31. DeWeese, M. S. and Hunter, D. C., Jr.: Vena cava filter for the prevention of pulmonary embolism. A five-year clinical experience. *Arch Surg, 86*:856-868, 1963.

32. Leather, R. P., Clark, W. R., Jr., Powers, S. R., Jr., Parker, F. B., Bernard, H. R. and Eckert, C.: Five-year experience with the Moretz vena caval clip in 62 patients. *Arch Surg, 97*:357-364, 1968.

33. Little, J. M. and Loewenthal, J.: Vena caval interruption for pulmonary embolism. Indications and technic. *Med J Aust, 2*:1119-1121, 1967.

34. Miles, R. M., Chappell, E. and Renner, O.: A partially occluding vena caval clip for prevention of pulmonary embolism. *Am Surg, 30*:40-47, 1964.

35. Spencer, F. C., Quattlebaum, J. K., Quattlebaum, J. K., Jr., Sharp, E. H. and Jude, J. R.: Plication of the inferior vena cava for pulmonary embolism. A report of 20 cases. *Ann Surg, 155*:827-837, 1962.

36. Whitcomb, J. G. and Mostyn, M.: Experience with vena cava sieve procedure for prevention of pulmonary emboli. *Am J Surg, 110*:767-771, 1965.

37. Cranley, J. J.: Discussion of paper by Adams and DeWeese. *Surgery, 57*:101, 1965.

38. Moran, J. M., Kahn, P. C. and Callow, A. D.: Partial versus complete caval interruption for venous thromboembolism. *Am J Surg, 117*:471-479, 1969.

39. DeMeester, T. R., Rutherford, R. B., Blazek, J. V. and Zuidema, G. D.: Plication of the inferior vena cava for thromboembolism. *Surgery, 62*:56-65, 1967.

40. Harjola, P. T., Scheinin, T. M., Standertskjöld-Nordenstam, C. G., Tahti, E. and Laustela, E.: Experiments on partial inferior vena caval interruption: Influence on pressure gradient, cinecavography, and on prevention of embolism. *Ann Med Exp Biol Fenn, 47*:217-221, 1969.

41. Annetts, D. L., Hoy, R., Ludbrook, J. and Tracy, G. D.: The effects of inferior vena caval plication and ligation on the lower limbs. *Med J Aust, 2*:703-707, 1968.

42. Crane, C.: Venous ligation in pulmonary embolic disease. In Sasahara, A. A. and Stein, M. (Eds.): *Pulmonary Embolic Disease.* New York, Grune and Stratton, 1965, pp. 277-282.

Chapter 28

THE INFERIOR VENA CAVA UMBRELLA FILTER*

KAZI MOBIN-UDDIN, JOE R. UTLEY, LESTER R. BRYANT AND MARCUS DILLON

THROMBOEMBOLIC DISEASE is a major cause of morbidity and mortality in hospitalized patients. Pulmonary embolism is one of the most common lethal processes found at autopsy. An estimated 50,000 deaths occur annually in the United States from pulmonary embolism and this same process contributes to death in many additional patients.

Barker and associates[1] have reported on the natural course of untreated thromboembolism in postoperative patients. Of 1,655 patients with pulmonary embolism, the first episode was fatal in 24.4 percent, and death occurred in 18.3 percent of the nearly one-third who had recurrent embolism. Despite anticoagulant therapy that has been considered adequate, recurrences of pulmonary embolism are not uncommon. Interruption of the inferior vena cava (IVC), by either ligation or plication, has offered good protection against recurrent embolism with the risk of a major surgical procedure and anesthesia. The operative mortality rate in patients with significant cardiopulmonary disease has been high[2,3,4] depending upon the severity of the underlying disease and the extent of obstruction to pulmonary blood flow.

To avoid general anesthesia and a major surgical operation, a simple transvenous catheter technique was developed for interruption of the IVC with an intracaval device of an umbrella design.[5,6,7,8,9] After satisfactory studies in dogs and an assessment of clinical results in the first 100 patients, the umbrella filter† (UF) was released for general clinical use in January 1970. The present report includes the results of clinical filter implants in 2,215 patients as reported by the evaluating physicians.

---

*This review would not have been possible without the assistance of many physicians. Drs. Samii Parviz of Jackson, Michigan and Albert M. Schwartz of Beth Israel Medical Center, N. Y., were among the many, who readily responded to our request for information.

†Edwards Laboratories, Santa Ana, California.

MATERIAL AND METHODS

The intracaval filter (Fig. 28-1) is of an umbrella design and consists of six spokes of stainless steel alloy* radiating from a central hub. A thin sheet of silastic† covers the metal on each side, but the spokes extend two mm beyond the silastic "body." There is a one-mm threaded hole in the center. There are eighteen fenestrations in the silastic body, each with a diameter of three mm. The threaded hole in the center provides fixation to the stylet for implantation. The original caval umbrella was twenty-three mm in diameter, but episodes of filter migration led to development of the twenty-eight-mm device. By virtue of its spring action, the large filter will adjust to all sizes of the IVC in adults. The catheter used for implantation of the umbrella consists of a No. 7 cardiac catheter with a metal capsule at the end. The capsule has a diameter of seven mm and a length of thirty-two mm. A threaded stylet fits inside the catheter and capsule for control of the filter.

The UF is threaded onto the end of the stylet and is unscrewed one-half turn (Fig. 28-2). Using a swab, the umbrella and the inner surface of the loading cone are lubricated with a sterile, water soluble lubricant (Lubrifax®, KY Jelly®, or Glycerine®) mixed with a few milliliters of heparin. The UF is pushed all the way into the distal portion of the loading cone and the applicator-capsule is advanced firmly into the loading cone. An assistant is particularly useful in holding the applicator capsule inside the loading cone. While maintaining the axial alignment, the stylet, with the help of a pin vise, is pulled back through the applicator, thus loading the UF into the capsule. The pin vise is advanced onto the luerlok hub of the applicator and retightened to prevent the umbrella filter from being accidentally ejected from the capsule or unscrewed from the stylet while manipulating the catheter.

Umbrella Filter Implantation

Under local infiltration anesthesia, a small incision is made at the right base of the neck and the right internal jugular vein is isolated between the two heads of the sternocleidomastoid muscle. A vascular clamp is applied proximally to occlude the vein and an umbilical tape tourniquet is put in place for distal control. The vascular clamp and tourniquet are very important for the prevention of air embolism and bleeding. The applicator-capsule containing the collapsed UF is inserted via a venotomy in the internal jugular vein (Fig. 28-3) and advanced under fluoroscopic control

---

*Elgiloy Company, Elgin, Illinois.

†Dow Corning Corporation, Midland, Michigan.

through the superior vena cava and right atrium in the IVC. The applicator is generally advanced to the level of the bifurcation of the IVC and it is then withdrawn so that the distal tip of the capsule is positioned at the

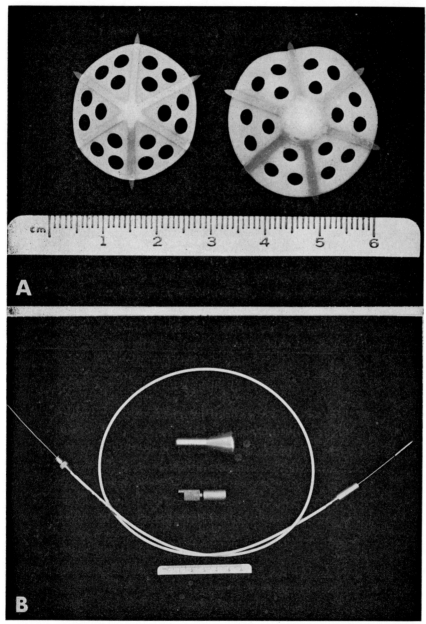

Figure 28-1. A. To the right is the 28-mm filter now recommended for use in all adult patients. The 23-mm filter may have application for recurrent embolism in adults up to 55 kg. body weight. B. Catheter used for umbrella filter implantation.

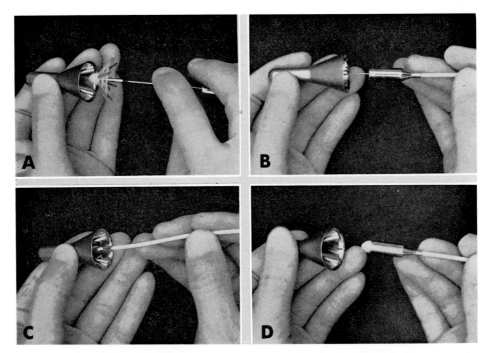

Figure 28-2. Demonstrates the technique of loading of the umbrella filter into the applicator-capsule.

level of the midpoint of the third lumbar vertebra. The pin vise is loosened, moved two cm proximally, and then retightened. After rechecking the position of the distal capsule under fluoroscopy, the stylet is advanced by pushing on the pin vise and the filter is ejected from the capsule. The filter should spring open and lightly fix in place at the intervertebral disc between the third and fourth lumbar vertebra. The pin vise is moved two cm proximal to the luerlok hub and retightened. Slight but firm upward traction is applied several times on the stylet to securely fix the filter into place. Slight upward traction is maintained while the stylet is unscrewed from the filter. The applicator is withdrawn from the vein, a vascular clamp is placed on the vein distally, and the vessel is repaired before wound closure.

TECHNICAL CONSIDERATIONS

The following operative details are emphasized: (1) Special care should be exercised in dissecting the adherent posterior wall of the internal jugular vein. The clavicular head of the sternocleidomastoid muscle may be divided to improve exposure. (2) The venotomy should be kept closed except during the actual insertion of the applicator capsule to avoid air embolism. (3) Occasionally, difficulty is experienced in advancing the

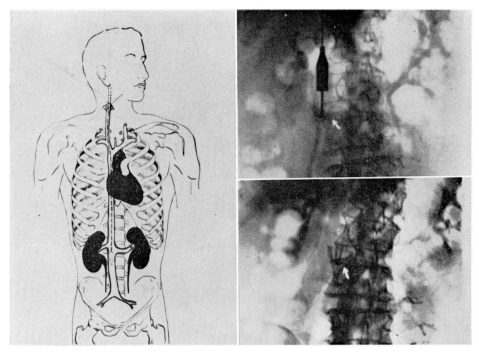

Figure 28-3. To the left, the applicator-capsule containing the collapsed umbrella filter has been inserted via the right internal jugular vein into the inferior vena cava below the renal veins. Top right, the filter has been ejected from the capsule into the inferior vena cava. Bottom right, the stylet has been unscrewed from the filter and the applicator has been withdrawn. Reprinted from: Mobin-Uddin, K., et al., Transvenous caval interruption with umbrella filter. *New Engl J Med, 286*:55-58, 1972.

applicator-capsule from the jugular vein into the superior vena cava. It usually hangs up in the vein under the clavicle. The following measures may prove helpful: handle the vein as little as possible to prevent spasm; allow the umbrella to protrude slightly at the end of the capsule to form a "bullet nose"; pass a suitable size Hagar dilator via the venotomy site and note the direction of opening into the superior vena cava; insert the applicator-capsule half-way into the vein, release the distal tape and apply slightly countertraction with the proximal tape, before advancing the applicator in the direction previously noted; do not use force to advance the applicator. Slight lubrication of the applicator-capsule may be helpful. (4) At times the applicator may not pass from the right atrium into the IVC, or it may pass preferentially into the right renal or hepatic vein. Under these circumstances, the applicator is withdrawn into the neck and a slight but gentle bend is made in the applicator catheter, just proximal to the capsule. The applicator can then be maneuvered by rotating it past the obstruction. Rarely, because of a prominent eustachian valve, the applicator-capsule cannot be advanced from the right atrium into the IVC. Under such circumstances, a guide wire is inserted via the jugular vein into the IVC. After turning the patient to one side, the applicator can then be easily manipulated into the IVC. (5) An inferior venacavogram made before umbrella insertion is a very valuable adjunct. It demonstrates the level of the renal veins and the size of the IVC, and it may reveal any unsuspected anatomical abnormalities of the IVC[10, 11] or the renal veins.[12] Any thrombus in the IVC that may interfere with placement of the UF can also be detected. (6) Accidental placement of the UF in the IVC above the renal veins can be corrected by displacing the filter downward by the applicator-capsule to a level below the renal veins.

Postoperative Management

Following UF implantation, anticoagulant therapy is withheld for twelve hours to minimize the possibility of retroperitoneal bleeding. Thereafter, intravenous heparin is resumed for seven to ten days, preferably by continuous infusion to maintain the partial thromboplastin time or the Lee-White clotting time at two times the control value. Oral anticoagulation with Warfarin sodium is started on the third postoperative day and continued for three months. Patients with continued predisposing factors such as cardiac failure and those with chronic obstructive airway disease associated with microemboli and cor pulmonale receive long-term anticoagulants after UF insertion. Elevation, elastic support, and early ambulation are employed to prevent or control peripheral edema.

Selection of Patients for Umbrella Procedure

Initially IVC interruption with the UF was used only in poor risk patients for whom surgical ligation or plication would have carried a higher operative risk. A large number of physicians who have gained experience with the umbrella procedure are now using it as the method of choice.

The UF has been used in patients who have recurrent pulmonary embolism despite adequate anticoagulation therapy, in those for whom anticoagulants are contraindicated, in patients with pulmonary embolism and shock (see Chapter 33), and following pulmonary embolectomy.[13] Prophylactic caval interruption with the UF has been used in high risk patients with recent deep venous thrombosis while awaiting a surgical procedure, in those with iliofemoral thrombosis that has not responded to medical management and in a controlled study group before hip nailing.[14]

Results

The results are summarized in Table 28-I. In seventy-one patients the UF could not be implanted mainly because of the inability to insert the applicator-capsule via the right internal jugular vein. In five of these patients, the left internal jugular vein and in one the right common femoral vein, was used to implant the UF.

TABLE 28-I

SUMMARY OF CLINICAL RESULTS IN PATIENTS TREATED
WITH THE UMBRELLA FILTER AS OF NOVEMBER 1973

| | No. of patients | | Total No. of |
	23 mm filter	28 mm filter	patients
Filter implants	1,981	234	2,215
Proximal filter migration	20	2	22-0.9%
Distal filter migration*	6	0	6-0.27%
Filter dislodgement without migration	20	0	20-0.9%
Misplacement of filter			
Right renal vein	7	0	7-0.3%
Right iliac vein	20	0	20-0.9%
Recurrent emboli			
Fatal	18	0	18-0.8%
Nonfatal	47	6	53-2.3%
Clinical edema	102	13	115-5.1%
Phlebitis	33	2	35-1.5%

*Following closed cardiac massage

Mortality and Recurrent Embolism

Of the 2,215 patients in whom the UF was implanted, recurrent embolism has been reported in 3.0 percent (fatal, 0.8%). For three patients, blood clot from the proximal surface of the UF was implicated as the source of recurrent pulmonary emboli.

Filter Migration

The clinical data of patients in whom filter migration occurred is summarized in Table 28-II. Filter migration has occurred in two of the 234 patients who have received the larger twenty-eight-mm filter. Of the 1,981 patients in whom a twenty-three-mm filter was used, proximal migration occurred in twenty instances. The filter lodged in a main branch of the pulmonary artery in thirteen patients, in the right ventricle in two, in right atrium in four, and in the IVC above the renal veins in three patients. Distal migration of the UF into the right iliac vein following closed cardiac massage has been reported in six patients.

Filter Dislodgement Without Migration

Partial dislodgement of the UF without migration has been reported in twenty patients. To prevent migration, the larger twenty-eight-mm filter

TABLE 28-II

CLINICAL DATA ON PATIENTS WITH UMBRELLA FILTER
DISLODGEMENT AND PROXIMAL MIGRATION

No. of patients	*Filter migrated to:*
13	*Pulmonary artery* 3 fatal—embolized with massive thrombus 7 removed—two died postoperatively 3 left in place—1 died few days later and 2 died after 3 months, death unrelated.
2	*Right ventricle* 1 removed on cardiopulmonary bypass 1 died six days later, no autopsy
4	*Right atrium* 1 fatal—embolized along with massive thrombus 1 found at autopsy, death unrelated 2 removed, 1 died postoperatively
3	*Supra-renal inferior vena cava* 1 died of cancer at 6 weeks 1 died of myocardial infarction 1 year later 1 alive and well. Venogram showed patency of IVC.

was implanted just above the previous filter in six patients. In the remaining patients, either nothing was done or surgical interruption of the IVC was performed with or without removal of the filter.

Misplacement of the Filter

The UF has been improperly placed in the supra-renal IVC, the right renal vein and the right iliac vein.

In three patients in whom the UF was accidentally extruded into the supra-renal IVC, the filters could be pushed downward with the applicator-capsule into the IVC below the renal veins. In two of these patients, a second filter was implanted proximal to the first because the latter became tilted as it was moved downward by the applicator-capsule.

Of the seven patients in whom the UF was inadvertently misplaced in the right renal vein, in three, the UF has been removed and IVC interrupted by direct surgical approach.

The UF was mistakenly placed in the right iliac vein in twenty patients. These have been treated either by removing the filter with interruption of the IVC or by implanting an additional filter in the IVC. In one patient, the applicator-capsule accidentally perforated the hepatic vein and the umbrella was extruded into the retroperitoneal space.

Significant retroperitoneal hematoma has been reported in five patients, right recurrent laryngeal nerve injury in two, and perforation of duodenum and ureter in one patient each. Air embolism during filter insertion has occurred in two patients (fatal in 1). Renal shut-down developed postoperatively in two patients in whom the UF was placed just below the renal veins. Exploratory laparotomy in one patient revealed an impingement on the blood flow from the left renal vein due to propagation of thrombus on the proximal surface of the UF. The right renal vein was not affected. The patient made an uneventful recovery after removal of the UF. Death occurred in the other patient without permission for autopsy. Postoperative septicemia led to removal of the UF in one patient on the seventh day after implantation. The organisms cultured from the blood and from the clot on the proximal surface of the UF were identical.

Statis Sequelae

Of the 2,215 patients with filter implants, 115 (5.1%) developed significant clinical edema and 35 (1.5%) experienced phlebitis of the lower extremities not previously present. Majority of these patients improved with the standard medical treatment.

DISCUSSION

Patients with nonfatal pulmonary emboli may be managed by the administration of anticoagulants, with or without interruption of the IVC. Unfortunately, there has been a wide variation in the reported results with anticoagulant therapy. Murray[15] notes a recurrence rate of only 2.6 percent nonfatal emboli in 149 patients, but Barker[16] recorded an incidence of 78.6 percent in a group of twenty-eight. Barritt and Jordan[17] had no fatal recurrences with anticoagulant therapy in fifty-four patients while Ochsner[18] and Byrne[19] reported fatal recurrent pulmonary emboli in 11.7 and 18.6 percent of their study groups, respectively. The reasons for such conflicting reports are not hard to find; as one analyzes these reports, one is struck with the variability in patient material, diagnostic and therapeutic criteria and interpretation of facts. DeBakey[20] in an exhaustive review of literature on venous thromboembolism pointed out that inconsistencies, conflicting findings and incompatible statistics keynote all phases of thromboembolism. The clinical diagnosis of venous thrombosis and pulmonary embolism is unreliable and the results of treatment will continue to vary. Diacoff and associates[21] diagnosed pulmonary embolism in only twenty-one of fifty-seven patients (36.8%) who had arteriography for suspected pulmonary embolism. It seems unrealistic to compare and evaluate the results of therapy when the very diagnosis of thromboembolism is uncertain. The Urokinase pulmonary embolism trial[22] phase I, a national cooperative study has provided an excellent opportunity to document the course of the

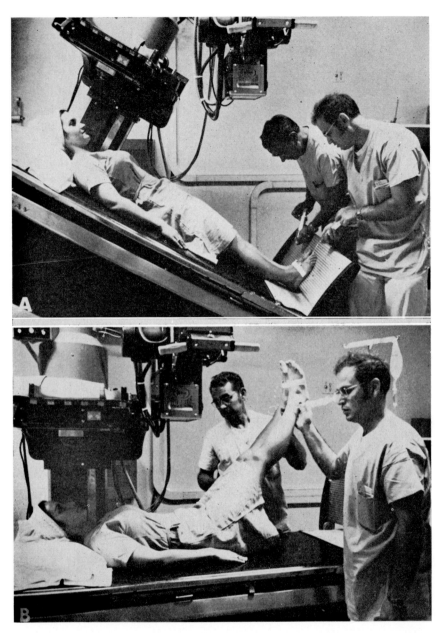

Figure 28-4.   A. The patient is placed supine on an X-ray tilt-table, with the head 45° from the horizontal. Fifty cc of 60 percent Hypaque is injected simultaneously in the subcutaneous veins of both feet with tourniquets above the ankle. Films of the leg and thigh region are exposed in rapid succession. B. Both lower extremities are raised to 45° and a film of the pelvis and abdomen is exposed. Intravenous fluids are administered to wash out the contrast media.

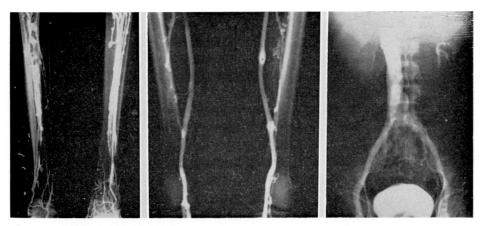

Figure 28-5.   Peripheral phlebograms, demonstrating the deep venous system of the lower extremities, the iliac veins and the IVC.

disease in patients with proven pulmonary embolism. The group reported 18 percent recurrence rate (fatal 9%) in sixty patients treated with adequate anticoagulation.

In analysis of the reasons for failure of anticoagulant therapy to prevent recurrent pulmonary embolism, it is apparent that heparin in adequate doses may prevent thrombus formation or propagation, but cannot prevent fragmentation and detachment of a nonadherent thrombus.

Nearly all emboli arise from the thrombi in the lower extremity or pelvic veins. Major or fatal emboli come from the large deep veins of the thigh or pelvis. Leg vein thrombi may become significant if thrombus extends into the popliteal vein or if thrombosis is extensive. Clinical evaluation detects less than one half the cases of deep venous thrombosis and pulmonary embolism is often the first manifestation of this disease.

Phlebography provides the most reliable evidence for the presence, and extent of venous thrombosis by demonstration of filling defects within the vein. A negative phlebogram essentially rules out significant deep venous thrombosis of the lower extremities. Phlebography has not been used widely in the past, largely because of technical problems and questions of interpretation. However, there now seems sufficient experience with this technique[23, 24, 25, 26] to warrant its use in selected patients with thromboembolism. At our institution, it is used routinely as part of work-up in patients with thromboembolic disease to determine the extent of residual venous thrombosis. The phlebographic technique used is described in Figure 28-4. Peripheral phlebograms gave adequate visualization of the major veins of the lower extremities and pelvis including the IVC (Fig. 28-5).

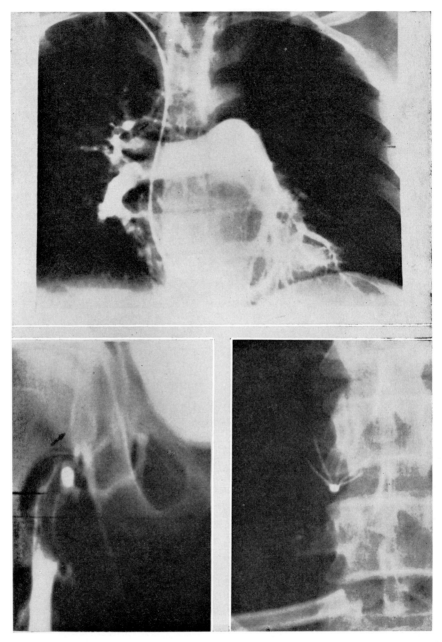

Figure 28-6. TOP—Pulmonary arteriogram in a patient demonstrating more than 50 percent embolic obstruction to pulmonary blood flow.

BOTTOM LEFT—Phlebogram demonstrating potentially lethal, non-adherent thrombus in iliofemoral vein.

BOTTOM RIGHT—Inferior vena cava umbrella filter in place for prevention of fatal pulmonary embolism.

In our experience, recurrent pulmonary embolism during "adequate" anticoagulation therapy has occurred most frequently in those patients in whom nonadherent thrombi were demonstrated by phlebography. A fresh nonadherent thrombus appears as a radiolucent defect within the vein with the contrast medium lining the vein wall (Fig. 28-6). It is our practice to recommend IVC interruption by the UF in those patients who have potentially lethal nonadherent thrombi in the iliofemoral veins.

As the physicians have gained experience with the use of UF, the complication rate has significantly decreased. The main causes of filter migration have been (1) exceptionally large IVC, (2) inadequate seating of the filter, (3) sudden embolic obstruction of the filter by a massive thrombus, resulting in dilatation of IVC, and permitting dislodgement and migration of the filter along with the embolus. With the introduction of the larger twenty-eight-mm UF, the incidence of migration has been reduced.

In an attempt to resist or prevent thrombus formation on the proximal surface of the filter, preoperative heparin impregnation of the UF by treating it with TDMAC/heparin complex[28] is being evaluated. Postoperatively anticoagulation therapy is continued for three months; if there is no con-

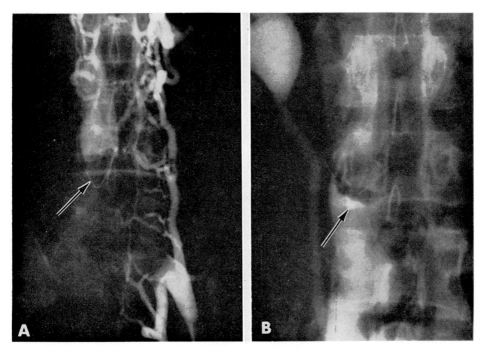

Figure 28-7. A. Angiogram of inferior vena cava in a patient five days after umbrella implantation. Note complete thrombotic occlusion of IVC and development of collateral circulation. B. Angiogram of IVC, three months after implantation of heparin-impregnated umbrella filter. Note free flow of blood through the filter.

traindication for its use. These measures may prevent thrombus formation (Fig. 28-7) and allow for endothelium to grow in between the fenestrations of the filter. Transvenous caval interruption by the umbrella filter has provided an effective means for prevention of pulmonary embolism with minimal risk to the patient.

REFERENCES

1. Barker, N. W., Nygaard, K. K., Walters, W., et al.: Statistical study of post-operative venous thrombosis and pulmonary embolism. Incidence of various types of operative procedures. Staff Meeting, Mayo Clinic, 15:769, 1940.
2. Crane, C.: Femoral vs. caval interruption for venous thromboemblism. *N Engl J Med*, 278:819, 1964.
3. Nabseth, D. C. and Moran, J. M.: Reassessment of the role of inferior-vena-cava ligation in venous thromboembolism. *N Engl J Med*, 273:1250-1253, 1965.
4. Moran, J. M., Criscitiello, M. G. and Callow, A. D.: Vena cava interruption for thromboembolism: partial or complete? Influence of cardiac disease upon results. *Circulation*, 39: Suppl 1:263-268, 1969.
5. Mobin-Uddin, K., Smith, P. E., Martines, L. D., Lombardo, C. R. and Jude, J. R.: A vena caval filter for the prevention of pulmonary embolus. *Surg Forum*, 18:209, 1967.
6. Mobin-Uddin, K., McLean, R., Bolooki, H. and Jude, J. R.: Caval interruption for prevention of pulmonary embolism; long-term results of a new method. *Arch Surg*, 99:711, 1969.
7. Mobin-Uddin, K., Bolooki, H. and Jude, J. R.: Intravenous caval interruption for pulmonary embolism in cardiac disease. *Circulation*, 41 (Suppl. 2): 153, 1970.
8. Mobin-Uddin, K., Trinkle, J. K. and Bryant, L. R.: Present status of the inferior vena cava umbrella filter. *Surgery*, 70:914, 1971.
9. Mobin-Uddin, K., Callard, G. M., Bolooki, H., et al.: Transvenous caval interruption with umbrella filter. *N Engl J Med*, 286:55, 1972.
10. Gray, R. K., Buckberg, G. D. and Grollman, J. H.: The importance of inferior vena cavography in placement of the Mobin-Uddin vena caval filter. *Diagnostic Radiol*, 106:277, 1973.
11. Meier, M. A., Burman, S. O., Hastreiter, A. R. and Long, D. M.: Interruption of double interior vena cava for prevention of pulmonary embolism. *Ann Surg*, 76:769, 1971.
12. Riggs, O. E.: Vena cavography relative to umbrella filter placement. *Radiology*, 105:450, 1972.
13. Huse, W. M.: Vena cava umbrella filter insertion during pulmonary embolectomy. *Arch Surg*, 106:737, 1973.
14. Fullen, W. D., Miller, E. H. and Steele, W. E., et al.: Prophylactic vena caval interruption in hip fractures. *J Trauma*, 13:403, 1973.
15. Murray, G.: Anticoagulants in venous thrombosis and prevention of pulmonary embolism. *Surg Gynecol Obstet*, 84:665, 1947.
16. Barker, W. F.: The management of venous thrombosis and pulmonary embolism. *Surgery*, 45:198, 1959.
17. Barritt, D. W. and Jordan, S. C.: Anticoagulant drugs in treatment of pulmonary embolism: Controlled trial. *Lancet*, 1:1309, 1960.

18. Ochsner, A., DeBakey, M. E., DeCamp, P. T., et al.: Thromboembolism. An analysis of cases at the Charity Hospital in New Orleans over a 12 year period. *Ann Surg, 134*:405, 1951.
19. Byrne, J. J.: Phlebitis; A study of 979 cases at the Boston City Hospital. *J Am Med Assoc, 174*:113, 1960.
20. DeBakey, M.: Collective review: Critical evaluation of problems of thromboembolism. *Int Abst Surg, 98*:1, 1954.
21. Diacoff, G. R., Ranninger, K., Moulder, P. V.: The diagnosis and management of massive pulmonary embolism. *Surg Clin North Am, 48*:71, 1968.
22. The Urokinase Pulmonary Embolism Trial, A national cooperative study: *Circulation, XLVII* (4): Suppl. 11, 1973.
23. DeWeese, J. A. and Rogoff, S. M.: Functional ascending phlebography of the lower extremity by serial long film technique. *Am J Roentgen, 81*:841, 1959.
24. Bergvall, U.: Phlebography in acute deep venous thrombosis of the lower extremity. *Acta Radiol [Diagn] (Stockh), 11*:148, 1971.
25. Nicolaides, A. N., Kakkar, V. V., Field, E. S., et al.: The origin of deep vein thrombosis: A venographic study. *Br J Radiol, 44*:653, 1971.
26. Rabinov, K., Paulin, S.: Roentgen diagnosis of venous thrombosis in the leg. *Arch Surg, 104*:134, 1972.
27. Grode, G. A., Falb, R. D. and Crowley, J. P.: Biocompatible materials for use in the vascular system. *J Biomed Mater Res, 3*:77-84, 1972.

Chapter 29

PULMONARY THROMBOEMBOLISM-THERAPY

Arthur A. Sasahara, *Moderator;* William W. Coon, James E. Dalen,

Jack Hirsh, Alton Ochsner, Kazi Mobin-Uddin

D R. SASAHARA: I think you've really heard the spectrum in therapy of
pulmonary embolism and you will hear more tomorrow, particularly
of massive embolism. I am sure the variety of approaches to treatment must
be confusing. Somehow if there were a universal therapeutic truth, there
would be a relatively narrow path to follow. Perhaps we can try to put
some of what's been said today into perspective. You've heard primarily
a surgical approach and you've heard also an anticoagulant approach. Because this is an area where only semihard data are available, with some
discussion, I hope that we will be able to come away with a little better
feel for appropriate therapy. Before we begin, I would like to have all the
panel members smile at each other, because perhaps at the end of the
half hour, they may not be able to do so.

Dr. Sasahara: I would like to begin with a question for Dr. Mobin-Uddin.
Dr. Mobin-Uddin, when you take into account massive, major and minor
pulmonary embolism, which account for 99 percent of pulmonary emboli,
and these patients receive your umbrella, who at the University of Kentucky received heparin therapy followed by long-term anticoagulation?

Dr. Mobin-Uddin: Here at this hospital once the patient experiences pulmonary embolism and also shows evidence of potentially lethal thrombi in
iliofemoral veins, caval interruption is performed prior to migration. I think
it is not fair for patients that you treat to let them have a recurrent embolus in the hospital and then you try to do a definitive procedure. The recurrent embolus may be fatal. Once a patient has shown the capacity to
embolize and phlebography demonstrates the presence of fresh nonadherent thrombi in the iliofemoral veins which could be fatal, it is imperative
that you protect the patient from recurrent pulmonary embolism.

320

Dr. Dalen: That's certainly the hard line. I knew that sooner or later I'd find some center where they are even more aggressive for surgical therapy than we are at our hospital and I have found it! When people say that they very rarely see heparin failure, what are they really saying? First of all, before I would be convinced, I've got to see a group of patients in whom the diagnosis of pulmonary embolism is confirmed by pulmonary angiography. The clinical diagnosis of pulmonary embolism is just not that good. I'm not convinced that if someone reports 700 patients with a clinical diagnosis of pulmonary embolism that all 700 had pulmonary embolism. The second thing is, how do you decide if a patient has had recurrent pulmonary embolism? It's up to the person doing the study. There have been very few studies where people really consistently look for recurrent pulmonary embolism. In fact, the only study that I know of where this was carefully done was the study that Dr. Sasahara mentioned, namely the Urokinase Pulmonary Embolism Trial. In this group of patients there is no question that we're talking about acute pulmonary embolism documented by scan and angiogram, that's the first criteria. Each patient had follow-up lung scans at periodic intervals independent of symptoms. When this was done, the recurrence rate of pulmonary embolism was about 15 percent and that is much higher than previous series reported by people using anticoagulants. All the patients were being treated with anticoagulants during the period of time that the 15 percent recurrence rate occurred. I think it is quite possible that the recurrence rate of pulmonary embolism on heparin therapy is much higher than we have been led to believe by earlier studies in which the original diagnosis of pulmonary embolism, and the diagnosis of recurrent embolism was a clinical diagnosis, not confirmed by angiography.

Dr. Sasahara: I think I should add that those urokinase data will be published in *Circulation*. Major recurrences of pulmonary embolism generally occurred when the anticoagulation regimen which was followed somehow broke down. It was necessary to use a standard regimen which does not permit individualization. Therefore, I think 16 percent may be too high. Would anyone else care to comment?

Dr. Hirsh: I don't think that a change in lung scan necessarily means that the patient has developed a recurrent embolism. One of the things we noticed when we were following patients with serial pulmonary angiograms who were treated with either heparin or streptokinase is that a large nonobstructing central embolus would sometimes move distally as it got smaller and become an obstructing embolus. This sometimes led to pulmonary infarction and frequently to a change in lung scan pattern. However, the patient didn't have a second embolus. I think that clinical symptoms and signs of pulmonary embolism supported by lung scan evidence or mortality may be more relevant to the issue in question than a changing lung scan in an asymptomatic patient.

Dr. Sasahara: Dr. Ochsner, you made a major point of trying to distinguish between phlebothrombosis and thrombophlebitis. I wonder if this is clinically important? In our series of proven pulmonary embolism, only about a third have thrombophlebitis with clear-cut signs that you described suggesting inflammation. Seventy percent have asymptomatic legs, yet by impedence or other objective tests, deep vein thrombosis is present. What would your comment be for that? From your initial comment I understood it to mean that if you have symptoms and signs in your leg, don't worry about it.

Dr. Ochsner: Patients with phlebothrombosis do not have symptoms and signs referable to the venous system. If, however, they are fortunate enough not to have a detachment of the nonadherent clot with the production of embolization, after a number of days the presence of a clot in the vein will produce an inflammatory reaction of the vein which will produce symptoms similar to those seen in thrombophlebitis, and incidentally, the clot will become attached.

It is possible for a patient with a thrombophlebitis to get a small embolus which is actually of no significance, however. This is the result of a coagulation thrombus in the relatively short segment on the cardiac side of the thrombophlebitic area in which the stagnant blood in the vein up to the next venous radical can become clotted. Since this is a coagulation thrombus and is nonadherent, it can become detached with the production of a small embolus.

Dr. Sasahara: No, I'm sorry, these were a series of patients with proven pulmonary embolism who presented with both chest pain and an acute leg.

Dr. Ochsner: I think originally they had a coagulation (bland) thrombus before they had their pulmonary embolism and it wasn't recognized.

Dr. Sasahara: Then subsequently developed a hot leg.

Question: What is the experience of the panelist on the use of low molecular weight dextran or rheomachrodex?

Dr. Coon: We ran a small clinical trial a number of years ago using clinical dextran (70,000 molecular weight). It has been shown the dextran with the higher molecular weight has a greater antithrombotic effect. From the clinical point of view this difference in antithrombotic effect may be less important because, after administration of "low" molecular weight dextran, the larger molecules are the ones which remain in circulation for twenty-four to forty-eight hours. We found a somewhat higher frequency of progression of leg vein thrombi during this therapy. We reserve the use of dextran for the treatment of nonembolic deep venous thrombosis in patients in whom anticoagulant therapy is contraindicated.

Question: Is there any contraindication for the use of the umbrella filter?

Dr. Mobin-Uddin: The umbrella filter procedure is recommended in all patients requiring caval interruption except in those with proven septicemia.

Dr. Ochsner: One of the indications for caval ligation is septicemia resulting from suppurative thrombophlebitis, as in suppurative thrombophlebitis in the pelvic veins with which we had a large experience in New Orleans, because we have a large Negro population. Until the introduction of the "pill" there was a large number of individuals admitted to the Charity Hospital in New Orleans who had had criminal abortions, many of whom had puerperal sepsis and an associated suppurative thrombophlebitis of the pelvic veins. The treatment of these individuals by the usually employed methods of supportive care and antibiotics was extremely disappointing—the mortality rate was as high as 80 percent. However, by interrupting the constant supply of septic emboli into the vascular system by ligating the venous drainage from the pelvis, the mortality rate promptly fell. This was accomplished by ligation of the inferior vena cava and the two ovarian veins. In males suppurative infections of the prostate and bladder occasionally are associated with suppurative thrombophlebitis and in these instances it is necessary to ligate the cava and the two spermatic veins.

Question: How do you deal with a patient who experiences recurrent pulmonary embolism via large collaterals after you have ligated the inferior vena cava?

Dr. Ochsner: I've never seen it. We've never had a pulmonary embolism after caval ligation.

Question. Do you do venograms after vena caval ligation?

Dr. Ochsner: We never do venograms. Venograms is a bastard word. It is half Greek and half Latin. We do phlebograms occasionally. We do not do them routinely.

Dr. Dalen: That's a very important point. Dr. Duncan Thomas reported in the *New England Journal* several years ago what he considered to be the recurrence rate of pulmonary embolism after IVC interruption. There are several important points about that paper that should be considered. It reported of patients referred because someone thought they had pulmonary embolism after they had IVC interruption by various surgeons at various hospitals. The main point that was made, I think, was that venograms demonstrated what one might expect if you tie off someone's IVC; that is, large collaterals. It has to work that way. The real issue is do patients, in fact, have significant pulmonary embolism via these collaterals? That's the point that needs to be proved and I agree with Dr. Ochsner; I think that it is quite uncommon. There is no question that the collaterals get big, but the key point is to prove that thrombi pass through these collaterals to cause pulmonary embolism. The only way I know how to get this information is to follow very carefully patients that have had IVC interruption and see how often they do get recurrence of pulmonary embolism. When we have done such a study at our hospital, the incidence of pulmonary embolism after the IVC interruption was about 1 percent. I personally believe that recurrence of pulmonary embolism via collaterals must be very uncommon and I'd look for proof that in fact it occurs.

Dr. Mobin-Uddin: In Miami, we followed 100 patients with caval interruption up to two years. Our recurrence rate was 2 percent.

Question: Dr. Mobin-Uddin, have you inserted the umbrella via the left internal juglar vein?

Dr. Mobin-Uddin: Yes, I have put it in one patient. The right internal jugular vein had been ligated previously, so I used the left internal jugular vein. I made a slight bend in the applicator just proximal to the capsule prior to insertion. It worked well.

Dr. Harrison (New Jersey): Do you perform the vena cava ligation just above the bifurcation or just beneath the renal veins?

Dr. Ochsner: We believe the caval interruption should be done as a life-saving procedure and I don't think it makes much difference where the interruption is done as long as it is done above the bifurcation and below the renals. Ligation can be done simply and usually takes about ten minutes. It is done through a muscle-splitting incision and performed extraperitoneally. All that is necessary is to mobilize the inferior vena cava enough to get an instrument and a ligature around it and simply tie.

Question: One of my patients, following application of Moretz clip, developed recurrent pulmonary embolism, three days postoperatively, proven at autopsy. I would like to ask the panel, could emboli passing through a three-mm clip be fatal?

Dr. Ochsner: This is well demonstrated by a splendid investigative work reported by Harjola et al. (Harjola, P. T., Scheinin, T. M., Standertskjold-Nordensta, C. G., Tähte, L., Lanstela, E.: Experiments on partial inferior vena caval interruption: Influence on pressure gradient, cinecavography, and on prevention of embolism. *Ann Med Exp Biol Fenn*, 47:217, 1969) in which the inferior vena cavae of dogs were interrupted by clips with apertures varying from 1.5 mm to 5.5 mm in diameter. Caval peak pressure gradiant was at most only slightly elevated by clip apertures exceeding 3.5 mm. Openings of 2.5 mm caused a significant pressure gradient and an aperture of 1.5 mm gave an elevation equal to that of the total caval obstruction. Vena cavography showed definite slowing of the flow of the contrast media if the diameter of the aperture was 3.5 mm or less. Openings of 1.5 mm gave total flow obstruction. Gelatin spheres and worm-like gelatin emboli passed unrestricted through 3.5 to 5.5 mm apertures. Openings of 2.5 mm offered only slight temporary obstacles to gelatin spheres two mm in diameter even when long gelatin emboli two mm in diameter passed through after a few seconds delay. The authors concluded: "Some proponents for caval plication procedure believe that small emboli escaping through four to five mm channels are too small to be significant. However, in recurrent pulmonary embolism, particularly if associated or coinciding with pulmonary hypertension, even small emboli may have disastrous consequences." I know that fatal pulmonary embolism has followed incomplete interruption of the vena cava, but I have had no experience with it. In our very limited experience, we have had no fatality but did have nonfatal pulmonary embolism.

Dr. Silver (Durham): Because heparin therapy remains the most widely used agent for managing pulmonary embolism, this audience should be aware of some unusual experiences that we have recently encountered while using heparin (*Surg Gynecol Obstet 136*:409-416, 1973.) Perhaps Dr. Coon would like to comment on our observations.

We have reported two cases and have seen two additional cases of heparin-induced thrombocytopenia with thrombotic and hemorrhagic complications. The first two patients had received heparin for pulmonary embolism and for a deep venous thrombosis. Both patients experienced myocardial infarctions during the heparin therapy. Both patients demonstrated low platelet counts (10,000 to 15,000 range), increased heparin tolerances and bleeding while receiving the heparin. After the heparin was stopped, their platelet counts quickly returned toward normal and their bleeding and clotting problems resolved. Our studies of these patients suggest that whenever heparin requirements increase, platelet counts fall, and new thromboses occur in a patient receiving heparin, the heparin should be stopped and a new mode of therapy begun.

Dr. Coon: I was very intrigued by those observations, Don. We haven't seen this entity as far as we know, but maybe we've been missing something. What brand are you using? We've seen some unusual sensitivity reactions to heparin once in a while, including the painful foot syndrome that disappears as soon as heparin is discontinued, but so far we haven't recognized the thrombocytopenia you described; I think it is a fascinating observation. I'm certainly going to look for it.

Question: I would like to know the incidence of recurrent pulmonary embolism on anticoagulant therapy. I am aware of the conflicting reports in the literature on this aspect.

Dr. Hirsh: I think that it is wrong to lump all the reports of heparin therapy in venous thromboembolism together when attempting to assess the efficacy of heparin therapy. The response of different individuals to heparin differs, some patients requiring as little as 10,000 units per twenty-four hours to maintain their clotting time at two to three times control levels or their PTT at one and one half to two and one half times control while others require up to 100,000 units to achieve this result. The majority of reports in literature on heparin therapy do not record the clotting time or PTT response to heparin and, indeed, many do not even record the heparin dose that was used. However, on careful review of the literature, the results have been uniformly good with an extremely low recurrence rate when heparin has been given in high doses or in doses sufficient to prolong *in vitro* tests of coagulation to within a defined therapeutic range. Therefore, before quoting results of effectiveness or lack of effectiveness of heparin therapy, it is important to take the heparin regimen used into account.

Question: Would any of the panelists comment on the use of antibiotics in pulmonary embolism in view of Dr. Altemeier's work?

Dr. Coon: We use antibiotics on a prophylactic basis to prevent secondary infection of pulmonary infarcts. I don't know anybody else who has documented Dr. Altemeier's studies on bacterial L forms and, until they do, I would not support the use of antibiotics in the usual case of deep venous thrombosis.

Question: Dr. Mobin-Uddin, how soon after umbrella insertion do you resume heparin therapy?

Dr. Mobin-Uddin: We do not give heparin for at least twelve hours following umbrella insertion. We prefer to administer heparin by continuous infusion method as we had many instances of bleeding by giving heparin by intermittent IV push method.

Question: Dr. Mobin-Uddin, in patients with prophylactic umbrella insertion prior to hip nailing or total hip replacement, when do you resume anticoagulant therapy?

Dr. Mobin-Uddin: I usually do not give anticoagulants to patients after hip surgery, as there is an increased incidence of postoperative bleeding.

Dr. Coon: We have persuaded some of our orthopedists to use the dextran prophylactic regimen. They are somewhat hesitant concerning the use of conventional anticoagulant therapy.

Dr. Hanway (New York): I am sorry that Dr. Simon and Dr. Rosenbaum are not here, but I got the idea this morning that they had a greater ability to diagnose pulmonary infarct by the plain chest film. It was my impression that even in retrospective studies, the correlation between the autopsy findings and the plain chest film taken within twenty-four hours of death was not very good.

Dr. Dalen: I frankly would not place too much emphasis on the plain chest film. We use the chest X-ray to look for pneumonia and to help us interpret the scan, but I can't get very worked up about trying to find an infarct, and following it every three to four days. I think there has been very poor correlation between the plain chest film and postmortem.

Dr. Hanway (New York): I would like to add that it is very difficult to differentiate pneumonia from an infarct by the plain chest film.

Dr. Dalen: I think one has to look at the total clinical picture. The chest X-ray is very important, because you have to compare it to the lung scan. If someone has the differential diagnosis of pulmonary infarction versus pneumonia, that's the hard one. You're absolutely right that one can look at the chest X-ray all day long and not be sure if the X-ray abnormality is an infarct or pneumonia. The important point is that there is an infiltrate. In our hospital, nearly everybody that has pulmonary embolism has bilateral pulmonary embolism as demonstrated by pulmonary angiogram. Most patients that have documented embolism have bilateral defects by scan. Therefore, if there is an infiltrate in one lung by X-ray, I would look very hard at the other lung by scan. If the other lung is normal by scan, and the only abnormality by scan is in the area of the infiltrate seen by chest X-ray, then the probability of pulmonary embolism decreases.

Dr. Sasahara: While we are on that subject, would you agree with the concept that in any patient in whom the physician seriously considers pulmonary embolism, a diagnostic work-up short of a lung scan is inadequate?

Dr. Dalen: I would almost agree with that. It depends on what his suspicion is based on. I mean sometimes suspicion is based upon pretty shaky findings like an elevated LDH or an S1Q3T3 pattern by EKG that has been there all the patient's life. Supposing that the patient's blood gases were absolutely normal, pO₂, let's say of 98 or 100, then one would look back at the evidence for pulmonary embolism and if it was pretty shaky, I might not do a scan. I would agree that in the vast majority of cases I would do a lung scan, but it depends upon what the clinical circumstances are that made you think of pulmonary embolism.

Dr. Santos (Chicago): Dr. Sasahara, what is the dose of urokinase and how is it administered? Aside from bleeding, was there any other significant complication with its use?

Dr. Sasahara: The dose was arbitrarily set at 2,000 units per pound per hour for twelve hours. That appeared to give a whole blood euglobulin lysis time within therapeutic range. Good lysis was achieved. The only significant complication was bleeding.

Dr. Pearlman (Boston): I would like to ask Dr. Coon with regard to application of the clip or ligature just below the renal veins by transperitoneal approach, and also comment on the prophylactic use of the clip in high risk patients during laporotomy.

Dr. Coon: Yes, this is the method we prefer, particularly in the good risk patients. We use the transperitoneal approach and very carefully make sure that either the clip or ligature or the Marion DeWeese filter is located just below the left renal vein so that we have good flow above it. This is an important element in preventing propagation of thrombus above the point of caval interruption. With regard to prophylactic caval interruption, one of our staff has been doing it routinely in conjunction with pelvic exenteration since these patients have a high risk of developing pulmonary embolism. We have also performed this procedure in some of our patients having a combined abdomino-perineal resection in whom we are worried about the risk of bleeding from anticoagulation in the postoperative period. We have been using clips under these circumstances.

The diverse opinions expressed regarding the primary therapy of pulmonary embolism requires some comment. On the one hand is the individual who will insert an umbrella or clip in almost every patient because he doesn't want a second emoblus to occur. Dr. Hirsh rarely utilizes this approach because his method of anticoagulation with heparin is effective; the incidence of recurrent embolism is very low. When you question clinicians regarding patients who have had recurrent emboli as to whether heparinization was adequate, they usually agree that it wasn't. It may well be that if you eliminate the cases in which the PTT was not maintained at two and one half to three times control, the rate of recurrent embolism would be extremely low. Perhaps our objective should be to teach the physician how to administer adequate amounts of heparin.

Dr. Ochsner: I am sure that anticoagulants will not prevent the detachment of an already present nonadherent clot. The clot in phlebothrombosis is similar to the clot that occurs in a test tube that can easily be detached. Not all patients with phlebothrombosis develop embolism, but certainly all of them are candidates for embolism and even fatal pulmonary embolism. The simplest way to be sure that a person will not develop embolism is to put a dam between the thrombus and the heart. This can be done best by interrupting the cava. Treating patients with phlebothrombosis with anticoagulants will not prevent the detachment of a clot but will give the physician a false sense of security. He believes that he is doing something for the patient, which indeed he is, but not necessarily something that will prevent him from having a pulmonary embolism. It is like playing Russian roulette.

Dr. Hirsh: I think statistics do help in making therapeutic decisions. The hospital mortality after ligation of inferior vena cava ranges in various studies from 3 percent to 12 percent in patients without severe heart disease but from 20 percent to 40 percent in patients with heart failure. In addition, follow-up of operated patients over a prolonged period of time indicates that the frequency of recurrent pulmonary embolism is considerable. On the other hand, Barritt and Jordan, in the only controlled study ever performed, showed that treatment with anticoagulants reduced the mortality in patients with established pulmonary embolism from 20 percent to 0 percent. In a recent publication we have also reported an extremely low recurrence rate and a zero mortality in patients with venous thromboembolism who were treated with adequate doses of heparin, that is enough heparin to prolong their partial thromboplastin time to at least one and one half times control value.

Question: Dr. Coon, how do you monitor patients on heparin therapy?

Dr: Coon: Although many clinicians are using the activated partial thromboplastin time, we prefer the thrombin time which is simpler and more reproducible in our hands. One may measure the prolongation of thrombin time by varying amounts of heparin and construct a curve which will reflect "units of heparin per milliliter of plasma." The Lee-White clotting time presents many problems in reproducibility and accuracy; most physicians have abandoned it for one of these other procedures.

Dr. Silver (Durham): If you were going to be anticoagulated with Coumadin, what level would you want to be kept at? My impression is 30 percent is worthless. I've always thought between 10 percent and 15 percent was ideal. What is your impression?

Dr. Coon: We've looked at all sorts of therapeutic ranges of prothrombin activity. The only way one can do this is by computer analysis of large numbers of patients. Our statistical studies have not shown any significant differences in thromboembolic complication rates in the range of 15 to 30 percent prothrombin activity. When prothrombin activity is below 15 percent, the rate of hemorrhagic complications increases markedly. I would rather maintain the patient in the 15 to 30 percent range to balance the risks of recurrent thromboembolism against the risk of a hemorrhagic complication.

Dr. Fullen: Dr. Mobin-Uddin, you mentioned that you were not too concerned about how close below the renal veins the filter was placed. Also in an answer to an earlier question, it was suggested that the recurrent embolization might be through the collaterals. Do you have any evidence to suggest that it is not from the superior aspect of the filter?

Dr. Mobin-Uddin: I usually keep patients anticoagulated for three months following insertion of the filter, to prevent thrombus formation on the proximal surface of the filter. This allows endothelium to grow in between the fenestrations of the filter. In patients in whom anticoagulants are contraindicated, there is a risk of clot embolization from the superior aspect of the filter. Fortunately, this does not occur frequently. We have only two case reports in which clot embolization from the proximal surface of the filter has been implicated. In an attempt to prevent or resist thrombus formation, we use filters which have been treated with the TDMAC/heparin complex.

Dr. Hirsh: Dr. Mobin-Uddin, you are in an ideal position to look at the recurrence rate on anticoagulants if you do repeated venograms on your patients following the insertion of the caval umbrella. Do you do venograms and, if so, in how many patients do you see thrombus distal to the umbrella?

Dr. Mobin-Uddin: It is very difficult to differentiate whether the thrombus distal to the umbrella originated at the filter or is a thromboembolus trapped by the filter. Moreover, we do a small number of cases, probably ten to twelve a year.

Dr. Hirsh: If you did venograms and found that the incidence of thrombosis distal to the umbrella was very small in patients who also had anticoagulants, perhaps this would indicate that there was no need for you to insert the umbrella in the first place. The umbrella is presumably inserted to prevent an embolus. Anticoagulants are given to prevent a thrombus from forming on the umbrella. However, if venography fails to demonstrate thrombosis distal to the umbrella, this indicates that the embolism has not occurred, perhaps because the patient is on anticoagulants, and that anticoagulants alone would have been sufficient to treat the patient.

Dr. Mobin-Uddin: Anticoagulant therapy may prevent further thrombus formation or propagation but will not prevent detachment and embolization of a thrombus that is already present. This is what Dr. Ochsner pointed out: that caval interruption is advised in those patients who harbor large, nonadherent potentially fatal thrombi in iliofemoral veins.

Dr. Hirsh: It is really a question of comparing theory with the fact. I think that what you say is theoretically very reasonable. However, these theoretical considerations have to be weighed against very good results that have now been reported for over thirty years with anticoagulant therapy alone.

Dr. Mobin-Uddin: One of my slides summarized the incidence of recurrent pulmonary embolism on anticoagulant therapy. The most recent being the Urokinase-Pulmonary Embolism Trial, Phase I, a national cooperative study which has provided an excellent opportunity to document the course of the disease in patients with pulmonary embolism. The group reported 18 percent recurrence rate (fatal 9%) in sixty patients treated with adequate laboratory control of anticoagulation.

Dr. Hirsh: However, you did not tell us what the dose of heparin was in these various studies, whether heparin was controlled by *in vitro* clotting tests and if so what the control was like. Unless these results are available, the reports shown on your slide are fairly meaningless.

Dr. Sasahara: I think the hour is up. Let me just summarize the consensus of the panel. I think it is marvelous that we all agree anticoagulation is the treatment of our choice!

MASSIVE
PULMONARY
THROMBOEMBOLISM

Chapter 30

THE MEDICAL TREATMENT OF MASSIVE PULMONARY EMBOLISM

Lester R. Bryant, Kazi Mobin-Uddin, Joe R. Utley and Marc Dillon

BEFORE DISCUSSING the medical, or nonoperative, management of acute massive pulmonary embolism, it is appropriate to define the authors' concept of this entity. Simply stated, acute massive pulmonary embolism is a clinical syndrome characterized by severe respiratory distress with sustained hypotension or shock. Most patients who suffer this catastrophe show complete or partial obstruction of at least 50 percent of the central pulmonary arterial bed when pulmonary arteriography is performed. In our opinion, however, the choice of intensive medical management versus pulmonary embolectomy should not be based on the degree of obstruction suggested by the pulmonary arteriogram. There are several reasons for this position. First, it is the pathophysiologic state which must be dealt with, and if recovery can be effected without a major surgical procedure, no one would question this choice. This is predicated on the knowledge that pulmonary embolization is largely reversible due to dissolution of the clot by the fibrinolytic system.[1,2] Second, single plane or biplane pulmonary arteriograms provide only an approximation of the degree of physical obstruction of the pulmonary arteries, and individual observers may arrive at different estimates of the percent overall obstruction. Finally, individual patients vary in their tolerance to major pulmonary vascular obstruction. This is related to the presence or absence of preexisting cardiopulmonary disease, to previous episodes of minor pulmonary embolism, and general health status.

Unfortunately, many patients who suffer acute massive pulmonary embolism will die within a few minutes after the onset of symptoms. In the autopsy series reported by Gorham, 44 percent died within fifteen minutes after symptoms began.[3] An additional 22 percent survived for only two hours. Because Gorham's study included only nonsurviving patients, it is reasonable to conclude that the study population was weighted in favor of the most massive forms of thromboembolism. Nevertheless, it serves to emphasize the great urgency in beginning treatment. While it is not the purpose of this communication to discuss differential diagnosis, it is pertinent to emphasize that the initial resuscitative efforts are just as appropriate for circulatory collapse from potentially lethal myocardial infarction as they are for massive pulmonary embolism.

The first step in medical management, then, is to initiate those processes which provide both *respiratory* and *circulatory* support. Table 30-I lists the essential steps of treatment in outline form. Nasal oxygen is started while preparations are made for endotracheal intubation and mechanical ventilation. An intravenous line is secured and a central venous catheter is put in place. If the peripheral signs of shock are present, or if the systolic blood pressure is below eighty mm Hg, an initial dose of intravenous metaraminol bitartrate should be administered. It is important to maintain the contractile force of the right ventricle and vasopressors are usually required to provide an adequate aortic pressure for coronary perfusion.

TABLE 30-I

AN OUTLINE OF MEDICAL MANAGEMENT FOR
MASSIVE PULMONARY EMBOLISM

  A. Respiratory support
    1. Nasal oxygen—intubation
    2. Mechanical ventilation
  B. Circulatory support
    1. Sodium bicarbonate
    2. Metaraminol bitartrate
    3. Isoproterenol
    4. Methylprednisolone
    5. Digoxin
  C. Monitoring
    1. Central venous pressure
    2. Hourly urine volume
    3. Arterial pressure line
  D. Anticoagulation
    1. Heparin sodium
  E. Contingency plan
    1. Pulmonary arteriogram
    2. Pulmonary embolectomy

According to the severity of the patient's circulatory failure, one or two ampules of sodium bicarbonate are given intravenously, and blood samples are drawn for serum electrolytes, blood urea nitrogen, and a complete blood count with hematocrit. Similarly, an initial arterial sample is drawn for blood gases, but the results are *not* awaited before deciding to institute mechanical ventilation. If respiratory distress and cyanosis have not been relieved by nasal oxygen, a nasotracheal or endotracheal tube is put in place and assisted ventilation is begun with 100 percent oxygen. While our own preference is for a volume-controlled ventilator (Bennett MA-1, Ohio 560), a pressure operated machine may serve adequately. In most patients, repeated small doses of intravenous morphine (3 to 5 mg) facilitate the acceptance of mechanical ventilation. Adjustments of flow rate and tidal volume should be made to provide the lowest possible mean intrathoracic pressure. Repeat measurements of arterial blood gases and pH are important in guiding adjustments of ventilator control.

The electrocardiogram should be monitored continuously, and measurements of central venous pressure should be made at frequent intervals. To achieve the most satisfactory circulatory support, it may be necessary to try several drugs in succession. If the patient's blood pressure responded to metaraminol, it may be satisfactory to continue with this agent. Our preference is to switch to an intravenous infusion of isoproterenol (1 to 4 mcg/min) if the heart rate does not exceed 120 beats per minute and if there is no significant cardiac arrhythmia. In the early stages of resuscitation, however, one or both of these conditions is frequently present. With failure of blood pressure response to either metaraminol or isoproterenol, an infusion of norepinephrine should be started through the central venous line.

Except for those few patients who recovered rapidly, we have administered large doses of intravenous corticosteroids to all cases of massive pulmonary embolism since 1968. The employment of these agents was suggested by the similarity of pulmonary embolism shock to the low cardiac output syndrome seen in some patients after cardiac valve replacement. An increased survival from this syndrome coincident with the use of corticosteroids has been documented by the reports of Dietzman and by our own clinical experience.[4, 5] Originally, hydrocortisone was given as a single intravenous injection of fifty mg/kg of body weight. More recently, methylprednisolone has been used in a dose of thirty mg/kg body weight. The corticosteriods should be administered as soon as it becomes apparent that the patient has a chance for survival with intensive treatment.

Rapid digitalization may offer some benefit in maintaining right ventricular output but the digitalis preparations are contraindicated in the presence of arrhythmias. Our policy has been to withhold digitalization until the serum potassium level has been obtained and the patient's response to vasopressors or isoproterenol has been determined. In the absence of continuing deterioration, digitalization is begun with 0.75 mg digoxin, intravenously. If the patient has shown a satisfactory response to continued medical management, two additional doses of 0.25 mg are given at four-hour intervals.

It is critical to prevent further embolization and to prevent build-up of clot on the thromboemboli already present in the pulmonary arteries. For these reasons, we administer an initial intravenous dose of 10,000 units of heparin and follow this with injections of 5,000 units at four-hour intervals. We have not used the technique of continuous intravenous heparin although it has theoretical advantages.[6]

Most patients who suffer massive embolism, even if they respond satisfactorily to medical management, will remain hypotensive or in shock for some hours. Therefore, the early insertion of a Foley catheter to monitor urinary output, and a radial artery catheter for continuous blood pressure monitoring is most important. The latter facilitates the repeated measurement of blood gases and is of practical importance during subsequent pulmonary arteriography. Elimination of the need to monitor blood pressure by the cuff method gives the angiographers better access to the upper extremities for cardiac catheterization. In addition, the angiographic equipment, respirator, and associated personnel leaves little space for someone to use a blood pressure cuff.

Because of the inherent delays associated with performance of pulmonary arteriography, the radiology department and the person responsible for angiography should be contacted simultaneously with the start of resuscitation. Similarly, the operating room and the cardiopulmonary bypass unit should be alerted for possible pulmonary embolectomy in the event the patient cannot be managed without operation. As soon as resuscitation is under control, the patient should be moved to the angiography laboratory for pulmonary arteriography. Confirmation of the diagnosis is critical for subsequent management. Because of distressing past experiences with patients who were found at operation not to have pulmonary embolism, most cardiac surgeons will not undertake embolectomy without arteriographic confirmation of the diagnosis.

Before injection of contrast material, the pulmonary artery and right ventricular pressures should be measured. In a review of fatal cases of pulmonary embolism, Del Guercio found that death was almost certain if right ventricular mean pressure exceeded twenty-two mm Hg in the absence of other causes for pulmonary hypertension.[7] On the other hand, Wechsler and his associates found no upper limits of mean pulmonary artery pressure or right ventricular end-diastolic pressure which precluded survival without pulmonary embolectomy.[8] In consideration with the response to treatment and the severity of obstruction demonstrated by pulmonary arteriography, the right ventricular pressure may be of value in the decision for subsequent management.

The injection of contrast material may be followed by a temporary worsening of the patient's condition which should be anticipated by those in attendance. If the arteriogram suggests less than 60 percent obstruction of the central pulmonary arteries, and the patient's condition is reasonably stable, continued respiratory and circulatory support are warranted. Figure 30-1 shows the pulmonary arteriogram of a patient with pulmonary embolism shock in whom there is severe partial obstruction of the right pulmonary artery and multiple segmental arterial occlusions in the left lung. Although the patient remained hypotensive with a central venous pressure above sixteen cm of water for six hours, he recovered without embolectomy. Isoproterenol was required for twenty hours, and mechanical ventilation was continued for approximately thirty-six hours. On the fifth day after the episode of massive embolism the patient underwent plication of the inferior vena cava. During that interval he received intravenous heparin in doses sufficient to maintain the Lee-White clotting time at greater than twenty minutes.

A point which should be emphasized is the lack of dramatic response to medical treatment after initial resuscitation in many patients. Systolic blood pressure may persist at levels of seventy to eighty mm Hg for several hours. In this situation, it is the trend of response which must guide the

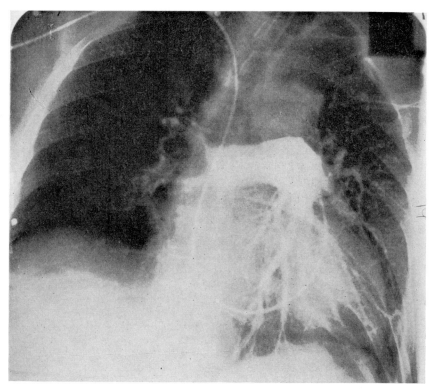

Figure 30-1. The pulmonary arteriogram of this fifty-one-year-old man shows severe partial obstruction of the right pulmonary artery with multiple segmental occlusions in the branches of the left pulmonary artery.

decision to persist with medical management, or to proceed with embolectomy. If the peripheral signs of shock recede, the administration of Mannitol produces a significant response in urine volume, and the arterial pH returns toward normal, the physician can conclude that cardiac output is improving even when hypotension persists. A lack of improvement, however, considered in association with arteriographic evidence of severe obstruction to pulmonary blood flow, should allow a prompt decision for surgical treatment. Figure 30-2 shows the pulmonary arteriogram of a thirty-eight-year-old man who had massive embolism six days after an automobile accident. Despite adequate treatment he remained in shock for more than two hours after embolization. Since the arteriogram suggested adequate perfusion of only one third of the lung fields, embolectomy was performed. His recovery was uneventful and a Mobin-Uddin vena cava filter was put in place on the third postoperative day.

The authors have had no experience with the use of intrapulmonary enzyme therapy (urokinase, streptokinase, fibrinolysin) as adjuncts to medical management.[9, 10] The results of the National Cooperative Trial of

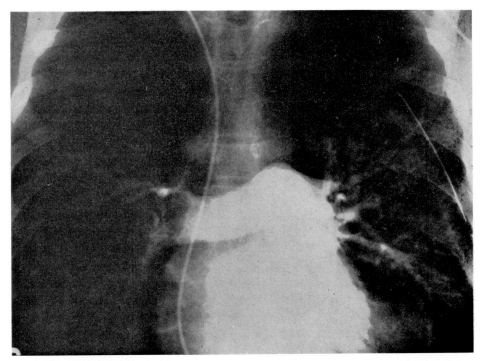

Figure 30-2. The diagnosis of massive pulmonary embolism was confirmed by pulmonary arteriography in this thirty-eight-year-old man. The right pulmonary artery is totally occluded and there is obstruction to blood flow in a large part of the left lung field.

Urokinase Therapy showed that this agent with subsequent heparin administration accelerated the resolution of pulmonary emboli when compared with heparin alone. Patients with massive pulmonary embolism treated with urokinase showed more frequent disappearance of dyspnea and of an accentuated pulmonic closure sound at twenty-four hours than did the patients who received only heparin. While the results of this national study suggest that urokinase may offer significant treatment benefit to victims of massive embolism, its prohibitive cost and general unavailability eliminate its practical use for the present.

REFERENCES

1. Sautter, R. D., Fletcher, F. W., Emanuel, D., Lawton, B. and Olsen, T. G.: Complete resolution of massive pulmonary thromboembolism. *JAMA, 189*:948-949, 1964.
2. Dalen, J. E., Banas, J. S., Jr. and Brooks, H. L.: Resolution rate of acute pulmonary embolism in man. *N Engl J Med, 280*:1194-1199, 1969.
3. Gorham, L. W.: A study of pulmonary embolism. *Arch Intern Med, 108*:76-90, 1961.
4. Dietzman, R. H., Ersek, R., Lillehei, C. W., Castaneda, A. R. and Lillehei, R. C.: Low output syndrome recognition and treatment. *J Thorac Cardiovasc Surg, 57*:138-146, 1969.
5. Dietzman, R. H., Castaneda, A., Lillehei, C. W., Ersek, R., Motsay, G. J. and Lillehei, R. C.: Corticosteroids as effective vasodilators in the treatment of low output syndrome. *Chest, 57*:440-453, 1970.
6. Martyn, D. T. and Jones, J. M.: Continuous intravenous administration of heparin. *Mayo Clin Proc, 46*:347-351, 1971.
7. Del Guercio, L. R., Cohn, J. D., Feins, N., Coormaraswany, R. P. and Mantle, L.: Screening for pulmonary embolism shock. *JAMA, 196*:751-756, 1966.
8. Wechsler, B. M., Karlson, K. E., Summers, D. N., Krasnow, N., Garzon, A. and Chait, A.: Pulmonary embolism: Influence of cardiac hemodynamics and natural history on selection of patients for embolectomy and inferior vena cava ligation. *Surgery, 65*:182-190, 1969.
9. The Urokinase-Pulmonary Embolism Trial: A national cooperative study. *Circulation, 47* (Suppl. 2) 7-12, 1973.
10. Kakkar, V. V. and Raftery, E. B.: Selection of patients with pulmonary embolism for thrombolytic therapy. *Lancet, 2*:237-241, 1970.

DISCUSSION

Question: Will you comment on the indication or contraindication to the treatment of the great anxiety that people have?

Dr. Bryant: Morphine is very important for allowing these patients to cooperate with the efforts at nonsurgical management. Six to ten milligrams is given as an initial dose, and an occasional patient will require as much as sixty mg per day to function with the respirator.

Dr. Bloomfield: Dr. Bryant, I must take issue with you over your statement about the slow recovery of these patients. I think it must be your modesty as a surgeon advocating the medical treatment. I think this is really a very rapid recovery in comparison with the recovery from myocardial infarction or a major operation.

Dr. Bryant: I say that deliberately to get some response. These patients do behave very differently from those who have need for assisted ventilation after major chest injuries or following major operations. The latter patients often relax and quickly fall asleep. Those who have a massive pulmonary embolism do not do that. It takes a number of hours for the patients to demonstrate that they are clearly out of trouble. As a matter of fact, we have watched some patients in the operating room during those several hours in which there is slow improvement.

Question: In regard to the use of Isuprel as a routine, would you comment on what you feel the hazards might be in case you were dealing with a myocardial infarction?

Dr. Bryant: The hazards of Isuprel are primarily those of arrhythmias. We use this agent so frequently in our patients with cardiac surgery that our group is familiar with the problem. The onset of ventricular premature contractions is a warning signal and I suspect the physician would have to be right on top of the situation if he suspected that myocardial infarction might be the more likely diagnosis. As a result of peripheral vasodilitation, the Isuprel may also produce a blood pressure drop and mandate volume replacement. In one of our patients, that circumstance forced us to provide significant volume replacement in the presence of acute right ventricular outflow obstruction.

Chapter 31

PULMONARY EMBOLECTOMY WITH PREOPERATIVE CIRCULATORY SUPPORT

Robert L. Berger

I N SPITE of repeated assertions that medical therapy is effective in massive
pulmonary embolism and that embolectomy is of little use, the disease
is still found to be the cause of death in 12 to 15 percent of all patients
examined postmortem.[4, 8] In an attempt to clarify this obvious paradox and
to formulate a rational therapeutic approach, a retrospective study was
carried out based on 252 patients who were subjected to pulmonary angiograms for suspected pulmonary embolism and 352 cases of pulmonary embolism found at postmortem examination.[1] The pertinent results of this
search revealed that (1) the mortality was influenced by the patient's cardiovascular status but correlated best with the extent of pulmonary vascular occlusion, (2) massive embolism ($< 50\%$ obstruction of the pulmonary
arteries) resulted in a 47 percent mortality, and (3) the mortality rose to
68 percent when massive embolism was associated with sustained shock.

The results of surgical therapy for pulmonary embolism were analyzed
by Cross and Mowlem[2] in a survey that included 115 embolectomies performed with cardiopulmonary bypass in twenty-eight institutions. Their
study revealed that embolectomy carried a 43 percent mortality. Although
these embolectomy results are disappointing, nevertheless they represent
an improvement over the outcome with medical therapy. In addition, a
closer look at the study suggests that the operative mortality could have
been further reduced by improvement in diagnosis and modification of the
operative approach. For example, pulmonary angiography, the most reliable method for the diagnosis of pulmonary embolism, was not performed
routinely, and nine patients in the series were operated upon with the
wrong diagnosis. Not one of them survived the operation. Another step
toward greater salvage would be the use of preoperative mechanical
circulatory support to prevent death from total circulatory collapse prior
to embolectomy. This technique was employed in only 35 percent of the

343

patients. Thus the routine employment of pulmonary angiography for diagnosis and the application of preoperative mechanical circulatory support would be likely to improve the results reported by Cross and Mowlem. In addition, early timing of the operation may also enhance the chances of success.

On the basis of the above information, pulmonary embolectomy in my view is indicated in the high-risk population, i.e., in those patients who have massive embolism associated with sustained shock. The diagnosis needs to be confirmed by pulmonary angiography, and the operation should be performed relatively early in the course and under the protective umbrella of preoperative circulatory support with the pump oxygenator.

CLINICAL EXPERIENCE

Twenty-one patients suspected of having massive pulmonary embolism were included in the present series. The diagnosis of massive embolism, or greater than 50 percent occlusion, was based on angiographic documentation of total or subtotal obstruction of at least the right or left main pulmonary arteries. Saddle emboli were encountered occasionally, but the most frequent presentation consisted of occlusion of one main pulmonary artery with multiple filling defects on the opposite side. In eighteen patients pulmonary angiograms were performed and confirmed the diagnosis. Three patients sustained cardiac arrest during or soon after the acute episode of suspected embolism, and time did not permit arteriography. Fourteen patients were in severe, sustained shock characterized by hypotension, peripheral vasoconstriction, oliguria and needed catecholamine therapy. Repeated attempts to discontinue catecholamine administration resulted in a fall of arterial pressure to shock levels. Seven patients with angiographic documentation of massive embolism did not develop overt circulatory failure or had only transient episodes of hypotension. The first three patients in this group underwent inferior vena cava interruption without any preparation for cardiopulmonary bypass, while in the last four patients the pump oxygenator was made available on a standby basis during the procedure.

The age range of the group was from thirty-eight to seventy-seven years. There were eleven women and ten men suffering from a variety of background diseases or conditions (Table 31-I).

As soon as the diagnosis of massive pulmonary embolism was suspected, heparin anticoagulation was instituted and an emergency pulmonary angiogram was obtained. Lung scan was done if shock was not present. Primary candidates for embolectomy (patients who had angiographic documentation of massive embolism plus refractory shock) were usually transferred from the radiology department directly to the operating room. The heart-lung machine was primed with crystalloid solutions. The femoral

TABLE 31-I

Case No.	Age (yr.) and sex	Associated diseases	Time* (hr.)	Angiography	Preoperative cannulation+	Preoperative mechanical circulatory support+	Procedure	Comment
1.	71,M	Postprostatectomy	6½	Yes	Yes	No	Embolectomy; IVCL**	Survived
2.	56,M	Postmitral valvotomy	½	No	Yes	Yes	Exploration	No pulmonary embolism, but myocardial infarction; died
3.	58,M	Guillain-Barre syndrome	8	Yes	Yes	No	Embolectomy, IVCL	Survived
4.	64,M	Postcolectomy	½	No	Yes	Yes	Embolectomy, IVCL	Late death
5.	38,F	? Pill	5	Yes	Yes	No	Embolectomy, IVCL	Survived
6.	64,F	Postcholecystectomy	2	Yes	Yes	Yes	Embolectomy, IVCL	Survived
7.	63,F	Postcolectomy	1½	No	Yes	No	Embolectomy	Survived
8.	67,M	? "Flu"	3	Yes	Yes	Yes	Embolectomy, IVCL	Survived
9.	68,F	Phlebitis	8	Yes	Yes	Yes	Embolectomy, IVCL	Survived
10.	53,F	Diabetes	5	Yes	Yes	Yes	Embolectomy	Caval tear, died
11.	61,M	Cerebrovascular accident	28	Yes	No	Late	Embolectomy	Died
12.	58,M	Phlebitis	5	Yes	Yes	Yes	Embolectomy, IVCL	Survived
13.	45,M	None	7	Yes	Yes	Yes	Embolectomy, IVCL	Shock during induction for IVCL; survived
14.	38,M	Paraplegia, empyema	8	Yes	Yes	Yes	Embolectomy, IVCL	Cardiac arrest during IVCL; survived
15.	77,F	Phlebitis	24	Yes	Yes	Yes	Embolectomy, femoral Vein ligation	Survived
16.	59,F	Pituitary adenoma—postop	6	Yes	Yes	Yes	Embolectomy, IVCL	Survived
17.	60,F	Postgastrectomy	6	Yes	Yes	Yes	Embolectomy, IVCL	Survived; hypotension during IVCL

*Between embolization and operation.

+Preoperative peripheral cannulation refers to the mere insertion of peripheral catheters for connection with the pump oxygenator. Preoperative mechanical circulatory support indicates that hypotension or cardiac arrest was encountered during induction of anesthesia of thoracotomy necessitating the prompt institution of partial cardiopulmonary bypass.

**Inferior vena cava ligation.

vessels were exposed under local infiltration anesthesia. The artery was cannulated first and connected to the outflow side of the heart-lung machine. The venous catheter was attached to the coronary suction line of the pump oxygenator and advanced from the femoral vein into the inferior vena cava under mild suction in order to retrieve any clots that might have lodged in the iliac vein or inferior vena cava. The blood removed from the patient during this maneuver was returned instantaneously through the femoral arterial line. The venous catheter then was transferred to the inflow side of the pump oxygenator, thereby completing the peripheral circuit for extracorporeal circulation. By-pass was not instituted, however, until hypotension deepened, cardiac arrest occurred, or exposure of the heart for embolectomy was completed. Anesthesia was induced, and the heart was approached through a sternum-splitting incision. The right atrium was flushed and explored digitally for intracavitary thrombi. Cannulation was completed by insertion of a catheter into the superior vena cava. Cardiopulmonary by-pass was instituted and the emboli were extracted through a longitudinal incision in the main pulmonary artery. Both lungs were massaged centripetally in order to dislodge peripheral clots and force them into a more accessible central location. The right ventricle was explored for residual clots. After completion of the embolectomy, appropriate venous interruption, usually inferior vena cava ligation or plication, was accomplished.

Right-sided pressures were measured in the open chest in seven patients after discontinuation of cardiopulmonary by-pass. In six patients seven postoperative right-heart catheterizations and pulmonary angiograms were performed two weeks to fifty-six months following embolectomy.

RESULTS

In fourteen primary embolectomies there were ten long-term survivors. The first death was in a patient with femoral thrombophlebitis who sustained cardiac arrest two weeks after mitral commissurotomy. The clinical findings and electrocardiogram were consistent with massive pulmonary embolism. Time did not permit angiography. The patient was transferred to the operating room, and femoral vein-to-artery circulatory support with the pump oxygenator was provided. On exploration there were no clots in the pulmonary arteries, and the patient could not be weaned from by-pass. At postmortem examination the pulmonary arteries were found to be patent and a large myocardial infarction was discovered.

The second death was in a patient who had a cardiac arrest minutes after massive pulmonary embolism. External cardiac massage was instituted and continued during transfer to the operating room and during cannulation of the femoral vessels for mechanical circulatory support. Embolectomy was performed, and the heart was resuscitated easily. Satisfactory cardiac and renal function returned, but the patient remained comatose. Because the brain damage was judged to be irreversible, respiratory support was discontinued on the tenth postoperative day and the patient died. It was assumed that the cerebral ischemia was sustained during the cardiac arrest and prior to embolectomy.

In the third death preoperative cannulation was not done, and the heart stopped during induction of anesthesia. Embolectomy was performed, but an effective heartbeat could not be restored. The fourth patient exsanguinated from a tear in the inferior vena cava during ligation of that vessel and following a successful pulmonary embolectomy (see Table 31-I).

The seven patients who sustained massive embolism but did not go into shock fell into two categories. The first three were treated by inferior vena cava interruption during the early stages of our experience when pump standby was not made available for this procedure in patients with massive embolism without shock. Two of three died during the operation. On the basis of this experience and similar observations by others,[6,7] subsequently the heart-lung machine was made available routinely on a standby basis during inferior vena cava ligation for massive embolism. Three of the next four patients went into shock during the procedure. They were immediately cannulated through the femoral vessels and supported with the pump oxygenator. Embolectomy was then performed, followed by caval interruption. All three became long-term survivors. In the fourth patient caval plication was accomplished without complication.

Intraoperative pulmonary artery pressure measurements in seven patients following embolectomy revealed a reduction from the preoperative levels. Three patients had right heart catheterization studies ten to fourteen days after their operation. All pressures were within normal limits. Simultaneous pulmonary arteriograms failed to show any evidence of residual clots in the pulmonary arteries. One of the three patients had recurrent thrombophlebitis with chest pain and underwent a third study two years after the operation. The pulmonary artery pressures were higher than at the previous study, reaching mild pulmonary hypertensive levels. On the pulmonary angiogram several underperfused areas were noted in both lungs. An inferior vena cava contrast examination demonstrated a patent vessel, indicating that the caval clip placed immediately after embolectomy must have slipped off, and it was concluded that the patient had recurrent small pulmonary emboli. Three additional right heart catheterization studies and pulmonary arteriograms carried out sixteen to fifty-six months after embolectomy showed normal pressures and patent pulmonary vasculature (Fig. 31-1).

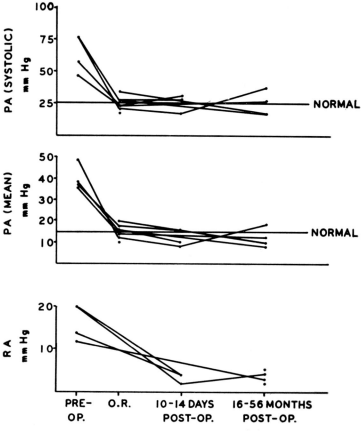

Figure 31-1. Hemodynamic measurements in patients with massive pulmonary embolism before, during, and after pulmonary embolectomy. (O. R. = intraoperatively, immediately after embolectomy; PA = pulmonary artery; RA = right atrium.)

COMMENTS

In the present series seventeen patients underwent embolectomy for massive embolism. There were thirteen long-term survivors and four deaths, or an uncorrected mortality of 23.6 percent. Three of the four deaths were due to misdiagnosis, irreversible cerebral ischemia sustained preoperatively, and exsanguination during inferior vena cava ligation, respectively, and they are not attributable to the embolectomy itself. Thus the corrected operative mortality is 5.4 percent. Although these results are more favorable than the mortality figures cited by Cross and Mowlem,[2] the reasons are easily explained once the pathogenesis of the disease is analyzed. Pulmonary embolism produces a number of physiological disturbances, but the dominating pathological feature appears to be mechanical obstruction to right ventricular outflow, which produces right ventricular strain, low output failure, and arterial hypoxemia. Removal of the block before the secondary physiological aberrations become irreversible should restore circulatory integrity and lead to total recovery. However, in order to accomplish this task successfully and to protect the patient from the stress of embolism and operation, a few critical steps in the overall management are mandatory.

Establishment of the correct diagnosis is one of the prerequisites for effective management. Massive pulmonary embolism presents as a catastrophic event, and at times it may be difficult to distinguish this disaster from other diseases with a similar clinical presentation. In our series one death was due to such an error, and in the survey by Cross and Mowlem[2] all nine patients in whom embolectomy was undertaken with an incorrect diagnosis died. The most reliable method for identification of pulmonary emboli is angiography, and therefore embolectomy should not be attempted without a contrast study. Exception to this rule is probably justified, but only under most unusual and desperate circumstances.

The importance of preoperative mechanical circulatory support with the pump oxygenator through peripheral cannulatation cannot be overemphasized. During massive pulmonary embolism life is maintained by maximal mobilization of physiological defenses, and even then circulatory compensation is only marginal. The stress of anesthesia or operation can easily upset this precarious balance, and they frequently precipitate circulatory collapse. Preoperative cannulation for mechanical circulatory support provides a most effective protection against fatal hemodynamic complications, and routine employment of this technique was largely responsible for the gratifying results in this series. The effectiveness of preoperative circulatory support is well substantiated in the literature, but the reports by Stansel, Hume, and Glenn[9] and Sautter[6] highlight this problem most poignantly. They encountered seven intraoperative cardiac arrests in eight patients when preoperative circulatory support was not provided and none in fourteen patients when preoperative pump oxygenator protection through peripheral channels was made available. Cannulation of the femoral artery and vein under local anesthesia is a simple matter, and in most cases it is imperative for a successful outcome.

Timing is another important determinant of the results of operation. Operative mortality can be lowered if the procedure is performed early and before far-advanced right ventricular failure, severe vital organ damage (e.g., of the brain or kidney), and irreversible metabolic derangements from persistent shock are established. If deterioration is allowed to progress and embolectomy is offered in the late stages of circulatory and metabolic decompensation, the mortality will be high, not from the operation, or, for that matter, not even from the embolism, but rather from the ill effects of uncontrolled secondary physiological disturbances. On the other hand it is equally true that in spite of the grave prognosis, some patients will survive without embolectomy, and therefore on the surface it may seem bold to decide in favor of an invasive approach that has been associated with a considerable risk in the past. The obvious task is to select the therapy that promises the best chance for survival. It would seem that with adherence to the protocol presented in this paper—and that includes relatively early timing—the outlook is far brighter with embolectomy than with nonoperative management. Early operation therefore is not only justified but is indicated. The appearance of sustained shock in massive pulmonary embolism heralds a poor prognosis, and a salvage operation with less than 10 percent mortality is certainly acceptable.

The use of pump standby during inferior vena cava ligation for massive embolism without shock was responsible for averting almost certain death in three patients. With extensive embolism, even in the absence of shock, circulatory compensation is frequently marginal. The stress of anesthesia and operation may upset the precarious balance and precipitate profound circulatory collapse. Deep shock or cardiac arrest occurred in five patients in this series during inferior vena cava ligation and was also reported by Sautter.[6] In this situation the availability of cardiopulmonary bypass for circulatory support facilitates a lifesaving definitive procedure. For this reason pump standby during vena cava ligation for massive embolism has been adopted as a routine practice in our institution. The approach to massive pulmonary embolism is summarized in Figure 31-2.

Although spontaneous lysis of pulmonary emboli has been documented, the process is time-consuming, unpredictable, and frequently incomplete. Dalen and his associates[3] studied fifteen patients with serial angiograms and found complete resolution in only three of the whole group. Walker and his co-workers[10] used serial lung scans to assess restoration of pulmonary perfusion following embolism in seventy-four patients. One-third showed almost complete resolution, one-third improved but the remainder failed to recover or became worse. In the national Urokinase Pulmonary Embolism Trial Study, the original lung scan defect persisted at the end of one year in 25 percent of the patients.[7] Phear[5] followed sixty-eight patients after pulmonary embolism for an average of 17.6 months. Six developed secondary pulmonary infection, eight had persistent atrial fibrillation, and twenty were left with dyspnea of varying severity. Ten patients exhibited clinical evidence of right heart failure, and three died. Two of these had postmortem evidence of residual pulmonary emboli. Thus incomplete lysis of embolized clots in the pulmonary arteries may result in long-term disability and represents an appreciable disadvantage of nonoperative management. The follow-up studies in this series suggest

PULMONARY EMBOLECTOMY
HEMODYNAMIC MEASUREMENTS

TREATMENT OF MASSIVE PULMONARY EMBOLISM

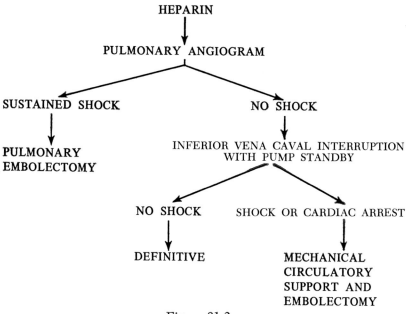

Figure 31-2.

that surgical removal of the embolus results in restoration of normal hemodynamics and normal pulmonary perfusion and thereby probably reduces disabling long-term complications.

REFERENCES

1. Berger, R. L., Gibson, H. and Ferris, E. J.: A reappraisal of the indications for pulmonary embolectomy. *Am J Surg, 116*:403, 1968.
2. Cross, F. S. and Mowlem, A.: A survey of the current status of pulmonary embolectomy for massive embolism. *Circulation, 35*:1, 1967.
3. Dalen, J. E., Barnes, J. D., Jr., Brooks, H. L., Evans, G. L., Pavaskos, J. A. and Deeter, L.: Resolution rate of acute pulmonary embolism in man. *N Engl J Med, 280*:1194, 1969.
4. Modan, B. and Sharm, E.: Factors contributing to the incorrect diagnosis of pulmonary embolic disease. *Chest, 62*:388, 1972.
5. Phear, D.: Pulmonary embolism: A study of late prognosis. *Lancet, 2*:832, 1960.
6. Sautter, R. D.: Massive pulmonary thromboembolism. *JAMA, 194*:104, 1965.
7. Sautter, R. D., Myers, W. O. and Wenzel, B. S.: Implications of the Urokinase Study concerning the surgical treatment of pulmonary embolism. *J Thorac Cardiovasc Surg, 63*:54, 1972.

8. Smith, G. T., Deeter, L. and Dammin, G. T.: Postmortem qualitative studies in pulmonary embolism. In Sasahara, A. A. and Stein, M. (Eds.): *Pulmonary Embolic Disease*. New York, Grune & Stratton, 1965.

9. Stansel, H. D., Jr., Hume, M. and Glenn, W. L.: Pulmonary embolectomy. *N Engl J Med*, 276:717, 1967.

10. Walker, R. H. S., Jackson, J. A. and Goodwin, J.: Resolution of pulmonary embolism. *Br Med J*, 2:135, 1970.

DISCUSSION

Dr. Mobin-Uddin: I noted in your presentation that three patients who were not in shock when you attempted ligation, developed shock during the procedure.

Dr. Berger: Well, this is where I enter your backyard and I suppose if we had used the umbrella filter without anesthesia, these patients might not have gone into shock and then would not have needed pulmonary embolectomy. However, some people still believe in surgical interruption of the inferior cava and this is why these people needed embolectomy.

Dr. Smith (Des Moines): Dr. Berger, on one of your earlier slides on some of the premises that you have had set up on one of the slides, it was right heart exploration.

Dr. Berger: Yes, we know of at least two cases where the patients re-embolized after embolectomy and after vena cava interruption. We assumed they must have had residual clots above the level of the vena cava interruption, and the heart was the source for reembolization. It is very simple to introduce a finger into the right ventricle and right atrium prior to embolectomy or during embolectomy and this way if there are clots in the cardiac chambers, you can get them out very easily indeed. In the present series, we retrieved a huge clot from the right ventricle during this maneuver.

Dr. Powell (Fort Knox): I came to this conference with a lot of questions. A few of them have been answered, most have been further muddled in my mind. I would like to ask, given the run of the mill pulmonary embolus patient with a small embolus definitely proven that you treat with anticoagulation. How long do you keep them on anticoagulation? And, how do you arrive at it?

Dr. Hanway (New York): Dr. Coon and his group have published a study in which they followed their patients in the hospital and postdischarge and they found if they stopped anticoagulants at the time of discharge, they had a 50 percent incidence of reemboli postdischarge. If they followed the patient to eight weeks, their incidence was in a very low range. Now I heard that he has now extended that to four months, but I think that this is the grounds on which the decision has been made purely on the basis of the incidence of reembolization following discharge.

Dr. Mobin-Uddin: I think the more important thing is to see if the patient has continuing predisposing factor such as congestive heart failure, or chronic obstructive airway disease with microemboli and cor pulmonale. These patients should be kept on long-term anticoagulant therapy. If they don't have a continuing predisposing factor, then probably about three or four months of therapy is sufficient.

Question: Dr. Berger, what precautions do you take to prevent knocking off a clot from iliofemoral vein when you go on partial, femoral vein to artery bypass?

Dr. Berger: First, we cannulate the femoral artery and this catheter is connected to the heart and lung machine. The venous cannula is introduced under coronary suction and the blood goes to the pump oxygenator, passes through the filtering system and is returned to the femoral artery. If there are clots in the iliofemoral system or inferior vena cava, usually we get them out with the venous catheter.

Dr. Mobin-Uddin: We inject contrast material into the femoral vein and make sure there are no clots in the iliac femoral system and inferior vena cava prior to introducing the femoral vein catheter.

Chapter 32

MASSIVE PULMONARY THROMBOEMBOLISM
FIBRINOLYTIC THERAPY

RICHARD D. SAUTTER, JEFFERSON F. RAY III AND WILLIAM O. MYERS

Introduction

SINCE EFFECTIVE thrombolytic agents have been at hand, there is and has been an attempt to identify those thrombotic conditions in which they would be useful. It would seem that if a disease process is initiated by thrombosis of a vessel, dissolution of the thrombus would restore homeostasis. This is not quite the case, as the restoration of homeostasis depends upon how quickly and completely dissolution can be affected and for what period of time the affected tissues can withstand anoxia without cellular death. For example, a thromboembolus to the superior cerebellar artery would have to be lysed within minutes for restoration of homeostasis to be complete. Conversely, a thromboembolus in a vessel supplying less specialized tissue, such as gut, could be lysed in hours after occurrence with expectation of complete restoration of homeostasis.

Massive pulmonary thromboembolism presents a unique opportunity for lytic therapy, as the lung has two separate circulations and there is little concern about tissue death. The problem is one of mechanical blockade of the pulmonary artery which, when severe enough, causes death. The patient's survival after an acute massive thromboembolus rests with the amount of obstruction within the pulmonary artery and that particular patient's cardiopulmonary reserve.

What the role of lytic agents in the treatment of massive pulmonary thromboembolism is does not have precise answers, as there is much unknown about the natural history of pulmonary thromboembolism, and the study of lytic agents is not yet complete. What follows is my personal opinion concerning the use of lytic agents in massive pulmonary thromboembolism based on personal experience, reports in the literature and, to some extent, prejudice.

For the purposes of this discussion, massive pulmonary thromboembolism is defined as 50 percent or more obstruction of the pulmonary arterial circulation.

THE COURSE OF PATIENTS WITH MASSIVE PULMONARY THROMBOEMBOLISM WHO RECEIVE SUPPORTIVE THERAPY

The mortality rate of patients with massive pulmonary thromboembolism who receive sodium heparin and intensive supportive therapy has been obscure. To investigate this area, we identified fifty-three consecutive patients from January, 1970, to July, 1972, who had the diagnosis of massive pulmonary thromboembolism confirmed by pulmonary arteriography (44) or pulmonary scan (9). All but three of the patients in this series received sodium heparin. In these three patients, sodium heparin therapy was contraindicated, but all three patients survived. All patients in this series received supportive therapy as required, i.e. oxygen, digitalis, inotropic agent, chronotropic agent. Seventeen patients had venous interruption to prevent further embolization. There were twelve patients who received lytic agents.

Seven deaths in this series are analyzed in Table 32-I. Three patients died suddenly, two suffered cardiac arrest, and one died fifteen minutes after the onset of symptoms. The two patients who suffered cardiac arrest underwent pulmonary embolectomy and represent the last two deaths in our embolectomy series. Of the four patients who died more than seventy-two hours after onset of symptoms, all had severe concomitant disease processes. The total mortality in this series was 14 percent. If, however, mortality is restricted to those patients who succumbed exclusively from the effects of the massive pulmonary thromboembolism (3), mortality was less than 6 percent.

TABLE 32-I

ANALYSIS OF 7 DEATHS

Consecutive patients with proven massive pulmonary thromboembolism	53
Sudden deaths	3
Male—76—cardiac arrest; died following embolectomy	
Male—78—cardiac arrest; died following embolectomy	
Male—61—died 15 minutes after onset of symptoms; had previous massive CVA	
Lingering deaths (death occurring more than 72 hours after onset of symptoms)	4
Male—58—post-operative triple coronary artery vein graft; occult CA of the lung; consumptive anticoagulopathy	
Male—71—diabetes; hemolytic anemia; upper GI hemorrhage	
Male—54—terminal Hodgkin's disease with pulmonary fibrosis secondary to cobalt treatment	
Female—61—terminal CA of esophagus	

During the study, an additional twenty-seven patients with massive pulmonary thromboemboli were found at autopsy but were not included in the mortality statistics. This is because the diagnosis was not suspected clinically and, lacking a pulmonary scan and pulmonary arteriography, the exact percentage obstruction of the pulmonary artery was not known. Obviously, the patients did not receive sodium heparin or other specific supportive measures. In a restrospective analysis of these patients, only four were found who would have been candidates for resuscitation had the diagnosis been suspected antemortem. The remainder would have been eliminated because of severe primary disease processes.

The time between the onset of symptoms and death in those patients who *will* succumb has been fairly well documented[1] (Fig. 32-1). Forty percent of those who will die do so in the first fifteen minutes, 60 percent within one hour. Following one hour, there is a slow decline in death rate over the next few days. How intensive supportive therapy would have affected those patients reported in this series who survived longer than one hour is unknown. There are no reports about coexisting disease processes present in patients who do not succumb immediately but ultimately die.

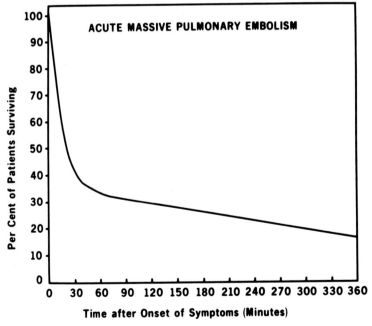

Figure 32-1. Graphic representation of survival time of patients with acute massive pulmonary thromboembolism from onset of symptoms. From Soloff, Louis A., and Rodman, Theodore: Acute pulmonary embolism. II. Clinical, *Am Heart J*, 74:829-847, 1967. (Reproduced with permission of author and publisher.[1])

An analysis of these two studies seems to indicate that (1) the majority of patients (86% in our study) who are clinically identified as having a massive embolus will survive if they receive sodium heparin and intensive supportive measures including venous interruption, (2) the majority of patients who die as a direct effect of the massive pulmonary thromboembolus do so immediately or within the first hour, and (3) those patients who survive the initial insult but ultimately die usually have additionally severe disease processes (five of seven patients in our study).

What happens to the thromboemboli in the pulmonary artery has been well documented. The fact that resolution is complete and universal is for the most part ignored by clinicians. A number of studies utilizing serial pulmonary arteriography demonstrate variability of spontaneous resolution of massive thromboemboli.[2-7] The resolution time *is* variable and the process *may* take months or as long as a year. But that there is complete lysis of a massive pulmonary thromboembolus by the natural intrinsic lytic process is established by the fact that occlusion of major pulmonary arteries by completely organized thrombi is never seen at the autopsy table. This has been confirmed in a personal communication from Dr. Jesse Edwards of the United Hospitals in St. Paul, Minnesota.[8] The only evidence of previous thromboemboli found by the prosector are fibrous bands and webs.

Evidence generated by the UPET[9] study regarding completeness of resolution requires explanation. One hundred five of the patients admitted to the trial had pulmonary scans one year following admission to the trial. Nineteen of these patients had a residual perfusion defect; seventeen patients in the group had a perfusion defect greater than 10 percent. Fourteen of these seventeen patients suffered a massive thromboembolus. These data would seem to indicate that there is a residual pulmonary deficit following massive pulmonary thromboembolism. However, these patients were *not* studied by pulmonary arteriography, nor were pulmonary function studies done. In reviewing these data, it is important to recall that Isawa[10] demonstrated sequential changes in pulmonary scans following acute thromboembolic episodes. These were best explained by change in the pulmonary arterial pressure and resistance in parallel circuits. He unequivocally demonstrated that by positioning the patient he could show normal perfusion by pulmonary scans in areas where a deficit had been demonstrated by the conventional techniques. Therefore, an abnormal pulmonary scan does not necessarily indicate compromised pulmonary function or obstruction of the pulmonary artery.

RATIONALE FOR FIBRINOLYTIC THERAPY

Fibrin is constantly being laid down on the endothelial surface and also constantly being lysed by the intrinsic fibrinolytic system. It is our concept that a depression of the lytic system allows fibrin to build up on susceptible endothelial surface, resulting in a thrombosis.

We and others have demonstrated that there is a depression of the fibrinolytic system immediately following major surgery.[11-13] It is this group of patients who are most prone to pulmonary thromboemboli. Lytic activity gradually returns to normal on or about the sixth postoperative day. If there is a depression of the system past the sixth postoperative day, there is a strong likelihood a thrombotic process has developed.

The whole blood euglobulin clot lysis time (WBELT) is one measurement of the natural lytic process, the normal ranging from forty-nine to 131 minutes. In 1965 we studied twelve patients with massive pulmonary thromboemboli proven by pulmonary arteriography. Their mean lysis time at the time of diagnosis was 235 minutes, indicating marked depression of the lytic system. Two of the twelve patients had values at the upper limits of normal. In all twelve patients plasminogen was sufficient to initiate lysis, should sufficient activator be present.

In a national collaborative trial (UPET), the mean lysis time of eighty-two patients with submassive and massive emboli was 200 minutes, indicating marked depression of the lytic system.[9] Mean plasminogen assay of this group was 2.11 CTA units, sufficient to initiate lysis should enough activator be present.

With this evidence it would seem reasonable that restoration or acceleration of the lytic process by the addition of activator to convert plasminogen to plasmin should benefit such patients.

RESULTS OF LYTIC THERAPY IN MASSIVE PULMONARY THROMBOEMBOLISM

In a 1965 pilot study of twelve patients with massive pulmonary thromboembolism, we administered eight-hour infusions of urokinase. There were no hospital deaths, but one patient did die at home of metastatic carcinoma.

Angiographic improvement was not uniform (Table 32-II), only half the patients showing moderate or marked improvement. The mean pulmonary artery pressure correlated well with the angiographic changes.

Of three patients who were in profound shock, two had marked improvement or near complete lysis and the third had moderate improvement. Although this series is too small for statistical significance, it does suggest that lytic therapy may benefit those patients most in need of help.

It is of interest that three patients had large saddle thromboemboli. One investigator has expressed concern about such lesions and has suggested that this represents an indication for pulmonary embolectomy.[14] This series, although small, does not support that contention.

TABLE 32-II

12 PATIENTS WITH PROVEN MASSIVE PULMONARY EMBOLI
TREATED WITH 8-HOUR INFUSION OF UROKINASE

Age range—29 years to 78 years	4 female
Mean—52 years	8 male

8 of 12 had undergone major surgery
Saddle emboli
2 right   1 left
Hospital deaths—0
(One patient died at home of metastatic carcinoma)

Angiographic improvement *24 hours after treatment*	*Mean pulmonary artery pressure (mm. Hg.)*	
	Preinfusion	*Postinfusion*
Marked 3 (2 patients in shock)	25	11
Moderate 3 (1 patient in shock)	35	22
Minimal 4	36	24
Worse 2	44	37

Two of the twelve patients did suffer reembolization in the first twenty-four hours of observation. Sodium heparin therapy was not started until forty-eight hours following lytic infusion in this group of patients. If, as in the UPET study, sodium heparin had been started as soon as the Lee-White clotting time returned to thirty minutes, these patients probably would not have reembolized. This reemphasizes the importance of sodium heparin in the treatment of pulmonary thromboembolism.

Several papers have described the use of lytic agents for the treatment of massive pulmonary thromboembolism.[15-23] These papers suffer the same defect as the above information in that there were no controls. On the other hand, the UPET study, a randomized double-blind trial which was rigidly controlled, pitted urokinase infusion against the heparin infusion. It is important to point out that sodium heparin therapy was rigidly maintained for at least five days following diagnosis, followed by six weeks of oral anticoagulant therapy. So, the *only* difference between the two groups of patients is that one received urokinase and one did not.

This study demonstrated unequivocally that urokinase accelerates lysis of pulmonary thromboemboli, that it does not alter the recurrence rate of pulmonary thromboemboli, and that bleeding is a hazard.

Of the 160 patients admitted to the trial, eighty-nine had massive thromboemboli, and resolution was greatest in this group. The most outstanding improvement was demonstrated in the eleven patients who were in shock, confirming our supposition that lytic agents benefit those patients most in need of help.

A closer look at these eleven patients is most appropriate to this discussion. None of them died from pulmonary thromboembolism. Two died later, one from central nervous system metastasis, the other from gastric bleeding. Seven patients received urokinase, four heparin.

The recurrence of pulmonary thromboembolism was nearly identical in both the urokinase and heparin-treated groups. Five patients were studied by venography before and after infusion of streptokinase or urokinase. Very little change in the peripheral thrombi was demonstrated. This would suggest that lytic agents will not supplant venous interruption in the prevention of recurrent pulmonary thomboembolism.

In the UPET study the reported incidence of bleeding during or following the use of lytic agents was 47 percent. However, this trial required many invasive procedures which would not be necessary except in a study protocol. Our incidence of bleeding during this period was five of thirty-seven patients (13.5%). In the UPET study, one institution avoided arterial puncture and has not had a severe bleeding episode in thirty-seven patients admitted to their group.[24] It is our opinion and the opinion of many people working with lytic agents that if the contraindications are observed and invasive procedures avoided before and during the lytic infusion, bleeding will be kept at a very acceptable level. The obvious contraindications to the use of lytic agents are the same as those for anticoagulants, one of the strongest being surgery less than ten days before the contemplated therapy.

By reviewing these data, a preliminary position can be arrived at concerning what lytic agents will, will not, and will probably do (Table 32-III).

TABLE 32-III

THROMBOLYTIC AGENTS

WILL

accelerate the lytic process (especially effective in massive pulmonary thromboembolism).
cause bleeding, unless contraindications are strictly observed.

WILL NOT

instantaneously lyse thromboemboli.
accelerate lysis of *all* thromboemboli.

WILL PROBABLY

not lyse more completely than normal lytic process.
not prevent recurrent pulmonary thromboemboli.

It is important to emphasize that currently there is no unequivocal evidence that lytic agents reduce the mortality in acute massive pulmonary thromboembolism.

PRIORITIES OF THERAPY FOR PATIENTS WITH A MASSIVE PULMONARY THROMBOEMBOLUS

The exact indication for the use of lytic therapy in those patients who have suffered a massive pulmonary thromboembolus is yet to be completely

Priorities of Treatment of Massive
Pulmonary Thromboembolism

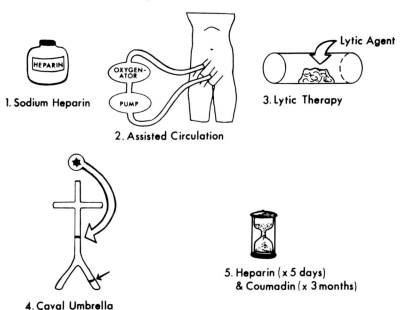

1. Sodium Heparin

2. Assisted Circulation

3. Lytic Therapy

4. Caval Umbrella

5. Heparin (x 5 days)
& Coumadin (x 3 months)

Figure 32-2.   Priorities of treatment for patients with massive pulmonary thromboembolism.

delineated. However, on the basis of current knowledge, lytic agents seem to be fairly well down the scale of priorities in therapy in these patients.

The priorities of therapy as we see them are (Fig. 32-2):

1. All patients should receive from 10,000 to 15,000 units of sodium heparin when the diagnosis is suspected. Not only does sodium heparin provide anticoagulant protection but it also reverses the effects of serotonin.
2. The patient should be supported or resuscitated by the use of cardiopulmonary bypass if the patient is in shock and imminent danger of death (not necessarily pulmonary embolectomy).
3. If lytic agents are to be used for the restoration of cardiopulmonary function, they need to be used at this point, prior to venous interruption, because of the hazard of bleeding.
4. Venous interruption, which requires only local anesthesia, is necessary in those patients who have potentially lethal thromboemboli demonstrated by venography. This can best be done by either the insertion of a Mobin-Uddin vena caval umbrella or plication of the femoral vein.

5. The patient should be maintained on sodium heparin therapy for at least five days and on oral anticoagulant therapy for at least three months.

Those patients who have suffered a massive thromboembolus and who are in shock or suffer a cardiac arrest can certainly be resuscitated or supported most effectively by the use of cardiopulmonary bypass. More rapid restoration of cardiopulmonary reserve may be possible by the administration of lytic agents while the patient is being supported in such fashion. Bleeding problems may be formidable but a cautious trial of such agents during cardiopulmonary bypass is indicated.

Summary

Although the exact role of lytic agents in the treatment of acute massive pulmonary thromboembolism has not yet been completely delineated, it is known that these agents will restore cardiopulmonary function more rapidly than will the natural lytic process and that they are most effective in acute massive pulmonary thromboembolization.

At present, lytic agents must be considered adjunctive therapy for the treatment of massive pulmonary thromboembolism, and the restricted availability of such agents should not handicap the physician in caring for a patient with this disease.

REFERENCES

1. Soloff, L. A. and Rodman, T.: Acute pulmonary embolism. II. Clinical. *Am Heart J, 74*:829-847, 1967.
2. Fred, H. L., Axelrad, M. A., Lewis, J. M. and Alexander, J. K.: Rapid resolution of pulmonary thromboemboli in man. *JAMA, 196*:1137-1139, 1966.
3. Dalen, J. E., Banas, J. S., Brooks, H. L., Evans, G. L., Paraskos, J. A. and Dexter, L.: Resolution rate of acute pulmonary embolism in man. *N Engl J Med, 280*:1194-1199, 1969.
4. Secker Walker, R. H., Jackson, J. A. and Goodwin, J.: Resolution of pulmonary embolism. *Br Med J, 4*:135-139, 1970.
5. Sautter, R. D., Fletcher, F. W., Emanuel, D. A., Lawton, B. R. and Olsen, T. G.: Complete resolution of massive pulmonary thromboembolism. *JAMA, 189*:948-949, 1964.
6. Sautter, R. D., Fletcher, F. W., Ousley, J. L. and Wenzel, F. J.: Extremely rapid resolution of a pulmonary embolus. Report of a case. *Dis Chest, 52*:825-827, 1967.
7. McDonald, I. G., Hirsh, J. and Hale, G. S.: Early rate of resolution of major pulmonary embolism. *Br Heart J, 33*:432-437, 1971.
8. Edwards, J. E., United Hospitals, St. Paul (written communication, March, 1973).
9. A Cooperative Study: Urokinase pulmonary embolism trial study group: Urokinase pulmonary embolism trial. Phase I Results. *JAMA, 214*:2163-2172, 1970.

10. Isawa, T., Wasserman, K., Taplin, G. V.: Variability of lung scans following pulmonary embolization. *Am Rev Resp Dis, 101*:207-217, 1970.
11. Sautter, R. D., Myers, W. O., Ray, J. F., III and Wenzel, F. J.: Relationship of fibrinolytic system to thrombotic phenomena in the postoperative patient. *Arch Surg*, in press.
12. Ygge, J.: Changes in blood coagulation and fibrinolysis during the postoperative period. *Am J Surg, 119*:225-232, 1970.
13. Mansfield, A. O.: Alteration in fibrinolysis associated with surgery and venous thrombosis. *Br J Surg, 59*:754-757, 1972.
14. McDonald, I. G., Hirsh, J., Hale, G. S.: Clarebrough, J. K. and Richardson, J. P.: Saddle pulmonary embolism: A surgical emergency? *Lancet, 1*:269-271, 1970.
15. Miller, G. A. H., Gibson, V., Honey, M. and Sutton, G. C.: Treatment of pulmonary embolism with streptokinase. A preliminary report. *Br Med J, 1*:812-815, 1969.
16. Clifton, E. E.: Treatment of pulmonary embolism with fibrinolytic agents. *Bull N Y Acad Med, 43*:267-281, 1967.
17. Hirsh, J., McDonald, I. G. and Hale, G. S.: Streptokinase therapy in acute major pulmonary embolism. *Am Heart J, 79*:574-578, 1970.
18. Hirsh, J., McDonald, I. G., O'Sullivan, E. F. and Jelinek, V. M.: Comparison of the effects of streptokinase and heparin on the early rate of resolution of major pulmonary embolism. *Can Med Assoc J, 104*:488-491, 1971.
19. Hirsh, J., et al.: Streptokinase in the treatment of major pulmonary embolism: experience with 25 patients. *Austr Ann Med, 19:Suppl, 19*:54-59, 1970.
20. Hirsh, J., Hale, G. S., McDonald, I. G., McCarthy, R. A. and Cade, J. E.: Resolution of acute massive pulmonary embolism after pulmonary arterial infusion of streptokinase. *Lancet, 2*:593-597, 1967.
21. Kakkar, V. V. and Raftery, E. B.: Selection of patients with pulmonary embolism for thrombolytic therapy. *Lancet, 2*:237-241, 1970.
22. Sasahara, A. A., Cannilla, J. E., Belko, J. S., Morse, R. L. and Criss, A. J.: Urokinase therapy in clinical pulmonary embolism. *N Engl J Med, 277*:1168-1173, 1967.
23. Sautter, R. D., Emanuel, D. A., Fletcher, F. W., Wenzel, F. J. and Matson, J. I.: Urokinase for the treatment of acute pulmonary thromboembolism. *JAMA, 202*:215-218, 1967.
24. Bell, W. R., Wagner, H. N. Jr., Johns Hopkins Medical Institutions, Baltimore (Oral communication).

Chapter 33

THE USE OF INTRACAVAL UMBRELLA FILTERS IN MASSIVE PULMONARY EMBOLUS

DENNIS A. BLOOMFIELD

Introduction

IN THE PAST, it has not been standard practice nor recommended therapy to interrupt the inferior vena caval blood flow as an emergency measure in the face of imminent demise from massive pulmonary embolus. This reluctance has been due to the well-recognized and not inconsiderable adverse effects of formal abdominal surgery under anesthesia in patients with an already heavily compromised cardio-respiratory system.[1, 2] The combination of shock, with cyanosis and acute right heart failure and the lack of preliminary preparation or work-up, constitutes an exceedingly high risk for any abdominal or thoracic surgery. On the other hand, there has been no lack of firm pathophysiologically supported indications for such an intervention and with the introduction of the umbrella filter and the subsequent ability to interrupt caval flow without hemodynamic alterations,[3] the indications and rationale for this procedure warrant reappraisal.

Although massive pulmonary emboli mechanically obstruct 50 percent or more of the pulmonary arterial bed,[4] this reduction, per se, may effect only minimal hemodynamic changes, as exemplified in the ability to resect one whole lung without producing pulmonary hypertension or right heart failure. Secondary reflexes, activated mechanically by the embolus or chemically by liberated breakdown products,[5] can produce pulmonary arteriolar constriction and it is believed that these are responsible for the pulmonary hypertension, the right heart failure, the intrapulmonary shunting and death.[6]

In the majority of patients, this demise occurs rapidly, before sophisticated medical or surgical help can be mobilized to aid the situation. However, between 33 percent[6] and 25 percent[7] of those patients who eventually die from massive embolism do so after the first one[7] or two[6] hours, at a time when the cardiovascular system has demonstrated its ability to main-

TABLE 33-I

HEMODYNAMIC SURVEY

Site	Before insertion		After insertion	
		Pressure (mmHg.)		
	Mean	Range	Mean	Range
Right atrium	8	5-15	7.5	4-20
Right ventricle		20-55		20-55
		5-20		5-20
Pulmonary artery	21	20-55	20	20-55
		10-25		5-20
Pulmonary wedge	7		7	
Brachial artery		76-130		100-150
		58-100		70-110
Cardiac output (1/min.)	3.7	2.3-5.1	3.9	2.8-5.0
Stroke volume (cc.)	33		31	

Hemodynamic data in four patients with massive pulmonary emboli before and immediately after umbrella filter insertion.

tain body perfusion adequate for survival. It appears likely then, that these delayed deaths are due to further episodes of embolization, evoking the reflexes detailed above and phlebographic studies such as that by Browse and associates[8] in patients immediately following pulmonary embolism, have revealed that 40 percent have fresh nonadherent residual thrombus in the legs and pelvis. If such thrombus migrations can be avoided during the critical postembolic period, life can be sustained and resolution of the initial embolus will afford eventual recovery. Interrupting this fatal cycle of recurrent embolization appears both a logic and effective intervention and for this purpose, umbrella filter implantation was undertaken on an emergency basis in patients who had survived a massive pulmonary embolus by one to two hours.

Analysis of this experience was directed towards two objectives—to ascertain that this procedure does not, in fact, produce detrimental hemodynamic conditions and that it does substantially increase survival in critically-ill patients.

Hemodynamic Effects of Filter Insertion

The hemodynamic effects of filter insertion were studied in the first twenty patients in this series. This goup comprised four patients with massive emboli and sixteen patients who had less severe emboli and were not in shock. The study, utilizing right heart and arterial catheterization, was carried out under local anesthesia and without premedication. Pressures were obtained in the right-sided cardiac chambers, the pulmonary wedge and a systemic artery. Cardiac output was measured by indicator dilution and arterial blood gases were analyzed. Pulmonary angiography was then performed, followed by filter insertion. Immediately after this, the complete hemodynamic survey was repeated. The prior and subsequent-to-insertion data for the four "massive emboli" patients are shown in Table 33-I.

The changes for the whole group are likewise insignificant, with right atrial mean and pulmonary artery systolic pressures rising only one mm Hg. Cardiac output, systemic arterial pressure and pulse rate varied in the whole group as in the critically ill subgroup of four, all rising slightly, but the changes are not statistically significant.

The trend towards increase in the systemic output and pressure probably reflects the effect of the pulmonary angiography and suggests a slight decrease in pulmonary vascular resistance. No detrimental hemodynamic effect was observed and it was concluded that filter insertion could be undertaken in critically-ill patients without further compromising their cardiovascular reserves.

RESULTS OF FILTER INSERTION

This report concerns the insertion of vena caval umbrella filters in twelve patients with massive emboli. While the pulmonary angiograms demonstrated extensive obstruction in all cases, the definition of massive embolus was not based on the quantitation of this investigation but on the extent of the hemodynamic derangement provoked by the embolus.

As an example of the critical condition of the patients in this group, the mode of presentation of the first four are summarized in Table 33-II.

The first patient, at sixty years of age, developed deep vein thrombosis following a stroke. Anticoagulants were withheld and subsequently she was admitted to the emergency room following a massive pulmonary em-

TABLE 33-II

Patient	Systolic pressure (mmHg.)			Pulse rate (min.)	pO_2	pCO_2	pH
1	0	$\rightarrow$	108*	120	70	30	7.49
2	0	$\rightarrow$	90*	150	42	30	7.50
3	$\frac{140}{110}$	$\rightarrow$	60*	130	92†	28	7.39
4	$\frac{190}{100}$	$\rightarrow 0 \rightarrow$	110*	100	100†	48	7.45

*On vasopressor agents.

†On 100% oxygen.

Massive pulmonary embolism—cardiorespiratory condition of patients on presentation. For explanation see text.

bolus. The blood pressure was unrecordable but with vasopressors, systolic blood pressure rose to 108 mmHg. at the time of the filter insertion. The second patient was admitted to the emergency room in a similar condition two weeks after thrombophlebitis complicating a bladder operation. The third was a seventy-seven-year-old-man, admitted for a nephrectomy, with a blood pressure of 140/110 mmHg. On the fifth postoperative day, he developed sudden chest pain, diaphoresis, shortness of breath and hypotension. The fourth patient was a seventy-eight-year-old hypertensive who was admitted with a stroke and, after six weeks in bed, suddenly developed symptoms and signs of a massive pulmonary embolus with shock. All patients had tachycardia and lowered pO_2, even on oxygen therapy.

Of the remaining patients who had filter insertions for massive emboli, two presented with cardiorespiratory arrests. Both had a further arrest during the procedure which, after resuscitation, was continued to a successful conclusion. A further patient had total obstruction of the left pulmonary

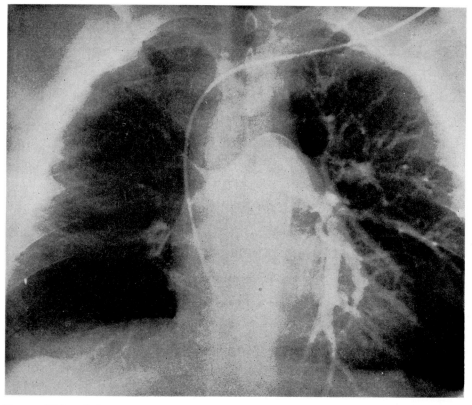

Figure 33-1. Pulmonary angiogram in massive embolus. Flow to the right lung is almost completely obstructed by an embolus at the bifurcation of the right pulmonary artery.

artery with continuing showers of emboli, one had recurrent emboli due to the combination of chronic bilateral thrombophlebitis and low cardiac output from pump failure following myocardial infarction, and one had multiple peripheral emboli complicating carcinoma with hepatic metastases. Prostatic surgery was the precipitating factor in one patient, chronic thrombophlebitis and obesity in another two. One of these patients developed severe retroperitoneal hemorrhage from heparin therapy. Twenty-four hours after cessation of this drug, an embolus almost completely occluded the right pulmonary artery (Fig. 33-1). All patients were confused, cyanotic, tachypneoic and hypotensive.

The hemodynamic data obtained at the time of implantation is presented in Table 33-III.

TABLE 33-III

Pressures (mmHg.)	Average	Range
Right atrium	10 mean	5-15
Right ventricle	54 systolic	27-80
Pulmonary artery	34 mean	16-50
Femoral artery	113 systolic	90-140*
Cardiac output (1/min.)	3.0	1.8-5.2
Rate (min.)	115	80-150
Blood chemistry (mmHg.)		
pH	7.46	7.39-7.50
pCO₂	32	24-48
pO₂	64	42-100†

*On vasopressor agents.

†On 100% oxygen.

Hemodynamic profile of patients with massive pulmonary emboli at the time of umbrella filter insertion.

Despite the critical condition of these patients, eight of the twelve made an uncomplicated and complete recovery, were discharged from the hospital and continue to do well. The details are presented in Table 33-IV.

Amongst the survivors, the longest follow-up time is twenty-eight months and the mean time is fourteen months. There has been no recurrence of pulmonary emboli in these patients. While it is not possible to demonstrate that this intervention saved their lives, it was the clinical impression that all the patients in this group were in critical condition at the time of filter insertion and were most unlikely to survive a further embolus.

Of the remaining four patients, one became apneic and asystolic between angiography and the filter insertion, which was completed during the eventually unsuccessful resuscitative attempts. The patient with liver metastases appeared to suffer a further pulmonary embolus thirty minutes after filter insertion and deteriorated over the following two hours. Both patients

TABLE 33-IV

RESULTS OF FILTER INSERTION

Patient	Age	Sex	Underlying disorder	Result of insertion	Long-term anti-coagulants	Months since insertion
AT	77	F	Nephrectomy	Well	Yes	23
AB	51	F	Cystolithotomy thrombophlebitis	Well	Yes	28
RR	60	F	Hemiplegia	Well	Yes	25
MD	78	M	Hemiplegia	Well	No	19
LW	73	M	Carcinoma with metastases	Died (2 hours) ? Further embolus	—	—
AR	49	M	Myocardial infarction	Died (7 days) acute myocardial infarction	—	—
MP	49	M	Myocardial infarction, congestive cardiac failure	Well (subsequently underwent cardiac surgery)	Yes	10
AB1	72	F	Thrombophlebitis, retroperitoneal hemorrhage	Well	Yes	7
SV	49	M	Unknown	Died during insertion	—	—
VP	67	M	Prostatic surgery, septicemia	Well	Yes	6
CD	79	M	Multiple injuries, fractured leg	Died (5 days) injuries	—	—
EJ	31	M	Thrombophlebitis	Well	Yes	1

The results of filter insertion in massive pulmonary embolism. For explanation see text.

who sustained cardiac arrests survived the procedure but eventually died —one at five days from the multiple injuries and fractures which had precipitated the pulmonary embolus, and the other at seven days from a second myocardial infarction in four months. In no patient was it felt that the filter insertion had contributed to death.

Complications were minimal in this series. One patient had continued fever associated with phlebitis, one has had persistent edema without phlebitis and the last patient, in whom a twenty-eight mm filter was inserted, felt sharp pain in the back aggravated by movement, on release of the filter. There was no bleeding, edema, renal dysfunction or fever in this patient; the filter was in an ideal location, and the pain quite suddenly subsided.

In the whole series of thirty-two patients, which includes the elective insertion patients as well as the emergencies of the massive emboli, there have been six instances of continuing hemoptysis or pleuritic pain. In no case was fresh pulmonary embolus demonstrated and no patient became shocked. In one patient at early reoperation and one at autopsy, the filters were occluded by thrombus on both surfaces but emboli on the under surface, as a primary cause of the obstruction, were not recognized. Such thrombus appears to be related to inability or contraindications to continue systemic anticoagulation, but does not appear to be completely avoided by these measures or by local heparin-bonding of the filter. Originally, great care was taken to place the filter exactly at the right renal vein-vena caval junction and this was achieved in both examined cases. It does not appear that even this maneuver affords adequate protection against the complication. Such thrombosis does not appear to lead to early embolization from the upper surface of the filter. Particularly if patients with massive emboli can be protected by systemic anticoagulation, no further pulmonary embolization has been observed in this study.

Filter insertion probably not only stops deterioration but may also have a positive beneficial effect. There is a rapid and physiologically inexplicable improvement that these patients experience in the first two-to-twelve hours after filter insertion. This suggests that subsequent and perhaps continuous embolization from residual thrombus is part of the natural history of massive embolism. As it is not reasonable to expect significant resolution of emboli in this time, one can hypothesize that beneficial circulatory adjustments can occur if the adverse reflex mechanisms are not activated by continuing embolization. This remarkable improvement can be documented by symptomatic relief and objective increase in arterial oxygen partial-pressure and systemic blood pressure maintenance without vasopressor agents. This improvement has also been observed by other workers and attests to the immediate effectiveness of the filter.

For the safety and efficacy of filter insertion in the critically ill, the standard technique needed to be slightly modified. Normally the visualization of the renal pelvis needed for filter placement is obtained by elective intravenous pyelography or observation of the excretion of the contrast used for the pulmonary angiogram. In these patients, however, the suddenness of the illness eliminates a prior investigational period and the angiogram contrast material does not opacify the renal pelvis quickly enough or in sufficient concentration, due to the low cadiac output and oliguria. Consequently, direct visualization of the renal vein-vena caval junction has been afforded by direct catheterization of the renal vein and a hand injection of five cc of Hypaque (Fig. 33-2). This is recorded on videotape and replayed at the time of positioning the filter.

Pulmonary angiography preceded deterioration in two patients. Consequently, small-volume, selective, hand-injections of contrast material have

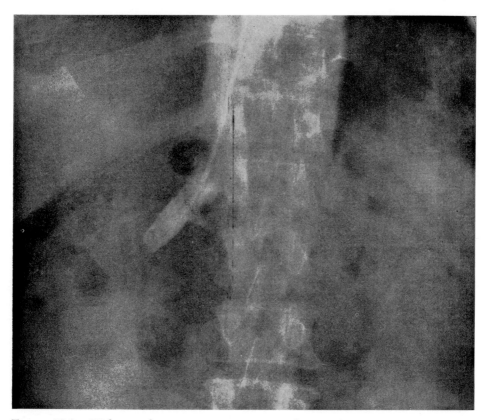

Figure 33-2. Right renal venogram in massive pulmonary embolus to identify the site of the vena caval-renal vein junction. Note the lack of "wash out" in the vein and the absent contrast material (from a previous injection) in the renal pelvis, resulting from poor renal blood flow and function.

been used to confirm the emboli if pulmonary artery pressures are exceedingly high, blood pressure is low or cyanosis is marked. A third problem, vagal syncope, during internal jugular vein dissection, occurred in two patients and has been countered by atropine premedication. With these modifications in technique it is concluded that inferior vena caval filter insertion is both practical and valuable in the management of cardio-respiratory collapse due to pulmonary embolus.

REFERENCES

1. Piccone, V. A., Jr., Vidal, E., Yarnoz, M., Glass, P. and LeVeen, H. H.: The late results of caval ligation. *Surgery, 68*:980-998, 1970.
2. Schowengerdt, C. G. and Schreiber, J. T.: Interruption of the vena cava in the treatment of pulmonary embolism. *Surg Gynecol Obstet, 132*:645-650, 1971.
3. Ahmed, S., Malhotra, J., Cerruti, M. and Bloomfield, D. A.: Hemodynamic effects of intracaval umbrella filter insertion. *Proc IX Interam Cong Cardiol, 61*, 1972.
4. Miller, G. A. H.: Massive pulmonary embolism—medical management. *Br Med J, 2*:777, 1970.
5. Comroe, J. H., Van Lingen, B., Stroud, R. C. and Roncoroni, A.: Reflex and direct cardiopulmonary effects of 5-OH-tryptamine (serotonin); their possible role in pulmonary embolism and coronary thrombosis. *Am J Physiol, 173*:379, 1953.
6. Gorham, L. W.: A study of pulmonary embolism. Part II. The mechanism of death; based on a clinicopathological investigation of 100 cases of massive and 285 cases of minor embolism of the pulmonary artery. *Arch Intern Med, 108*:189, 1961.
7. Donaldson, G. A., Williams, C., Scannell, J. G. and Shaw, R. S.: Reappraisal of application of Trendelenburg operation to massive fatal embolism: Report of successful pulmonary-artery thrombectomy using cardiopulmonary bypass. *N Engl J Med, 268*:171, 1963.
8. Browse, N. L., Thomas, M. L., Solan, M. J. and Young, A. E.: Prevention of recurrent pulmonary embolism. *Br Med J, 3*:382, 1969.

DISCUSSION

Question: Both from this presentation and Dr. Sautter's comments earlier today about trying to position it as close to the renal vein, I wonder if threading a catheter along with the umbrella or perhaps having another lumen in the introducer for the injection of dye at the same time wouldn't be in order.

Dr. Bloomfield: I tried strapping a catheter to the side of the introducer for a few cases but it is just as simple, with the vein open in the neck, to slip in a straight catheter that goes down to the inferior vena cava just as readily as does the introducer. It takes longer to strap a catheter on to the side of the introducer.

Question: When you put the inserter in, do you often enter in the right renal vein?

Dr. Bloomfield: Yes. I've occasionally gone into the right renal vein. I've also had trouble getting through into the inferior vena cava and in both these circumstances, I have withdrawn, put a gentle bend in the inserter so I could direct the tip and reintroduced it. It is obviously very important to recognize the fact that you can and have entered the right renal vein.

Dr. Fullen: We kept track of the number of times this happened and in nearly a third of eighty attempts our catheter entered the right renal vein. We don't bend it because somebody tried that and ruined one inserter. We have found that simply turning the patient a few degrees to the opposite side will let it pass, but in that group of patients it gives a nice localization of where the right renal vein is, so that it saves the problem of catheterizing it. We have not been very happy with vena cavagrams because the renal veins are not seen very well unless enormous quantities of dye are injected at high pressure. Therefore, we've used straight catheterization of the vein with a small amount of dye as you have and been very happy with it.

Dr. Bloomfield: We would look to identify that vein before putting the introducer in, so we would have that information already. In a patient in whom I feel almost definitely sure that we are going on to the umbrella insertion, I do the whole precedure through the neck. I will do the pulmonary angiogram and then while the films are being developed, pull the catheter back to the right atrium and then advance to the renal vein, record the venogram on video tape and we're ready to go as soon as the films confirm the embolus. It doesn't cost any more time and we have two introducers so it doesn't matter if we bend one!

AUTHOR INDEX

SUBJECT INDEX